The Mommy MD Guide

to Pregnancy and Birth

Tips That 60 Doctors Who Are
Also Mothers Use During
Their Own Pregnancies and Births

By Rallie McAllister, MD, MPH
and Jennifer Bright Reich

MOMOSA
PUBLISHING

© 2010 by Momosa Publishing LLC

Printed in Hong Kong

Illustrations by Carrie Wendel

Book design by Leanne Coppola

2   4   6   8   10   9   7   5   3   1   paperback

Library of Congress Control Number: 2010926116

ISBN 978-0-9844804-0-1

The Mommy MD Guides

Motherhood is a journey.
Mommy MDs are your guides.

MommyMDGuides.com

Best Wishes for a healthy Happy Pregnancy!
[signature] MS Sanders, MD

To my sister Gayle Santich
—RM

To Mike, Tyler, and Austin
—JBR

Contents

PART III: YOUR THIRD TRIMESTER

PART IV: YOUR BABY'S BIRTH

Acknowledgments

My deepest thanks go to my friend and partner, Jennifer Bright Reich, who worked tirelessly and cheerfully to design, develop, and deliver this book. It was her vision to create a guide that would allow moms-to-be to fully enjoy their pregnancies, while keeping themselves and their babies as healthy as possible. It was a joy for me to help her transform her vision into reality.

My sincere gratitude goes to all of the wonderful Mommy MD Guides who bared their souls and shared some of the most private moments of their lives. Reading their funny, heartwarming—and occasionally heart-wrenching—stories about pregnancy, labor, and childbirth will undoubtedly bring joy and comfort to many moms-to-be who are about to make the most exciting and unforgettable journey of their lives.

As always, I'm grateful for the love and support of my family: my husband, Robin, my two younger sons, Oakley and Gatlin, and my oldest son, Chad, his wife, Lindsey, and their beautiful new baby, Bella. There is no greater treasure in life than a loving family.
—*Rallie McAllister, MD, MPH*

∽◦

First and foremost, thank you from the bottom of my heart to Rallie McAllister. This book would not have been possible without you, and I will forever be grateful. I'm so lucky to get to work each day with such a dear friend.

Thank you to the dozens of smart, kind doctors who shared their stories and their wisdom with us for this book. Talking with you was both an honor and a delight, and I'm so happy for the opportunity to share your experiences and wisdom with our readers.

Many thanks also to the Mommy MD Guides team. I'm so fortunate to work with such a talented group: editor Amy Kovalski, consultant Jennifer Goldsmith, designer Leanne Coppola, layout designer Susan Eugster, indexer Nanette Bendyna, publicity consultant Mary

Lengle, illustrator Carrie Wendel, photographer Allison M. Gulsby, and Magnum Offset Printing sales manager Alice Fan.

I am very grateful to Drew Frantzen, who designed our Mommy MD Guides logo, establishing the very tone and style of our brand.

Thank you to my mentors and friends who have shared their wisdom and advice: Susan Berg, Tim Foster, Elly Phillips, Joey Green, Anne Egan, David Umla, Linda Hager, Larry Chilnick, Barbara Sellers, and Buddy Lesavoy.

Most of all, thank you to my family—Mike, Tyler, and Austin Reich and John R. Bright, Mary L. Bright, Robyn Swatsburg, and Judy Beck—for all of your support, encouragement, and love and for making my life so rich, rewarding—and fun.

—*Jennifer Bright Reich*

Meet the Mommy MD Guides

The idea for this book began with a cry in the night. Well, many cries in the night, actually. My sons both had acid reflux as babies, and they didn't sleep well. They cried—a lot. The record number of wakings was 11 in one night, or at least that's when I stopped counting.

In desperation, I talked with their pediatrician, Rima Strassman, MD, a wonderful doctor and also a mother of four, including twin babies at the time. Dr. Strassman called me one night after work and talked with me for more than a half hour, explaining how she had solved her own twins' sleep problems. Her method would call for more tears on my sons' part, and more tears on mine, but it had worked for her, she explained. Her reassurance and her experience gave me the courage to try it, and it worked for me too.

Over the years as a writer, I've interviewed hundreds of doctors. Every now and then, a doctor would say, "When my kids were little, I . . ." That always piqued my interest. If a physician juggling a busy practice and a hectic home life or a resident working 110 hours a week used a tip, no doubt it worked. And I figured that if it worked for her, it'll likely work for me too.

In 2008, I had the incredible good luck to meet Rallie McAllister, MD, MPH. That year, we worked together on a few projects. Then in early 2009, we decided to join forces to publish the Mommy MD Guides, a series of books filled with tips that doctors who are also mothers use for their own families. To accompany the book series, we also created the website MommyMDGuides.com.

To create this book, the first book in our Mommy MD Guides series, we spoke with 60 doctors who are also mothers—Mommy MD Guides. We spoke with many Mommy MD Guides who are still in the trenches with their babies. Some of them were even pregnant when we talked. We also spoke with Mommy MD Guides whose babies are grown up with babies of their own. They're Grammy MD Guides!

Combined, these doctors have centuries of experience as physicians, and among them they have 146 babies.

Because doctors so often see the things that can go wrong, they try to do everything as right as they can for their own health and for that of their families. Physicians are a healthier group than the whole. Even though women physicians sometimes will just suffer with things that take time and that affect them alone, pregnancy is different. Most doctors go the extra mile to take care of their own bodies while they're carrying their babies.

The tips and stories in this book are presented in the Mommy MD Guides' own words, and each tip is clearly attributed to the doctor who *lived* it. Most of these stories contain kernels of advice. This is what doctors who were becoming mothers did to make it through pregnancy and birth. Other stories in this book are just that—true stories. The implied advice is: I made it through this pesky problem, and you can too!

Even though this book is filled with advice from a select group—all Mommy MD Guides—you'll find that they hold vastly differing opinions. Pregnancy and birth are filled with issues that people feel very strongly about. Should your baby sleep with you or in the next room? Should you breastfeed or bottlefeed? Should your baby boy be circumcised or no? We've presented many different viewpoints—but not with the intent to confuse or to offer conflicting advice. Instead, we wish to present many different options so that you can choose what's best for you and your family.

As you read this book, keep in mind that every person is different, and in fact every pregnancy is different. Women experience different symptoms at different times. We encourage you to use the index at the back of this book as a resource, in addition to reading week by week.

Welcome to the Mommy MD Guides! Best wishes for a happy, healthy pregnancy and birth!

—*Jennifer Bright Reich*

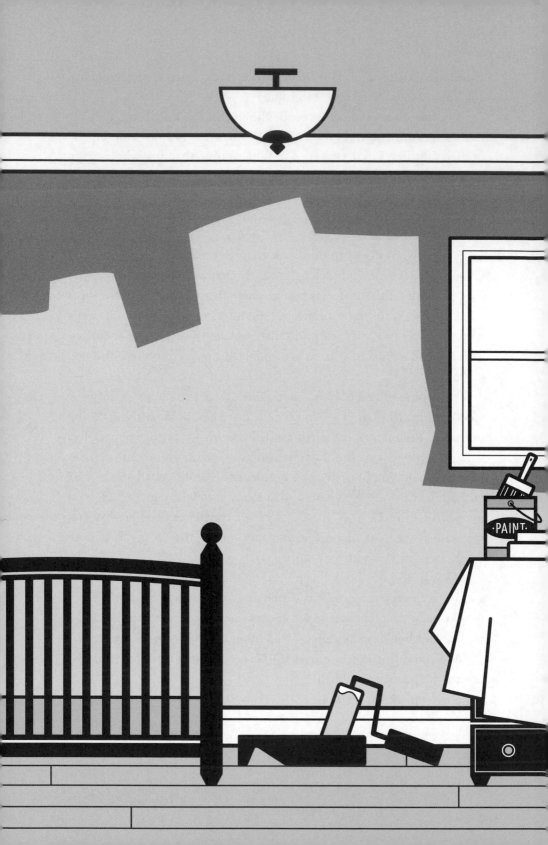

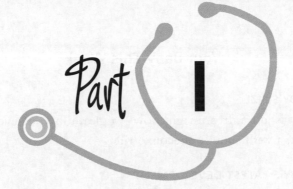

Part I

YOUR FIRST TRIMESTER

Chapter 1
Week 1

Your Baby This Week

YOUR BABY'S SIZE
Your baby is just a dream right now—a gleam in your eye, a song in your heart, a wish about to become true.

YOUR BABY'S LATEST DEVELOPMENTS
Right now, your "baby" is just one tiny cell. The egg that will join with your partner's sperm is being released from one of your ovaries, around day 14 of your menstrual cycle.

YOUR LATEST DEVELOPMENTS
Not pregnant yet, you don't feel any different, physically. But you might be able to discern some signs of ovulation. Just before you ovulate, you might notice an increase in clear, egg white–like, slippery vaginal discharge.

Also, if you track your basal body temperature—first thing in the morning—you'll notice that your temperature will increase by 0.4 to 0.6 degree Fahrenheit when you ovulate. Your body temperature increases to provide a warmer, more fertile environment for the egg. Some women feel a mild cramping or pain when they ovulate.

Also, you might experience a dizzying array of feelings: excitement, fear, joy.

JUSTIFICATION FOR A CELEBRATION
You're about to embark on one of the most exciting journeys of your life. Sit back and hold on. It's going to be a wild ride!

Hoping to Get Pregnant

Perhaps you've been hoping for a baby for weeks, months, or even years. Or maybe you've just been bitten by the "baby bug." You notice pregnant women everywhere, and just the thought of a baby of your own makes you smile.

༄

When I was just 22 years old, I was ready to have a baby, despite the fact that I didn't have a partner! I was living on a spiritual commune called the Farm at the time, and I remember a cute baby dress coming in a bag of stuff and thinking, *Oh, that's cute!* I kept that dress. I think my subconscious mind was saying, *It's time!* My daughter was ready to come through.

—*Stacey Marie Kerr, MD, a mother of two grown daughters, a family physician with strong roots in midwifery, and the author of* Homebirth in the Hospital, *in Santa Rosa, CA*

༄

My husband and I tried for quite a while, hoping to get pregnant. Ironically, it was when we *stopped* trying that we got pregnant. Even though I had some ovulation issues, I ended up with four kids! There's lots of hope!

—*Karen Heald, MD, a mom of four boys and a board-certified family physician in private practice outside Atlanta, GA*

༄

I was an infertility patient, and all of my children were conceived through in vitro fertilization. I was very nervous about pregnancy loss, but I was so very excited about trying to get pregnant. I had spent many years and a lot of money trying to conceive, and so I was really hoping to get pregnant.

—*Kelly Campbell, MD, a mom of three and an ob-gyn in private practice at Women's Healthcare Physicians in West Bloomfield, MI*

༄

I'm from a family of seven, and I'm extremely maternal. I got married at age 22, and my husband and I had to put off having children for a bit because medical school was so rigorous. But I was longing for a baby. I remember talking with my husband about it when I was in my senior year of medical school.

"I don't know if I can put having a baby off any longer," I said.

My husband looked at me like I had lost my mind. "Your maternal yearnings are superseding your objective thinking," he said.

I knew he was right, and we decided to wait until a more practical time. But things didn't go quite as planned . . .

—*Ann Kulze, MD, a mother of four children, ages 20, 19, 18, and 14, a nationally recognized nutrition expert, motivational speaker, physician, and the author of the critically acclaimed book* Dr. Ann's 10-Step Diet: A Simple Plan for Permanent Weight Loss and Lifelong Vitality

∽

My husband and I married very young. I had just turned 20, and he was 22. We put off having kids for a while to finish college, and then my husband went on to law school and I went on to medical school.

When I was in my third year of medical school, I took an elective in infertility. It terrified me! I was convinced I was infertile and would never get pregnant. I came home one day and told my husband, "It's now or never!"

I'm sure he thought, *Okay, what the heck.*

To both of our surprise, I got pregnant that first month.

—*Ann LaBarge, MD, a mom of four children, ages 16 to six, and an ob-gyn in private practice at the Midwest Center for Women's Healthcare in Park Ridge, IL*

∽

We had infertility issues, and it took us about three years to get pregnant. For me as a doctor, going through that experience helped me to relate to what my patients go through. It's so hard every month trying to get pregnant, and then feeling the disappointment when your period comes. We tried to get pregnant on our own for around two years, and then we went to an infertility specialist. We went through some frustrating infertility testing, and then we did in vitro fertilization, which is how we have our twins.

If you're struggling with infertility, be patient. The majority of my patients who struggle with

? When to Call Your Doctor or Midwife

If you're younger than age 35 and you've been trying to get pregnant for a year, consider seeing a specialist for an infertility workup. If you're 35 or older, consider seeing a specialist after trying for six months.

infertility do ultimately conceive. Don't get lost in the feeling of "It's not going to happen for us." For the majority of women, it *does* happen!

—*Jennifer Gilbert, DO, a mom of three-month-old twins and an ob-gyn at Paoli Hospital in Pennsylvania*

Starting a Pregnancy Journal or Scrapbook

Having a baby truly changes everything, and you're probably noticing changes in your life and in yourself already. Now is a wonderful time to reflect on those changes and to capture them in a journal or scrapbook.

⋘

With my daughter, I kept a baby book. I carefully recorded my thoughts and experiences, such as stories about my baby shower.

When I was pregnant with my two sons, instead of a baby book, I blogged about my experiences online. This began as a way for me to convey my thoughts and experiences to my husband, who's an Army surgeon and was deployed. But I kept up my blog even after my husband got home because I enjoyed it so much.

—*Lezli Braswell, MD, a mom of one daughter and two sons and a family medicine physician currently working in an emergency room fast track in Columbus, GA*

⋘

When my husband and I found out I was pregnant, we were so excited. Right away, I started to keep a journal. I think a lot of people hesitate to journal because they fear that it will become a huge, time-consuming process and they won't be able to keep up with it. But all I did was keep a steno pad on my nightstand. Here and there throughout my pregnancy, I wrote down my thoughts to my baby. I didn't pressure myself to write something every day; I wrote when I had something to say.

For example, I wrote to my baby after I saw her on the ultrasound; I wrote how I reacted when I first felt her moving; and I told her how much I love her. I kept a journal for each of my children during the pregnancies and still do to this day. When my children were little, part of the reason why I journaled was I realized that those first five years are the most important years of their lives as far as learning and emotional development. If something happened to me before they were old enough, would they remember me at all?

I still write in my kids' journals, describing how I felt the first time they told me that they love me and what my hopes and dreams are for them. I plan to give each of my children their journal when their first child is born.
—*Kelly Campbell, MD*

I've always journaled. It's been a place I go whenever there's been a major event in my life. I write down my thoughts about events I've been moved by.

Mommy MD Guide-Recommended Product
Digital Camera

Parenthood is one big photo opportunity. Babies change and grow quickly, and they do so many funny, adorable things that you'll want to capture every silly moment, step, and smile.

Digital cameras are perfect for photographing babies and kids because each snap is free. You pay only for the photos that you print. With digital photography, you can adjust color and contrast and crop photos on your computer, e-mail the photos to your friends and family, and print them out at home or at a store or upload them to an online photofinisher. Companies such as **www.Shutterfly.com** allow you to store, share, and print photos easily and inexpensively.

Digital cameras range in price from less than a hundred dollars to thousands of dollars. They range in size as well: Subcompacts can fit in a pocket, and compacts fit in a purse. The leading manufacturers are Canon, Fujifilm, HP, Kodak, Nikon, Olympus, and Sony. Some digital cameras are easy to use; others should come with a six-week training course.

When you're considering the cost of a digital camera, factor in any extras you'll need, such as a case, memory cards, spare batteries, battery recharger, and tripod. Before you step into a camera shop or a big-box store to buy a digital camera, check out some reviews online. If you Google "digital camera reviews," you'll find plenty of opinions! Then at the store, ask to hold the cameras you're considering in your hand and press a few buttons. Get a sense of how easy a camera is to operate and how the camera feels to you.

I'm not a disciplined journaler. I don't write diary entries every day. But I did journal a lot during my pregnancies.

Pregnancy is a really important time for reflection. During my pregnancy, I reflected a lot. It's important to think about what has happened in your life—both the celebratory moments and the times that might have been somewhat tragic. It's helpful to reflect on those events. Think about how you managed them, and then ask yourself how you want life to be different for your newborn baby coming into the world.

—*Nancy Rappaport, MD, a mother of two teenaged daughters and a teenaged son, an assistant professor of psychiatry at Harvard Medical School, an attending child and adolescent psychiatrist in the Cambridge, MA, public schools, and the author of* In Her Wake: A Child Psychiatrist Explores the Mystery of Her Mother's Suicide

Taking Prenatal Vitamins

When you're pregnant, your need for certain nutrients, including folic acid, calcium, and iron, increases. Taking prenatal vitamins is one of the most important things you can do to prevent neural tube defects, which are birth defects of the brain and spinal cord, such as spina bifida. Research has shown that getting enough folic acid before and during pregnancy can prevent most neural tube defects. Because the baby's neural tube develops so early in pregnancy—during the first four weeks—the U.S. Public Health Service recommends that all women of childbearing age take 400 micrograms of folic acid each day. Some experts, however, recommend that all women take 800 micrograms a day.

Prenatal vitamins are available both over the counter and by prescription. Talk with your doctor or midwife before taking prenatal vitamins.

The one thing I did to prepare for pregnancy was start taking folic acid. That's one of the most important things you can do to decrease the risk of serious birth defects in you baby.

—*Ruth D. Williams, MD, a mom of twins—a boy and a girl—and another boy, and an ophthalmologist in private practice at the Wheaton Eye Clinic in Wheaton, IL, who specializes in the diagnosis and treatment of glaucoma*

Before getting pregnant, I took prenatal vitamins. I took prescription ones because my husband is an Army surgeon, and my doctors on the Army base gave me the prescription vitamins right at my appointments. But the over-the-counter ones are just as good.

—*Lezli Braswell, MD*

∾

I was more compulsive with my first baby, and I started taking folic acid several months before I got pregnant. With my second baby, I was much more relaxed, and I started to take it when I found out I was pregnant.

With both pregnancies, instead of taking prenatal vitamins, I took regular multivitamins, which have the same amount of folic acid as most prenatal vitamins (400 micrograms), with fewer gastrointestinal side effects. They're gentler on your stomach.

—*Michelle Paley, MD, PA, a mom of a six-year-old daughter and a two-year-old son and a psychiatrist and psychotherapist in private practice in Miami Beach, FL*

∾

I began taking a prenatal vitamin at least three months before I started trying to get pregnant. Taking prenatal vitamins increases the chance of a healthy pregnancy. They help to prevent some diseases, and at least you can cover those.

Any brand of prenatal vitamins is fine, and over-the-counter vitamins are as good as the ones that need a prescription. The most important part of the vitamin is the folic acid. Make sure your vitamins have 800 micrograms of folic acid.

It can be hard to take vitamins if you have morning sickness. I found it helped to take my vitamins with a meal during the day.

—*Aline T. Tanios, MD, a mom of three and a general pediatrician and hospitalist who treats medically complex children at Arkansas Children's Hospital in Little Rock*

∾

One thing I did to prepare my body for pregnancy was to take prenatal vitamins. I had morning sickness, so it was hard to take them, but I made sure to do it because I knew it was an important aspect of having a healthy baby.

I took the vitamins with apple juice or orange juice to mask the medicine taste.

—*Diane Truong, MD, FAAP, a mom of one daughter and one son and a pediatrician in a multispecialty group practice in Southern California*

ᘓᕈᓍ

Vitamins are no good to you if you throw them up. One trick if you have morning sickness and can't choke down your prenatal vitamins is to chew a children's Flintstones Vitamin instead. Flintstones Complete vitamins, for instance, contain 400 micrograms of folic acid, which is what most experts recommend pregnant women get each day.

—*Ashley Roman, MD, MPH, a mom of two daughters, ages three years and six months, and a clinical assistant professor in the department of obstetrics and gynecology at the New York University School of Medicine in New York City*

ᘓᕈᓍ

I started taking prenatal vitamins long before I got pregnant. I actually took sample prescription prenatal vitamins, but the over-the-counter ones are just fine. However, some of them are quite large and have an odor. If you have a hard time taking them because of morning sickness, try one with a different coating. Some of the prescription vitamins are smaller and coated to mask the odor. Prescription vitamins can be expensive, but generics are cheaper.

—*Diane Connelly, MD, a mom of a six-year-old daughter and an ob-gyn in HMO practice in Riverside, CA*

ᘓᕈᓍ

For my first and second pregnancies, I took prenatal vitamins and didn't have a problem. But for some reason, during my third pregnancy they started to give me migraine headaches. I discovered that it was the niacin in the vitamins that was causing them.

I had to stop taking the prenatal vitamins, and then I became anemic and felt really awful. That made me realize how helpful those prenatal vitamins are!

—*Patricia S. Brown, MD, a mom of two daughters, ages nine and seven, and a three-year-old son and a psychiatrist at Columbia-New York Child and Adolescent Telepsychiatry and in private practice in Cresskill, NJ*

Getting More Calcium

Milk: It does a *pregnant* body good. Calcium is critical for keeping your bones and teeth healthy and strong. Calcium is also required for muscle contraction, blood vessel expansion and contraction, secretion of hormones and enzymes, and transmitting impulses throughout your nervous system.

When you're pregnant, it's very important to get 1,000 milligrams of calcium each day. The average woman gets only 700 milligrams of calcium a day—not enough. If you don't get enough calcium, your body steals it from your bones. Over time that loss can lead to osteoporosis.

During your second and third trimesters, and if you're breastfeeding, your body actually absorbs more calcium from your food than it usually does when you're not pregnant. But still, if you don't take in enough calcium from food and supplements, your baby's needs will come out of *your* bones.

The prenatal vitamin you're taking likely contains calcium. But check the label. It might not offer as much calcium as you think. You need to make up the rest in your diet. The best sources of calcium are low-fat dairy products, such as milk, cheese, and yogurt. Many beverages and foods are fortified with calcium, such as orange juice and breakfast cereals. There's no need to worry about getting too much calcium. Your body can absorb only around 600 milligrams of calcium at a time.

If you're buying a separate calcium supplement, don't take one that contains bone meal or dolomite. They might also contain arsenic, lead, mercury, and other toxic substances.

⌒⌒

I'm really good about drinking milk every day. I drink one glass each day with breakfast, and I eat yogurt frequently. So I was confident I would get enough calcium in my diet during my pregnancy.

—*Sadaf T. Bhutta, MBBS, a mom of a three-year-old daughter and 18-month-old triplets and an assistant professor and the fellowship director of pediatric radiology at the University of Arkansas for Medical Sciences and Arkansas Children's Hospital, both in Little Rock*

I don't like milk, but during my pregnancies I made myself drink it. I knew that I—and my baby—needed the calcium.

—*Patricia S. Brown, MD*

∽

When I was pregnant, I was living on a farm. I remember one day, my husband went down the road and got a gallon of ice-cold whole milk that had been milked from the cow just that morning. I chugged about half of that gallon. I will never forget the feeling of that milk going down and knowing that this is what my body needs—*badly*.

—*Stacey Marie Kerr, MD*

∽

I don't normally like ice cream, but I ate a lot of it when I was pregnant. I like milk, but I don't normally drink a lot of it. When I was pregnant, I had a taste for ice cream and milk.

I'd like to say it was so that I could get more calcium, and that was a nice side benefit, but the truth is I just craved milk and ice cream during all three of my pregnancies.

—*Lezli Braswell, MD*

∽

During my pregnancy, I snacked a lot on low-fat dairy foods like cheese and yogurt. That was very helpful to get extra calcium.

—*Stephanie Ring, MD, a mom of two sons, ages six and two, and an ob-gyn at Red Rocks Ob-Gyn in Lakewood, CO*

RALLIE'S TIP

I've never been able to tolerate dairy products very well, because I'm a little lactose intolerant. Plus when it comes to taking calcium in the form of those gigantic horse pills, I'm a wimp! Fortunately, I found a brand of liquid calcium at my health food store. A couple of tablespoons a day gave me all the calcium I needed without upsetting my stomach.

Improving Your Diet

Whatever you put into your mouth—chips and candy or carrots and cauliflower—nourishes your baby as well. Common sense says you'd rather grow your baby on healthful foods than junk.

As a guideline, the March of Dimes recommends that you strive to eat six ounces of grains (such as breads, cereal, pasta, and rice), 2½ cups of vegetables, 1½ to 2 cups of fruits, 3 cups of milk products (such as milk, yogurt, and cheese), and 5 to 5½ ounces of protein (such as meat, poultry, fish, peanut butter, and eggs) each day. (See "Thinking about Food Safety" on page 20.)

During pregnancy, it's also important to drink enough fluids. By the time your baby is born, your blood volume will increase by up to 50 percent. Your heart works 40 percent harder than before you were pregnant to keep all of that blood moving. It's important to drink plenty of water (or other noncaffeinated beverages such as milk and juice) to stay hydrated.

∽

Before I got pregnant for the first time, I really overhauled my diet. I've never eaten as well in my entire life as I did during that pregnancy. I ate tons of greens and vegetables.

—*Sadaf T. Bhutta, MBBS*

∽

Before I got pregnant and during my pregnancies, I tried to eat more healthfully. I tried to stick to what I call the pregnancy diet, which is eating well with a little bit of everything, a generally well-balanced diet. I tried to eat fish three times a week, and I ate some protein at every meal, including breakfast. I was all about my bacon-and-egg sandwiches.

—*Ashley Roman, MD, MPH*

∽

I've always been a healthy eater, and I always tended toward whole, real, fresh foods. I focused on eating those foods while I was pregnant, and I remember avoiding empty calories like chips, doughnuts, and fast food. I knew those were not foods the baby needed!

If I had known what I know now before I got pregnant, I would have been even *more* diligent in my nutrition choices. It's that important.

—*Ann Kulze, MD*

∽

When I was pregnant with my first baby, I was living on a spiritual commune called the Farm. We grew all of our own organic food, and we ate only what we grew. For example, we grew soybeans, harvested them, and then made soy milk and tofu.

When I was pregnant with my last baby, I was no longer living on the commune. In fact, I was in residency training, working 110 hours per week! But I continued to focus on eating reasonably healthy. If there are 27 ingredients on the box and you can't pronounce them, you probably shouldn't be eating whatever is in that box.

—*Hana R. Solomon, MD, a mom of four, ages 35 to 19, a board-certified pediatrician, the president of BeWell Health, LLC, and the author of* Clearing the Air One Nose at a Time: Caring for Your Personal Filter

∽

Before I got pregnant, my husband put together a laminated card of the foods I was supposed to eat. Being so restrictive about what I should be eating made it even harder to eat well. Absolute guidelines often send us running in the other direction. My husband's plan for me was a dismal failure.

I think that good nutrition is a matter of common sense and moderation. When I was pregnant, I tried to eat more healthy foods than not, and I tried to eat all foods in moderation.

—*Ellen Kruger, MD, a mom of two teenagers and an ob-gyn in an academic and clinical practice in New Orleans, LA, with Ochsner Health System*

Chapter 2
Week 2

Your Baby This Week

YOUR BABY'S SIZE
This week, your baby begins as just a single egg.

YOUR BABY'S LATEST DEVELOPMENTS
Once the egg is released from your ovary, it's caught by the fingerlike ends of the fallopian tube and drawn into the tube. Then the egg journeys down the fallopian tube toward your uterus. Along the way, the egg encounters the sperm that have made it to your fallopian tube. Their numbers dwindled quickly after ejaculation. Only the strongest, hardiest, and *luckiest* have made it this far. Of the 200 to 400 million swimmers that your partner ejaculated, many spill out. Others are lost along the way. But some sperm burst through the mucus secreted by your cervix, cross through your uterus, and swim into the fallopian tube. Around 200 sperm make it to the egg. One (two if you're becoming pregnant with twins!) sperm unites with the egg. The cell begins to divide—again and again and again . . .

YOUR LATEST DEVELOPMENTS
You still don't feel pregnant because the egg hasn't yet begun to implant into your uterus. Perhaps you feel a bit of anxiety and excitement, wondering if . . . maybe . . . you might be pregnant.

JUSTIFICATION FOR A CELEBRATION
Perhaps egg and sperm have met and joined!

Getting into Shape and Adjusting Your Weight

Despite what we see on sitcoms and in the movies, pregnancy isn't an all you can-eat buffet. Your body actually only needs an additional 300 calories each day, about the number in a tall glass of fat-free milk.

It's important to be at a healthy weight when you get pregnant because either being overweight or underweight can affect your pregnancy. One way to check your weight is by using a measurement called body mass index (BMI). If you Google "BMI," you'll find charts and calculators online.

You might want to make a note of your weight and your bust, waist, and hip mesurements to refer back to in the months ahead.

✑

I didn't prepare to get pregnant because it was a surprise. But I was in the Army at the time, so I was very physically fit. That's a great way to start your pregnancy.

> —*Patricia S. Brown, MD, a mom of two daughters, ages nine and seven, and a three-year-old son and a psychiatrist at Columbia-New York Child and Adolescent Telepsychiatry and in private practice in Cresskill, NJ*

✑

I think it's very important to get to a healthy weight before getting pregnant. Before I started trying to get pregnant, I made sure I was at the lower end of my weight comfort range. That's best for a healthy pregnancy, and also it's better to start at the lower end of your range because it's shocking enough when you get on a scale during pregnancy.

> —*Mary Mason, MD, a mom of a nine-year-old girl and six-year-old boy, an internist, and the chief medical officer for a multi-state managed care company that coordinates care for about 70,000 pregnant Medicaid moms a year*

✑

Before I got pregnant the first time, I got into the best shape of my life. I lost some extra weight, and I ran three miles every day. I wanted my body to be as healthy as possible before I got pregnant.

> —*Sadaf T. Bhutta, MBBS, a mom of a three-year-old daughter and 18-month-old triplets and an assistant professor and the fellowship director of pediatric radiology at the University of Arkansas for Medical Sciences and Arkansas Children's Hospital, both in Little Rock*

The time when you're thinking about getting pregnant is a great time to clean up your act. I'm an older mom, and I can say from experience that if you're having kids later in life, you really need to get yourself into the best shape possible. Pregnancy seems to be more physically taxing for older moms. Take charge of your health now and get yourself in shape so you can have a healthy pregnancy.

Think you're too busy and that you don't have the time? Just wait until you have the baby! I found that the investments I made in my health before and during pregnancy paid off after I became a parent. Kids require so much energy, and if you're in good shape and good health, you'll be better able to keep up. I didn't really appreciate my own health until I had kids.

—*Stephanie Ring, MD, a mom of two sons, ages six and two, and an ob-gyn at Red Rocks Ob-Gyn in Lakewood, CO*

Before I started trying to get pregnant with my second baby, I actually became a little *less* restrictive with caloric intake. Normally, I choose small portions of healthful food, and I have a slender figure. By avoiding a stingy diet, I easily became pregnant with both of my sons.

—*Amy J. Derick, MD, a mom of one 15-month-old son who is 17 weeks pregnant with her second son. Dr. Derick is a dermatologist in private practice at Derick Dermatology in Barrington, IL*

Weaning Off of the Bean

There's a reason Starbucks franchises are multiplying like rabbits: We're a nation of caffeine fiends. But while coffee in general and caffeine in particular offer many health benefits—such as helping to protect you against type 2 diabetes, liver cancer, and Parkinson's disease—during pregnancy, you can definitely have too much of a good thing.

Most experts recommend that during pregnancy you limit your caffeine intake to 200 milligrams a day. That's about the amount in one 12-ounce cup of coffee. Bear in mind that's *not* the serving size typically handed out a drive-thru window.

Besides coffee, caffeine is also found in lesser amounts in tea, chocolate, and soda—and of course Red Bull and other energy drinks. If you drink tea, it's best to avoid green tea and herbal teas. Many herbs have medicinal effects, and it's not known how they might affect pregnancy.

⁓

During my pregnancy, cutting back on caffeine was easy because I developed an aversion to coffee! I couldn't stand the smell of it, let alone the taste.

—*Ann Kulze, MD, a mother of four children, ages 20, 19, 18, and 14, a nationally recognized nutrition expert, motivational speaker, physician, and the author of the critically acclaimed book* Dr. Ann's 10-Step Diet: A Simple Plan for Permanent Weight Loss and Lifelong Vitality

⁓

When I got pregnant, I was working in an emergency room. I lived on caffeine. But as soon as I found out I was pregnant, I quit drinking coffee right away.

I thought that it would be difficult, but it wasn't. It was amazing that as soon as I found out I was pregnant, my baby's needs were paramount. I couldn't drink coffee anymore because I couldn't do anything that might hurt her.

—*Christy Valentine, MD, a mom of one, a specialist in pediatrics and internal medicine, and the founder of the Valentine Medical Center in Gretna, LA*

⁓

I drink a *significant* amount of coffee—four or five cups a day. You can drink one or two cups of coffee daily during pregnancy, so during my pregnancies, I made a pot with half decaf coffee and half regular. That way, I could still *drink* four cups, but I'd only get two cups of caffeinated coffee each day.

—*Gina Dado, MD, a mom of two daughters and an ob-gyn with Arizona OBGYN Affiliates, Paradise Valley Branch, in Scottsdale, AZ*

⁓

In preparation for getting pregnant, I was careful to be as healthy as possible. For example, prior to getting pregnant, I had been drinking quite a lot of coffee. Before I started trying to get pregnant, I cut back to one cup a day. I couldn't get down to zero, but I did cut back significantly.

—*Siobhan Dolan, MD, MPH, a mom of three, a consultant to the March of Dimes, and an associate professor of obstetrics and gynecology and women's health at Albert Einstein College of Medicine/Montefiore Medical Center in the Bronx, NY*

Before getting pregnant, I tried not to drink a lot of extra caffeine. But I didn't totally cut caffeine out of my diet because I like it!

I'm a middle-of-the-road sort of person when it comes to my diet, not really too radical. So I just always simply tried to do all things in moderation.

—*Lezli Braswell, MD, a mom of one daughter and two sons and a family medicine physician currently working in an emergency room fast track in Columbus, GA*

I did have caffeine now and then during my pregnancies. I think moderation is the key. I believe that if it was dangerous to have a little caffeine in pregnancy, we'd know it by now.

You don't want to be a lab rat and drink six cups a day. But I think that a cup or so a day should be just fine. Overindulgence is bad; moderation is good.

—*Ellen Kruger, MD, a mom of two teenagers and an ob-gyn in an academic and clinical practice in New Orleans, LA, with Ochsner Health System*

The one thing I did in preparation for pregnancy, especially with my third and fourth babies, was cut back my enormous caffeine habit. In my second pregnancy, a surgeon in medical school told me that I drank more coffee than any pregnant woman he had ever seen.

Unfortunately, my second daughter was born nine weeks premature and very small. According to the March of Dimes, there's a very loose possible association between caffeine intake and premature birth. I decided that it probably wasn't worth the risk, especially if it was easy for me to quit.

—*Kristie McNealy, MD, a mom of seven- and four-year-old daughters and a two-year-old son, who's pregnant with another son, and a blogger at www.KristieMcNealy.com, in Denver, CO*

I drank coffee during all of my pregnancies. I drank one or two cups of coffee each day with my first two pregnancies, and I drank one or two grande nonfat lattes each day during my third pregnancy.

I believe that moderation is the key. If you live your life in balance, it all works out.

—*Jennifer Kim, MD, a mom of three girls, ages eight, five, and four; an ob-gyn in private practice in Evanston, IL, at the Midwest Center for Women's Healthcare; and a clinical assistant professor at the University of Chicago, Pritzker School of Medicine*

Talking with Your Doctor or Midwife about Medications

"Just say no" takes on new meaning during pregnancy. Experts recommend that pregnant women avoid both over-the-counter and prescription drugs as much as possible. While a tiny handful of medications have been deemed safe for pregnant women, some drugs have been found to be dangerous during pregnancy, and many medications simply haven't been tested enough to know for sure.

According to one study, about 80 percent of pregnant women take over-the-counter medications while pregnant. But an estimated 10 percent of birth defects result from the mom's exposure to drugs.

The Federal Drug Administration breaks all medications into safety categories from A to X. A is the safest, while X indicates that a drug is dangerous in pregnancy. If your doctor has prescribed a medication, ask the doctor or your pharmacist which category the medication falls in.

Talk with your doctor or midwife as soon as possible about any medications you take, both over-the-counter and prescription. Also discuss any vitamins and supplements you take, such as vitamin C and omega-3 fatty acids.

At this time, it's also a good idea to talk with your doctor or midwife about any preexisting medical conditions you have, such as diabetes or asthma. Your health care provider will help you to develop a strategy to manage your condition effectively. Pregnancy can impact every aspect of your health.

~

Especially because I was an older mom, I talked with my doctor about the over-the-counter and prescription medications I was taking before I started trying to get pregnant. It's important to minimize medications—or better yet, avoid them entirely—during pregnancy.

—*Stephanie Ring, MD*

When I first found out that I was pregnant, I was concerned because I was in the Army at the time, and I had just gotten a bunch of immunizations in preparation for being deployed overseas. I talked with my doctor right away about them, and thank goodness, it was all fine. I had great medical care in the Army.

—*Patricia S. Brown, MD*

⤫

I didn't have to worry about talking with my doctor about medications because I've never been on any medications in between my pregnancies.

However, if I had been taking any medicine, I definitely would have checked with my doctor either before or as soon as possible after finding out I was pregnant to make sure that everything was safe for me to take while pregnant.

—*Kristie McNealy, MD*

Thinking about Food Safety

During pregnancy, both you *and* your baby are very vulnerable to foodborne illnesses. You're more at risk than usual because during pregnancy your immune system is weakened. This makes it harder for your body to fight off harmful microorganisms such as salmonella bacteria. Foodborne illnesses put your baby at risk because her immune system isn't developed yet.

Following these five simple steps will help to protect both you and your baby from foodborne illnesses. First, wash your hands thoroughly with soap and warm water before preparing and eating food and after using the bathroom and handling pets. Second, wash cutting boards, dishes, utensils, and countertops with hot water and soap. Rinse raw fruits and vegetables thoroughly under running water. Third, think of raw meat, poultry, and seafood as potentially contaminated and keep them away from ready-to-eat foods. Fourth, cook foods thoroughly to kill bacteria. You'll find handy charts online that list the temperatures specific foods need to reach to be considered safe. (See also "Mommy MD Guide–Recommended Product: Pampered Chef Digital Pocket Thermometer on opposite page.) Fifth, chill food properly. Your fridge thermostat should register 40°F. It's important to discard any perishable food that's been left at room temperature for more than two hours.

There's a short list of foods that you should pass on to protect yourself against a bacteria called listeria: raw (unpasteurized) milk, refrigerated smoked seafood unless it's in a cooked dish such as salmon and lox, pâtés or meat spreads, soft cheeses such as feta and brie, and hot dogs and luncheon meats—unless they have been heated to steaming hot.

You should also avoid fish and seafood that might contain methylmercury. At high levels, this metal can be harmful to your baby's developing nervous system.

According to the FDA, pregnant women should be sure to avoid eating fish with the highest mercury levels (including orange roughy, grouper, and king mackerel), limit fish containing high levels of mercury to three 6-ounce servings per month (including canned white albacore tuna, halibut, and lobster), and limit seafood containing low levels of mercury to six 6-ounce servings a month (such as snapper, blue and snow crab, and canned chunk light tuna).

Mommy MD Guide-Recommended Product
Pampered Chef Digital Pocket Thermometer

Food poisoning is never fun. But it takes on a whole new element when you're pregnant. Just think about it: morning sickness plus food poisoning. Once your baby is born, you'll want to be extra cautious about food safety to keep her from getting sick.

One way to prevent food poisoning is to make sure that your food is cooked to a high-enough temperature to kill any bacteria. Before serving your food, check it with an instant-read thermometer.

You can buy them online and in many stores. Look for a shatterproof dial with easy-to-read numbers.

One to consider is the Pampered Chef Digital Pocket Thermometer. It features an easy-to-read display and a protective sheath with a temperature guide for desired doneness, so you always have that critical information at your fingertips.

There are so many do's and don'ts regarding diet that it can drive you crazy.

I absolutely avoided raw food. If you pick up a parasite during pregnancy, it can be difficult to treat. Food that has passed quality controls for big national companies and the FDA is probably safer than your husband's buddy's deer sausage.

—*Ellen Kruger, MD*

As soon as I found out I was pregnant, I stopped eating sushi. The risk of infection with bacteria and the mercury levels in raw fish can be dangerous during pregnancy.

It's amazing when you're pregnant how you start taking such good care of yourself—the way you should do all the time!

—*Christy Valentine, MD*

Before I got pregnant, I started to limit the amount of certain types of fish that I ate. Although fish is very nutritious and a great source of healthful things such as omega-3 fatty acids, fish can also contain mercury, which can affect a baby's brain development and nervous system.

—*Monica Lee-Griffith, MD, a mom of one, an ob-gyn, and senior staff, Henry Ford Health System in metropolitan Detroit*

Quitting Vices

If you smoke, you've never had a better reason to quit. Today.

Smoking nearly doubles your baby's risk of having a low birth weight. Babies born to women who smoke are more likely to have birth defects, particularly congenital heart defects.

Babies whose mothers smoked are up to three times as likely to die from sudden infant death syndrome (SIDS) as babies of mothers who didn't smoke. Also, babies whose mothers smoked appear to be more jittery and difficult to soothe. They seem to go through withdrawal-like symptoms, similar to babies of mothers who used street drugs.

Smoking doubles your risk of placenta previa, which is a low-lying placenta that covers part or all of the opening of the uterus, and placenta abruption, in which the placenta peels away from the wall of your uterus before delivery.

In addition to not smoking, it's important to avoid *secondhand* smoke as well. Research suggests that babies of moms-to-be who were regularly exposed to secondhand smoke during pregnancy might have slowed growth. These babies might also be more likely to be born at low birth weights.

Along the same lines, it's critical that women planning to get pregnant avoid alcohol. The position of organizations such as the March of Dimes and the American Pregnancy Association is clear: There is no safe amount of alcohol to consume while you are pregnant

Alcohol passes through the placenta, so when you drink, so does your baby. And alcohol is a teratogen, which is a substance known to be harmful to human development. Alcohol is broken down much more slowly in a fetus's body than in an adult's. Because of this, the baby's blood alcohol can remain higher, longer than the mother's blood alcohol.

During pregnancy, drinking alcohol can cause a range of both physical and mental defects. Each year in the United States, up to 40,000 babies are born with fetal alcohol spectrum disorders, which is a term used to describe the problems associated with alcohol before birth. According to the March of Dimes, the birth defects caused by drinking alcohol are the most common type of preventable birth defects.

The consequences of a mom-to-be drinking can affect her baby for a lifetime. But sadly, women aren't getting the message. U.S. government surveys suggest that about one in a dozen pregnant women drinks during pregnancy. That's one in a dozen too many.

∽◦

Before my husband and I started trying to get pregnant, I cut out alcohol. I think when you're planning a pregnancy, the best policy is to act as if you *are* pregnant.

—*Stephanie Ring, MD*

∽◦

I don't drink very often, but two days after I found out I was pregnant, I went on a previously planned trip with some friends to Mexico. One of my friends asked me to have a cocktail with her.

When we sat down and I ordered a lemonade, she looked at me and asked, "Are you pregnant?" I hadn't planned on telling anyone that soon, but she guessed!

—*Monica Lee-Griffith, MD*

ᔐ

When I was trying to get pregnant, I limited the amount that I drank, and once I knew I was pregnant, I cut alcohol out entirely.

—*Ashley Roman, MD, MPH, a mom of two daughters, ages three years and six months, and a clinical assistant professor in the department of obstetrics and gynecology at the New York University School of Medicine in New York City*

ᔐ

During my second pregnancy, my husband was in the Army, and we were living in Germany. Because of Germany's central location, we could take day trips to four different countries, and we enjoyed lots of wonderful food. I love wine, but I don't drink during pregnancy. I remember missing out on all that good French wine.

—*Ann Kulze, MD*

ᔐ

When I was trying to get pregnant, I was a resident physician. So I was especially careful to do all of the things you're supposed to do to make sure your body is as healthy as possible.

For example, I took prenatal vitamins religiously. Also, I didn't drink alcohol, and I certainly didn't take any drugs. But the truth is that it wasn't really an issue for me because I didn't do any of those things prior to getting pregnant anyway!

—*Siobhan Dolan, MD, MPH*

ᔐ

I think that in terms of getting healthy, even in the preconception period, I felt it was important to have my body as healthy as possible. So even before I was pregnant, I wasn't drinking or taking prescription or nonprescription drugs, and I was taking prenatal vitamins. I wanted the environment for my baby to be as good as it could be. You can't control a lot, but you must control the things that you can.

A number of birth defects can occur during the first six weeks, even before many women know they are pregnant. If you wait to stop smoking until after your pregnancy test comes back positive, you may have already done something.

—*Sharonne N. Hayes, MD, a mom of two and the director of the Women's Heart Clinic at Mayo Clinic in Rochester, MN*

RALLIE'S TIP

I have been very fortunate to have adopted very few vices—at least in terms of substance abuse—during my life. I have struggled with caffeine since I began medical school, but in the grand scheme of things, that's really a minor problem.

I have worked with many women who have struggled with addictions to alcohol, tobacco, prescription pain medications, and illicit drugs, such as cocaine, heroin, and marijuana. These addictions can be extremely difficult to overcome even in the best of circumstances. The good news is many women are able to avoid using these substances the entire time they're pregnant, even if they never were able to avoid using them for more than a few days at a time during previous attempts when they were not pregnant.

The emotions of motherhood are incredibly powerful, and there's something about pregnancy that seems to give many women the strength they need to steer clear of substances of abuse that will harm their babies. Although many of these women might not have been motivated to seek help with addiction for themselves and their own personal safety and well-being, they are often driven to seek treatment for the safety and well-being of their unborn babies.

Overcoming any addiction is rarely easy, but it's always possible, especially with the love, help, and support of caring family members and the assistance of trained, compassionate professionals. Moms-to-be will never, ever regret avoiding substance abuse during pregnancy, but they may have a lifetime of regret if they expose their babies to these toxins.

I always encourage pregnant women who struggle with substance abuse to tap into every resource available to them, including physicians, counselors, employee assistance programs (EAPs) at work, members of the clergy, friends, and hospital- and community-based programs. For every pregnant woman who struggles with addiction, there is help, and there is plenty of reason for hope.

Chapter 3
Week 3

Your Baby This Week

YOUR BABY'S SIZE
This week, your baby is only a group of cells about the size of the head of a pin, about 0.006 inch.

YOUR BABY'S LATEST DEVELOPMENTS
The embryo is growing rapidly, dividing over and over. The developing ball of cells is called a zygote. As the zygote begins to accumulate fluid, it forms into a tiny blastocyst. As the cells divide, the blastocyst journeys through your fallopian tube to your uterus, arriving three to seven days after fertilization. For the next few days, the blastocyst floats freely around in your uterus, growing and developing. This week, the fluid in the center of the ball divides the ball into two groups. The cells on the inside will form your baby, and the cells on the outside will form your baby's placenta.

At some point this week, the cell ball will stop floating freely, and it will come to rest on the surface of your uterus. Once the cell ball attaches, it begins to receive protection, oxygen, and nutrients from you.

YOUR LATEST DEVELOPMENTS
You won't feel any pregnancy symptoms yet. But that probably won't stop you from watching for early signs of pregnancy.

JUSTIFICATION FOR A CELEBRATION
Your baby has arrived at his "home" for the next nine months.

Preparing for Pregnancy—Or Winging It

Some women prepare for pregnancy for a long time, taking vitamins, reading books, checking their schedules, and dreaming about their babies-to-be for months or even years. Other women become pregnant completely by surprise, with no planning or preparations at all. These are two very different ways to begin the same adventure.

※

Well before conception, I tried to make my life as stress free as possible to get my body ready to conceive. I was ever-mindful of maintaining low stress while working in my practice. I consciously kept myself from getting frustrated over little things. Before becoming pregnant, I was mentally and physically ready.

—Amy J. Derick, MD, a mom of one 15-month-old son who is 17 weeks pregnant with her second son. Dr. Derick is a dermatologist in private practice at Derick Dermatology in Barrington, IL

※

I was in the Air Force and had just come home from a deployment to Somalia for Operation Restore Hope. I decided that was a good time to start trying to get pregnant.

I had always been fairly good about nutrition and exercise, and my husband and I were both triathletes BC (before children). But I always like to practice what I preach, and so I took extra good care of my body at that time.

—Susan Wilder, MD, a mom of an older daughter and twin girls, a primary care physician, and CEO and founder of Lifescape Medical Associates in Scottsdale, AZ

※

Plan your pregnancies if you can. I planned mine, and they came out fairly close to the plan. I timed mine so that even though I was in training, I would be pregnant at a time when I wouldn't be exposed to a lot of radiation at work. My husband and I had been married for five years, and he wanted to get started, but I wanted to wait until after my training was over, so we compromised.

—Sharonne N. Hayes, MD, a mom of two and the director of the Women's Heart Clinic at Mayo Clinic in Rochester, MN

I was totally unprepared for pregnancy! I was working at my first job after completing my residency, and I wasn't planning on having a baby then. So I didn't do anything to prepare. I was very surprised to find out I was pregnant!

—*Christy Valentine, MD, a mom of one, a specialist in pediatrics and internal medicine, and the founder of the Valentine Medical Center in Gretna, LA*

My daughter was a honeymoon baby, so I hadn't done much to prepare. I became pregnant during my third year of residency, which was doable but not really the most ideal time.

Knowing what I know now, I wouldn't have done that. I would have taken more time to prepare for pregnancy, and I would have waited until things settled down in my life a bit.

I was able to prepare more before getting pregnant with my son, as my life was more settled. Consequently, I was able to enjoy his baby phase. My daughter grew up in the blink of an eye, and I missed her infancy.

—*Diane Truong, MD, FAAP, a mom of one daughter and one son and a pediatrician in a multispecialty group practice in Southern California*

I didn't do anything to prepare for pregnancy. I got pregnant within the first six months of my marriage.

It was my first year in practice; I was adjusting to being married. I half ignored my pregnancy. I was working crazy hours and on call every two or three nights. But fortunately pregnancy usually goes pretty well despite the circumstances around us.

—*Jennifer Kim, MD, a mom of three girls, ages eight, five, and four; an ob-gyn in private practice in Evanston, IL, at the Midwest Center for Women's Healthcare; and a clinical assistant professor at the University of Chicago, Pritzker School of Medicine*

I didn't do a single thing to prepare for pregnancy. I don't think it is fully possible to prepare for pregnancy. Pregnancy and motherhood are immense and transcendent experiences. They are by nature wonderfully overpowering. Feeling overpowered and helpless in the face of something "bigger than you are" is part of the picture. You have to just go with it.

Of course, you'll feel better if you have some control over the basics—if you're in good physical health and if you have financial security and a devoted partner. I was lucky to have *this kind* of preparation in place.

—*Elizabeth Berger, MD, a mom of two, a child psychiatrist, and the author of* Raising Kids with Character

Watching for Early Signs of Pregnancy

Some women go through their first month of pregnancy with no symptoms at all. But 70 percent of women develop some early clues that they're pregnant.

Quite possibly, you aren't feeling symptoms yet. But you might be on the lookout for the classic pregnancy symptoms of nausea, fatigue, dizziness, frequent urination, breast tenderness, and an odd metallic taste in your mouth.

❧

The first trimester of pregnancy feels like a hangover. It takes a while for the placenta to get its act together and take over the metabolism of waste from your liver. For the first 12 weeks or so of pregnancy, you feel tired. Smells and bright lights bother you, and you feel nauseated.

Just like people vary in how bad their hangovers are, women vary in how bad their first trimester symptoms are. I was fortunate. My hangover-like symptoms weren't too bad.

—*Ellen Kruger, MD, a mom of two teenagers and an ob-gyn in an academic and clinical practice in New Orleans, LA, with Ochsner Health System*

❧

I was so excited to get pregnant I took a home pregnancy test as soon as it was possible to test positive—before I had even missed my period. I didn't wait around to look for any early signs.

The first clue I was pregnant was the positive pregnancy test.

—*Lezli Braswell, MD, a mom of one daughter and two sons and a family medicine physician currently working in an emergency room fast track in Columbus, GA*

In my second and third pregnancies, I knew I was pregnant because I felt a sleepiness unlike anything I'd felt at any other time. A dreamy sensation would come over me in the middle of the day. I would give anything to lie down and take a nap.

—*Ann Kulze, MD, a mother of four children, ages 20, 19, 18, and 14, a nationally recognized nutrition expert, motivational speaker, physician, and the author of the critically acclaimed book* Dr. Ann's 10-Step Diet: A Simple Plan for Permanent Weight Loss and Lifelong Vitality

The first sign I was pregnant was nausea and carsickness that has never gone away. To this day, I have to be the driver in a car; I can't be a passenger. I could talk myself into being carsick right now if I wanted to. Pregnancy resets something in your system.

—*Stacey Marie Kerr, MD, a mother of two grown daughters, a family physician with strong roots in midwifery, and the author of* Homebirth in the Hospital, *in Santa Rosa, CA*

It's amazing how every pregnancy is so different. With my first daughter, the first indication I was pregnant was the fatigue! I was so tired. With my second, the thing I remember most is that my breasts became huge. I started off heavier than I was before my first pregnancy. I thought to myself, *This is ridiculous. I'm as big as a house!*

—*Janet Lefkowitz, DO, a mother of two girls and an ob-gyn in private practice in Rhode Island*

Researching Your Family's Health History

Before getting pregnant or early in your pregnancy is a great time to have a conversation with your family, and your partner's family, about their health. If certain conditions run in your family, or worse, in both of your families, it's better to know. You might consider searching online and talking with your doctor or midwife about it as well.

If you Google "family health history," you'll find many helpful resources to help you to compile your own medical family tree.

You might want to talk with your mother, grandmother, and sisters about their birthing experiences. While not entirely predictive of your experience, they'll certainly be interesting.

❧

Before I got pregnant, my husband and I talked a bit about each of our family's history. As a doctor, I knew that the major risk for Caucasians is cystic fibrosis. Because I knew that didn't run in either of our families, I wasn't too worried about our genetics. My doctor did screen me for cystic fibrosis, and the test was negative.

❧

It's easy to search online for your family heritage and "genetic risks" to find out if there are certain conditions someone from your background might be at risk for. Or you could ask your doctor about it.

—*Lezli Braswell, MD*

❧

I didn't talk with my family about their health history when I was pregnant, but in hindsight, it would have saved me a lot of worry.

After my daughter was born, she was having seizures. Her doctor and I were terribly worried that the seizures were caused by problems with her delivery. When my mother-in-law came to visit, she matter-of-factly mentioned that *everyone* on her side of the family has seizures in their first six months of life. Then they outgrow it. I breathed a huge sigh of relief after that.

Find out your family history ahead of time. Situations like mine aren't as anxiety provoking if they're not a surprise.

—*Ellen Kruger, MD*

❧

My husband and I probably should have done more researching into our families' health history than we did. My husband's mother died suddenly when he was four years old, and it wasn't clear why. I didn't really go hunting for the details about it. We didn't have a strong genetic bias or history, so we didn't worry too much.

> —*Nancy Rappaport, MD, a mother of two teenaged daughters and a teenaged son, an assistant professor of psychiatry at Harvard Medical School, an attending child and adolescent psychiatrist in the Cambridge, MA, public schools, and the author of* In Her Wake: A Child Psychiatrist Explores the Mystery of Her Mother's Suicide

As a doctor, I was already very aware of my family's health history. There was no need for me to research it. But for someone who isn't aware of their family health history, it's very important to check into.

—*Ashley Roman, MD, MPH, a mom of two daughters, ages three years and six months, and a clinical assistant professor in the department of obstetrics and gynecology at the New York University School of Medicine in New York City*

It's good to have a conversation with your mom and any sisters who have had children about their birth experiences. I knew my mother and sister had short labors. I think some families are blessed with easier childbirths than others. Although that's not totally predictive of your birth experiences, it was nice to know ahead of time.

—*Melanie Bone, MD, a mom of four "tweens" ages 15 to 12, a gynecologist, the founder of the Cancer Sensibility Foundation, and the author of the syndicated column* Surviving Life *and the book* Cancer, What's Next?, *in West Palm Beach, FL*

It's normal to be scared and worry what the pain of labor will be like. I think it's helpful to talk to your mother and ask her what her labor was like.

I didn't do this. Instead, after my baby was born, I asked my mother why she didn't tell me what labor was like!

"If I had told you, you wouldn't have had a baby," she said.

But the truth is that pain is very subjective. If you feel reassured and can remain calm, you can get through labor with minimal perception of pain.

—*Erika Schwartz, MD, a mom of two and the director of www.DrErika. com, who's been in private practice for more than 30 years in New York City, specializing over the past 15 years in women's health, disease prevention, and bioidentical hormones*

Choosing a Doctor or Midwife

You likely already have a doctor you see for your routine care, and perhaps you have another doctor you see for gynecologic issues. But where do you want to go for your care during your pregnancy?

You might choose an obstetrician, which is a doctor who specializes in the management of pregnancy, labor, and birth. They're commonly called ob-gyns—or even just obs. About 80 percent of pregnant women choose obs. An obstetrician who's specially trained in the care of high-risk pregnancies is called a maternal-fetal medicine specialist.

Or you might consider a certified nurse-midwife. They are registered nurses with advanced training and experience taking care of pregnant women and delivering babies.

Another choice that many women might not think of is a family practice doctor. These doctors are trained in *all* aspects of health care, for every member of your family. A family physician can be your doctor during and after pregnancy, and then also your baby's doctor, and in fact your whole family's doctor.

Whichever avenue you choose to take, check with your insurance company to make sure the provider is covered. Consider what hospital the provider is affiliated with—is it covered by your insurance company and convenient to your home? And find out who covers when the provider is away and who handles phone calls and after-hour emergencies.

Most important, talk with the provider and spend some time in the office. Pay attention to how you feel about the provider, the office, and the staff. You'll be spending a lot of time there in the months ahead.

⌒⊘

Really take your time choosing an ob or midwife. You never know what's going to happen. I ended up having a C-section, and throughout the entire procedure, my lovely ob—whom I adored—sat and held my hand. She was sick as a dog with the flu, and her colleague performed my C-section, but she hung in with me!

—JJ Levenstein, MD, FAAP, *a mom of one son in college and a pediatrician in private practice in Southern California*

⌒⊘

I think that the most important thing to look for when choosing a doctor or midwife is to find someone you trust. You need to find a person you trust to make the best decision for you.

This came into play for me when I was in labor, and my ob-gyn made the call that I needed to have a C-section. It wasn't at all what I had expected to happen, but I trusted completely that she was making the right decision for me and my babies.

—*Jennifer Gilbert, DO, a mom of three-month-old twins and an ob-gyn at Paoli Hospital in Pennsylvania*

≈⁓

I had a unique situation during my pregnancy because my dad is an ob-gyn. Even though my dad had decades of experience, I decided not to go to him for my prenatal care or to have him deliver my babies.

It's a very personal decision, but I think it's important not to have a friend or family member deliver your baby just in case things don't go as planned. You don't want to feel that those people are responsible.

—*Debra Luftman, MD, a mom of a teenaged daughter and a teenaged son, a board-certified dermatologist in private practice, a coauthor of* The Beauty Prescription, *the developer of the skincare line of products Therapeutix, and a clinical instructor of skin surgery and general dermatology at UCLA*

≈⁓

I wanted to have an obstetrician deliver my baby. Especially because she was my first child, I knew I would feel more comfortable delivering with an obstetrician in a hospital.

—*Christy Valentine, MD*

≈⁓

Obstetricians delivered all three of my babies. I think it's very important to take the time to find an obstetrician who's really a good match for you. You want to find someone you're comfortable with and who shares your philosophies about birth. The relationship between a woman and her obstetrician is very special.

For myself I chose an obstetrician in solo practice, rather than a doctor in a group practice. It was very important to me to know who was going to deliver my babies. Pregnancy is such a special time, and I really enjoyed the relationships I had with my obstetricians. I think that when you know and trust your doctor, you'll be much calmer in the delivery room.

—*Ayala Laufer-Cahana, MD, a pediatrician, mother, artist, serious home cook, and the founder of Herbal Water Inc., in Wynnewood, PA*

≈⁓

One option to consider when choosing your practitioner is a family doctor. In my mind, that's the best choice. I chose a family doctor to deliver my older daughter. A family doctor will see you through your pregnancy and then pick up your new baby's care from the very beginning.

As a family doctor myself, I feel a strong heart connection to babies I've known from the beginning when they were just blips in their mother's belly. I've helped them to grow from tiny seeds.

—*Stacey Marie Kerr, MD*

‿⁄◦

At the hospital where I was going to give birth, there is a large midwifery group. Most of the deliveries at that time were done by midwives. Only the complicated cases and C-sections were done by doctors. The logic was, if things are going well, let the labor progress as naturally as possible. I had to see an ob-gyn, though, because I had a complicated pregnancy.

—*Ellen Kruger, MD*

‿⁄◦

For my first baby, I had a midwife. I thought that they spend more time getting to know their patients than some doctors are able to. But we moved before my second pregnancy, and I couldn't find a midwife group near our new home. I found an ob instead, and he turned out to be fabulous.

—*Sonia Ng, MD, a mom of seven-year-old and one-year-old sons and a pediatrician and expert in sedation at Children's Hospital of Philadelphia Pediatric Care at Princeton Health Care System in Princeton, NJ*

‿⁄◦

It's very important to find the best medical care provider for you, whether that's a midwife or physician. My first two babies were delivered by midwives, and my last two were delivered by a family doctor who is still my 19-year-old's doctor. I looked for a doctor who understood that I wasn't diseased, only pregnant. He was willing to be there during my deliveries just in case he was needed—not to intervene.

—*Hana R. Solomon, MD, a mom of four, ages 35 to 19, a board-certified pediatrician, the president of BeWell Health, LLC, and the author of* Clearing the Air One Nose at a Time: Caring for Your Personal Filter

‿⁄◦

When I was in medical school, a nurse-midwife came and spoke to our class. She addressed some of the differences between ob care and the way her group of midwives practiced. For me, it seemed like the midwives were the better way to go—as long as everything was going smoothly and progressing normally.

For two of my babies, I delivered with midwives. My second baby was born nine weeks early, so that was a lot more complicated. I had a whole team of practitioners for that delivery!

For my first baby, I was especially glad to have gone with the midwives. I pushed with that kid for three hours, and the midwife was super patient. She allowed me to keep going without any intervention until we reached the point where the baby either needed to be born or I needed to have a C-section. The midwife used a vacuum, and my daughter was born.

After my baby was born, I told the postpartum nurse how long I had pushed. The nurse said, "If you had an ob, you would have had this baby hours ago by C-section."

—*Kristie McNealy, MD, a mom of seven- and four-year-old daughters and a two-year-old son, who's pregnant with another son, and a blogger at www.KristieMcNealy.com, in Denver, CO*

⌒

Midwives delivered both of my babies—at home! My father was an MD, so I was raised around standard medical care, and I have an appreciation for it. But I wanted a different approach during my pregnancies. Birth is not a new experience to the human body. If our ancestors could deliver at home, in a more natural place where the birth process was honored with patience, that was where I wanted to be. I didn't want to give birth in a hospital where it might feel that birth was a medical emergency or an illness.

To me, the birth process is very normal and natural. I felt much more comfortable with midwives, who are highly trained in the process of vaginal births. At the end of the day, my fellow obstetricians are trained surgeons. They are excellent at what they do, but it was important for me to try and have a natural birth if I could. I feel it is healthier for us, and for our children. I wanted to avoid medical intervention unless my midwife thought it was important.

You can have a wonderful birth wherever you go, but while we have made such incredible technological advances in obstetrics care these days, it's ironic that there's a high rate of birth dissatisfaction among the majority of my patients who deliver in hospitals. We've gotten away from the normal rhythms of the body, and birth is one of them.

A hospital is a place of business. The staff works within a time frame that might not necessarily suit your own biological clock and birth rhythm. For example, during my second pregnancy, my water started to trickle on a Tuesday night at 11 pm. I called my midwife to say I think my water broke. My midwife asked if I had a fever, which is a sign of infection. Because my temperature was normal, my midwife told me to go to sleep and take long walks the next day. Around 26 hours after that first trickle, I went into labor naturally and gave birth 3 hours later, at home.

If I had been with a doctor instead of a midwife, I probably would have ended up on Pitocin at the very least. The second your water breaks, many doctors start looking at the clock and thinking about inducing labor, and if labor doesn't progress, this could lead to a C-section.

I feel very blessed that I was able to have my children the way nature intended. My birth experiences were fine: no IV, no vaginal tears, no stitches. Sure it was painful! It's called labor because it's laborious! But you need to have the pain; that's how you get the baby out!

—*Lauren Feder, MD, a mom of two sons, a nationally recognized physician who specializes in homeopathic medicine, and the author of* Natural Baby and Childcare *and* The Parents' Concise Guide to Childhood Vaccinations, *in Los Angeles*

Trying to Relax

Studies rank pregnancy at number 12 on the list of life's most stressful events. And of course the rest of your stress isn't going away anytime soon.

It's perfectly natural to worry about your growing baby. In fact, it's great training for parenthood. You might worry about your new role as a mother, how having a baby will impact your relationship with your partner, or how you'll pay for college in 2028.

But stress isn't going to do you any favors in pregnancy. Ironically, stress can worsen just about every pregnancy symptom: aches and pains, headaches, heartburn, hives, and nausea. Plus, stress will suppress your immune system, which is already weakened by pregnancy. (Hello, cold and flu!)

There are many ways to decrease stress, such as taking deep breaths, listening to music, going for a walk, talking with a friend, sipping (decaf!) tea, reading a book, gazing at a sunset, and having a massage. Take a moment to come up with a list of your top three stress relievers. If possible, come up with some you can do at the same time, such as listening to your favorite artist while taking a bubble bath and doing some deep breathing. Then when you feel stressed, that's your go-to place.

❧

When I was pregnant with my first baby, I was living at the Farm, a commune in Tennessee. They have been delivering babies there with midwives for more than 35 years, and they have a C-section rate of less than 2 percent. We expected birth to go right, and so it did. I think that is key: When you expect something to go right, it more likely will.

—*Stacey Marie Kerr, MD*

❧

Meditation is a huge part of my life. It gives me a buffer from reality. I have a fairly intense life, and I do a lot of listening. Sitting quietly in meditation allows my brain to rinse out like clothes in a washing machine. The chance to sit quietly and to learn to be an observer is a helpful skill in pregnancy—and also in parenting. It helps you to be more receptive to what your kids are trying to say.

—*Nancy Rappaport, MD*

❧

When I got pregnant with my first child, I was in my residency training. My husband and I weren't actually planning to get pregnant at that time.

Because I was in the second year of a three-year residency program, I wasn't able to alter my work schedule. But I did try to rest as much as I could and take the best care of myself possible.

Having a little time to myself is the best stress reliever for me. So I made time to exercise even if it was just taking a walk or doing yoga. That was very relaxing for me.

—*Elissa Charbonneau, DO, a mom of an 18-year-old son and a 16-year-old daughter and the medical director of the New England Rehabilitation Hospital in Portland, ME*

❧

During my pregnancy, I tried not to worry too much about anything. This approach has served me very well.

My approach to life is that I don't like having huge expectations. I like for life to surprise me! So before I got pregnant, I didn't try to imagine what it would be like to be pregnant, and before my baby was born, I didn't try to imagine what it would be like to be a mother. I figured I'd know soon enough.

—*Ayala Laufer-Cahana, MD*

During my pregnancies, I tried to minimize sources of anxiety as much as possible. One important thing that I did to help ease anxiety and relax during my pregnancies was to choose practitioners I felt could best serve me and meet my needs. I placed myself in the hands of people I felt most confident with in terms of their professionalism, clinical skills, and bedside manner.

A lot of women become anxious about their deliveries and worry if their needs will be met. For example, if women see doctors in a large group practice, they aren't sure who exactly will be delivering their babies. I chose a midwife, and so I knew who would be delivering my baby. That took away one source of stress.

—*Lauren Feder, MD*

? When to Call Your Doctor or Midwife

During pregnancy, your emotions might be on a wild roller-coaster ride. It's normal to have worries, doubts, and fears. More than 70 percent of pregnant women experience mood swings while they're pregnant, especially during the first trimester.

However, if you feel depressed for more than two weeks, call your doctor or midwife.

Chapter 4
Week 4

Your Baby This Week

YOUR BABY'S SIZE

Your baby right now is just a cluster of cells called a blastocyst. She is around 0.014 inch to about 0.04 inch, about the size of an "o" on this page. Your baby is growing at an amazing rate. During the first month alone, she increases in size by 40 times.

YOUR BABY'S LATEST DEVELOPMENTS

This week, the implanted blastocyst is embedded more deeply into the lining of your uterus. Spongelike fingers from the blastocyst's outer cells burrow into the lining to link up with your blood vessels. You and your baby are now joined.

This week, three different layers of cells begin to develop, each with its own important job. The ectoderm, which is the outer layer, forms the hair, skin, nipples, nails, tooth enamel, eye lenses, nervous system, and brain. The mesoderm, which is the middle layer, will become the reproductive organs, heart and blood vessels, skeleton, and muscles. The endoderm, which is the inner layer, becomes the digestive and respiratory systems, urinary tract, and bladder. Arm and leg buds begin to form this week, although they don't look anything like arms or legs yet.

The placenta is forming. Your body creates the placenta—a completely new organ—to nourish your baby. It's the placenta that is producing a hormone called human chorionic gonadotropin (hCG) that might be creating early pregnancy symptoms in you.

The umbilical cord is beginning to form, and the amniotic sac is in the earliest stage of formation. The amniotic sac is a bag of fluid inside your uterus where your baby develops and grows.

YOUR LATEST DEVELOPMENTS

You haven't gained any weight. You don't look pregnant, and you might not even *feel* pregnant.

On the other hand, you might feel some nausea due to the hormonal changes going on in your body. The tiny blastocyst produces chemical messengers that send signals to your body to keep your period from starting. Even though your period isn't coming, you might feel bloating and cramping similar to what you usually feel before your period. You might also feel some pressure in your lower abdomen. This could be caused by an increase in blood circulation or by your uterus already beginning to stretch. Some women have backaches and headaches.

Your breasts might feel tender, tingly, or sore. And they might be getting larger. These developments are caused by the increased levels of progesterone and estrogen in your body. Amazingly, these changes are already setting the stage for breastfeeding.

Your mood might be going amok, which is also caused by the increasing levels of hCG, estrogen, and progesterone. You might feel overemotional and tearful. You might suddenly feel very tired because of the increased hormones. Plus, your body is working very, very hard.

You might have some implantation bleeding right around the time your period would have been due, or perhaps a little before. This can look like light pink, red, or brown spotting or yellowish discharge.

Also because your levels of the hormone hCG are rising, this week you might get a positive result on an at-home pregnancy test. The test is more likely to be positive if you take it first thing in the morning, when your urine is more concentrated, and later in this week.

JUSTIFICATION FOR A CELEBRATION

You're probably expecting your period at the end of this week, but when it doesn't come, you might suspect you're pregnant. A positive pregnancy test is cause for celebration indeed!

Taking a Pregnancy Test—Or Ten

Visit any grocery store, drugstore, or Target, and you'll find a dizzying array of home pregnancy tests. But amazingly, they all work the same way. They detect hCG hormone, which is only in your urine when you're pregnant. Your body starts to make hCG when the fertilized egg implants into your uterus. It's like a switch is turned on. The amount of hCG in your body rapidly increases with each passing day of your pregnancy.

Home pregnancy tests are highly accurate—if you use them correctly. Some tests promise that they can tell you if you're pregnant on the first day of your missed period. But they can't always detect the low level of hCG that's present at that time. Most tests can accurately tell you that you're pregnant about one week after your missed period. But just try to wait that long to take one…

∽

When I thought I might be pregnant, I took a home pregnancy test. Actually, I took a lot of home pregnancy tests. When the first one came back positive, I worried perhaps there was something wrong with the test. So I took another. It was positive too. But I took another one the next day just to be sure. I took about four of them before it was all said and done.

—*Kerri A. Daniels, MD, a mom of one toddler daughter and an instructor in the department of pediatrics at the University of Arkansas for Medical Science in Little Rock*

∽

I was so tired all of the time, and I suspected I might be pregnant. So I went to a drugstore and bought a pregnancy test. It came back positive. I went back to the drugstore and bought two more tests, and they were positive too. Then I was convinced!

—*Christy Valentine, MD, a mom of one, a specialist in pediatrics and internal medicine, and the founder of the Valentine Medical Center in Gretna, LA*

∽

My husband and I tried for a while to get pregnant, and I was so surprised and thrilled when I found out. I saved that pregnancy test. In fact, I think I still have it in a drawer in my bedside table.

—*Diane Connelly, MD, a mom of a six-year-old daughter and an ob-gyn in HMO practice in Riverside, CA*

When I found out I was pregnant the first time, I took two tests just to be sure. I think it's a good idea to check it twice.

I found out I was pregnant the second and third times during my annual exams. It was coincidental that I had doctor's appointments. In both cases, my period was a week late. I thought it was because of stress. When I mentioned it to my gynecologist, she gave me a pregnancy test, and sure enough I was pregnant. My doctor was very happy to give me the good news!

—*Aline T. Tanios, MD, a mom of three and a general pediatrician and hospitalist who treats medically complex children at Arkansas Children's Hospital in Little Rock*

Discovering That You're Pregnant

There are few moments in life like discovering that you are pregnant. It's as if you're striding confidently down one path in life and suddenly a giant gust of wind blows you off of that path—and onto a new one. When that stick turns blue, your life is dramatically, irreversibly changed.

∽◇

When I found out I was pregnant, I felt wonder, joy—and terror.

—*Elizabeth Berger, MD, a mom of two, a child psychiatrist, and the author of* Raising Kids with Character

∽◇

Getting pregnant—and then becoming a mother—changes your whole outlook on life. It changes everything about your life. People say that all of the time, but you can't really understand it until you've gone through it on your own.

    —Jennifer Gilbert, DO, a mom of three-month-old twins and an ob-gyn at Paoli Hospital in Pennsylvania

⤨

Even though my husband and I were trying to get pregnant, when I saw that positive test, I thought, *Oh my God. What have I done?* We spend our whole lives contracepting, and then suddenly when you get pregnant, it hits you that you're going to be someone's mother. Anyone with half a brain is going to panic at first when she sees that positive pregnancy test.

    —Ellen Kruger, MD, a mom of two teenagers and an ob-gyn in an academic and clinical practice in New Orleans, LA, with Ochsner Health Systems

⤨

When I found out I was pregnant, I was terrified. I thought, *Oh, God, what have we done? How are we going to make this work?*

    I was in medical school, applying for residency programs, and my life was about to get crazy busy. But quickly, my husband and I got used to the idea of having a baby. We knew we could make it.

    —Ann LaBarge, MD, a mom of four children, ages 16 to six, and an ob-gyn in private practice at the Midwest Center for Women's Healthcare in Park Ridge, IL

⤨

When I got a positive on my pregnancy test, I was in my second year of a four-year residency program, and my husband and I had been married for a year and a half. We had bought a house, and we were doing exactly what everyone says you're supposed to do.

    I remember being scared to death. I thought, *What have we gotten ourselves into?* I wasn't worried about our finances because we both had jobs and bright futures. But I was terrified of the responsibility of it all.

    I went into a small room off of the labor room at the hospital and shut the door. I needed some time to collect myself and contemplate what lay ahead. Even when you have all of your ducks in a row, finding out you're pregnant is still terrifying.

    —Kathie Bowling, MD, a mom of three grown sons and an ob-gyn in private practice in Providence, RI, who's also on the clinical faculty at the Warren Alpert School of Medicine at Brown University

When my pregnancy test came out positive, at first I was surprised. Then it hit me, *Oh my goodness, what am I going to do?* It really hit me at that moment that I was now responsible for another person. That was a defining moment in my life. My daughter brought my life into focus.

—*Christy Valentine, MD*

⁂

For several years after my husband and I had been married, I squelched my yearnings for a baby. We were both training to be physicians, and it wasn't the right time.

In the spring of my senior year, I started having some stomach discomfort. I took Zantac and tried to ignore it. Then my period was late. Lo and behold, I found out I was pregnant, a month or two before beginning what was going to be the most demanding, exhausting time of my career—my internship.

—*Ann Kulze, MD, a mother of four children, ages 20, 19, 18, and 14, a nationally recognized nutrition expert, motivational speaker, physician, and the author of the critically acclaimed book* Dr. Ann's 10-Step Diet: A Simple Plan for Permanent Weight Loss and Lifelong Vitality

⁂

My husband and I had been married for a few years when we started trying to get pregnant. I was in medical school at the time. I figured that we were as ready as we ever would be!

I assumed that it would take a long time to get pregnant, so when I suddenly became very, very fatigued, it didn't dawn on me that I might be pregnant. I went out for my birthday and joked about what a lightweight I was because I was so exhausted.

When I missed my period, at eight weeks, I took a pregnancy test. I was quite surprised to find out I was pregnant!

—*Janet Lefkowitz, DO, a mother of two girls and an ob-gyn in private practice in Rhode Island*

⁂

I didn't take a test to find out I was pregnant until I was 10 weeks into my pregnancy. My husband had convinced me that all of my symptoms were caused by stress. I was finishing my residency at the time, and we were moving from Illinois to Georgia. We had a lot going on.

I was so happy to find out that I was pregnant! My husband was happy too, once he got over his shock.

—*Karen Heald, MD, a mom of four boys and a board-certified family physician in private practice outside Atlanta, GA*

∽⊙

When I got pregnant with my son, I was an intern. My husband and I weren't planning to start a family at that time, but we were open to having children at any point. We were living in separate states then and seeing each other on weekends, so pregnancy wasn't really on my radar.

I was so busy and tired that I didn't have much time to think about myself. I was too busy taking care of other people and worrying about how *they* were feeling. I didn't find out that I was pregnant until later in my first trimester. It sort of snuck up on me! Discovering that I was pregnant was a very welcome surprise.

—*Julie Silver, MD, a mom of a 17-year-old son and 13- and 9-year-old daughters, a Boston-area physiatrist, and the award-winning writer of more than a dozen books, including* After Cancer Treatment: Heal Faster, Better, Stronger

∽⊙

The first time I got pregnant really easily. But I had a much more difficult time the second time. I was working in a residency program at the Mayo Clinic. I was exhausted and burned out. I was in premature menopause. A friend of mine who's also an infertility specialist said that my only chance of getting pregnant again was with a donor egg. I didn't want to get on that roller coaster, so I tried to put it out of my mind.

A few months later, I sprained my ankle really badly. In reflexology, the female reproductive system is localized near the Achilles tendon. Next thing I knew, I was pregnant with twins! Reflexologists might say that the increased blood flow to the area of the body focused on reproduction might have helped me overcome my infertility issues.

When I found out I was pregnant and told my friend, she was shocked. My husband told her, "This is your fault! You don't tell my wife she can't do something, because she will show you that you're wrong."

—*Susan Wilder, MD, a mom of an older daughter and twin girls, a primary care physician, and CEO and founder of Lifescape Medical Associates in Scottsdale, AZ*

Telling Your Partner the Good News

Finding out that you're pregnant is a moment you'll remember forever. Telling your partner the news will also become a cherished memory. How will you remember this moment?

⤠⤙

I took my pregnancy test at the hospital, and my med school classmates knew that I was pregnant before my husband did. When I took the little stick home with the positive sign, I just rang the bell and stood there with it in front of my face. My husband's jaw dropped, and then he just smiled!

—*JJ Levenstein, MD, FAAP, a mom of one son in college and a pediatrician in private practice in Southern California*

⤠⤙

I told my husband that I was pregnant as soon as I found out. He shared my excitement, and he liked the idea of having two sons. He's so in love with our older son that he's eager to double the fun.

—*Amy J. Derick, MD, a mom of one 15-month-old son who is 17 weeks pregnant with her second son. Dr. Derick is a dermatologist in private practice at Derick Dermatology in Barrington, IL*

⤠⤙

When I found out I was pregnant with my oldest daughter, my husband and I were living in New York City. We were going out to dinner that night to celebrate his birthday. I put the ultrasound photo into a frame that said "Daddy and Me," and I hid it in my purse.

When my husband asked if I wanted to order wine, I said, "I think you should open your last present first." He knew what it was right away, and he ordered a martini and I got iced tea.

—*Marra Francis, MD, a mom of three daughters and an ob-gyn who's based in The Woodlands, TX*

⤠⤙

I took my first pregnancy test at night when my husband was asleep. I knew that he would be excited if I thought I was pregnant, and I didn't want him to be disappointed if I wasn't.

When the test came back positive, I didn't want to wake my husband, so I planned to wait to tell him until the morning. That lasted about five minutes, and then I woke him up and told him. He wasn't totally with it at first, and he said rather formally, "Congratulations!" But then a few minutes later, he woke up the rest of the way, and his excitement set in.

—*Kerri A. Daniels, MD*

RALLIE'S TIP

My third pregnancy caught me completely off guard. My second son was just four months old when I realized I was expecting again. I wanted my husband to experience the joyous surprise the same way I had, so I wrapped the pregnancy test strip in a small box and gave it to him on Father's Day. It took my husband a minute or two to understand the meaning of his gift, but when he figured it out, he was just as surprised—and just as happy—as I had been when I watched the "positive" indicator appear on the test strip a few days earlier.

Not Panicking about Implantation Bleeding

Most women think of pregnancy as a time when they won't be having their periods. This is true because you won't be menstruating.

Being pregnant doesn't mean you won't have any bleeding, though. Studies show that between 20 and 30 percent of women experience bleeding during early pregnancy. One cause of early bleeding is implantation bleeding. This can happen anywhere from six to 14 days after conception. As the embryo burrows into your uterine wall, you might notice some bleeding, or some yellow or brown discharge.

This type of bleeding is usually spottier and lighter in color than a period, and it doesn't last as long.

∽

I didn't have any implantation bleeding with my first son, but I did with my second. It was just a little blood, but of course I was motivated to do some research to determine the cause: implantation bleeding or my period. No period. I was pregnant.

—*Amy J. Derick, MD*

∽

Although bleeding in the first trimester is scary, I wouldn't have been too worried because even if you have some, there's a very good chance the pregnancy will continue and be just fine. Bleeding combined with cramping is more of a concern.

—*Gina Dado, MD, a mom of two daughters and an ob-gyn with Arizona OBGYN Affiliates, Paradise Valley Branch, in Scottsdale, AZ*

Coping with Morning Sickness

Morning sickness is so common in pregnancy that it almost seems like a rite of passage. But while more than half of all pregnant women experience morning sickness, not all of them do! The nausea and vomiting usually begin around the sixth week of pregnancy and last until around the 12th week, but morning sickness can begin as early as week four, and it can linger long after week 12.

Despite its name, morning sickness can strike any time—day or night. It's caused by the increase in estrogen, progesterone, and hCG hormones, which support your pregnancy. Stress, fatigue, and a poor diet can make morning sickness worse. Many doctors consider morning sickness to be a positive sign, because it indicates that the placenta is developing well. But if you're one of those women who don't experience it, don't worry. Be grateful instead.

One of the first clues I was pregnant was morning sickness. It came on out of nowhere. I'd be out walking the dog, and all of a sudden I'd have to stop to throw up. The dog would turn around and look at me like, *What the heck was that?*

—*Susan Wilder, MD*

❧

I got pregnant during my ob-gyn rotation. Every morning as I was puking, at least I was around people who understood. I did my fair share of vomiting until I was 12 weeks pregnant.

I think it's helpful to surround yourself with supportive people at a time like this when you're pretty miserable. It's also helpful when your partner brings you Ritz crackers and orange slices cut "just so" to alleviate the morning sickness.

—*JJ Levenstein, MD, FAAP*

❧

Fortunately, I didn't have a lot of nausea in my pregnancy. The only time I felt sick was in stop-and-go traffic. I tried to avoid that as much as possible.

—*Kerri A. Daniels, MD*

❧

For my entire life, I could ride in a car and read with no problems. One day, I was riding in the car and all of a sudden, trying to read made me sick. That was the first clue I was pregnant. To this day, I cannot read and ride. Having a baby truly changes everything.

—*Karen Heald, MD*

❧

With both of my pregnancies, I had terrible morning sickness. It was bad with my daughter, but with my twins it was unrelenting. I think that was because with twins, you have double the amount of hormones. My nausea was so bad that I had to take prescription medication for it. I didn't want to, but I had to be able to function on some level.

I had an especially rough time when riding in a car. I found that Sea-Band wrist bands helped. It helped a lot if I was the driver, and I refused to ride in the backseat! (See "Mommy MD Guide-Recommended Product: Sea-Band Antinausea Bands" on page 55.)

—*Kelly Campbell, MD, a mom of three and an ob-gyn in private practice at Women's Healthcare Physicians in West Bloomfield, MI*

During my first pregnancy, I was an intern. I had to be at work by 7 am, so I didn't have time for morning sickness.

Instead, I vomited when I had time, at night. I believe that your body will adjust to your circumstances—if you allow it to. I found that eating salty things, such as saltine crackers, made me feel better. Thank goodness, after around my third month, my "night" sickness went away.

— *Erika Schwartz, MD, a mom of two and the director of www. DrErika.com, who's been in private practice for more than 30 years in New York City, specializing over the past 15 years in women's health, disease prevention, and bioidentical hormones*

I'm a mountain mama kind of person. My parents were Holocaust survivors, and I was raised by a single mom in a ghetto in Brooklyn. During my pregnancy, when I felt a little sick to my stomach, I put crackers near my bed and drank 7-Up. I dealt with it. It's no big deal. It is all in your perspective; you choose how to perceive the experience—torture, tolerable, pleasant, etc.

— *Hana R. Solomon, MD, a mom of four, ages 35 to 19, a board-certified pediatrician, the president of BeWell Health, LLC, and the author of* Clearing the Air One Nose at a Time: Caring for Your Personal Filter

I had such terrible nausea and vomiting that I thought pregnancy was the best diet in the world. I had morning sickness with all three of my pregnancies. I was able to adjust my work so that I didn't do surgery in the first trimester.

One thing that tasted good that I could keep down was a Slurpee from 7-Eleven. Fortunately, the morning sickness ended after the first trimester.

— *Judy Dudum, MD, a mom of three, an ob-gyn, and a senior staff physician at Henry Ford Health System in Detroit, with interests in nutrition and adolescent gynecology*

I was a terrible pregnant person, sick from conception on. I had awful morning sickness, and I wasn't eating well. During my pregnancy, I was living on a spiritual commune called the Farm. We were such strict vegetarians that we didn't even wear leather.

All I wanted to eat was fried potatoes; anything else made me sick. My first baby was grown on fried potatoes, and my second was grown on Lord knows what! I never figured out that *eating* was what made the nausea go away.

—*Stacey Marie Kerr, MD, a mother of two grown daughters, a family physician with strong roots in midwifery, and the author of* Homebirth in the Hospital, *in Santa Rosa, CA*

During the first few months of my pregnancy, I was drooling all of the time. I had way too much spit. (This feeling of having too much saliva is known as ptyalism.) I thought I was going to have to wear a bib by the end of pregnancy. Nothing helped. It was very annoying.

—*Sonia Ng, MD, a mom of seven-year-old and one-year-old sons and a pediatrician and expert in sedation at Children's Hospital of Philadelphia Pediatric Care at Princeton Health Care System in Princeton, NJ*

I never got a chance to wallow in my fatigue and nausea because my husband was 1,000 miles away for the first four months of my pregnancy. Luckily, I only vomited three times the entire pregnancy.

At some point in the pregnancy, I stopped being able to tolerate flat liquids of any kind—even water. Seltzer water always came to my rescue. It worked best during those times when I was at a restaurant and I felt the nausea wave coming. If you don't like plain seltzer, try one with fruit flavoring.

Grab some oatmeal bars or snack bars and put them in your pockets so you can nibble on them when you're hungry. The South Beach Diet bars taste yummy even though they're low-fat and low-carb.

—*Tyeese Gaines Reid, DO, a mom of one, an emergency medicine resident physician at Yale New Haven Hospital in Connecticut, and the author of a time management book,* The Get a Life Campaign

During my first pregnancy, I had intense morning sickness 24/7. Thank goodness, I had finished my senior year of medical school, and I had a few months off before I began my internship. I spent the entire time on the couch. I was so sick that I couldn't eat. I lost 15 to 20 pounds, and I was practically the size of a refugee.

I tried everything you can imagine to feel better: prescription drugs that made me sleepy, pressure bands on my wrists, you name it. I discovered one thing that was amazingly effective: chopped, fresh ginger. It was a godsend for me; it enabled me to function.

I took a thumbnail-size piece of fresh gingerroot, chopped it fine, and steeped it like you would tea in hot water, for two to three minutes. I'd sip that all day long and chew up the ginger at the bottom of each mug. Afterward, my nausea was decreased by about 50 percent. Nothing else, not even prescription drugs, was as effective as the ginger tea.

Thankfully, the nausea abated just in time for my internship. At that point, it was helpful that I was so busy because it distracted me from thinking about the miserable nausea. I couldn't think about myself because I was so busy taking care of patients.

—*Ann Kulze, MD*

I had morning sickness with all four of my pregnancies. It wasn't until around 20 weeks that I felt better. Eating small, frequent meals helped. Eating eased the sensation that I was going to throw up. I tried to avoid throwing up at all costs because one of the many ironies of pregnancy is that when you throw up, it doesn't make you feel better.

In my third pregnancy, I also discovered that an over-the-counter sleep medicine called Unisom helps ease morning sickness. It's an antihistamine, and it's not habit-forming. But of course it does make you sleepy, so I took half a pill in the morning and then a full pill at night. It takes the edge off morning sickness, and plus you sleep better. (Talk with your doctor or midwife before taking this or any medication.)

—*Ann LaBarge, MD*

? When to Call Your Doctor or Midwife

You should call your doctor or midwife immediately if you have lost more than two pounds, vomit bright red or black blood, vomit more than four times in one day, or can't keep fluids down for more than a day.

Less than 1 percent of pregnant women develop a condition called hyperemesis gravidarum—nausea and vomiting that is so severe the mom-to-be isn't able to consume enough nutrients and calories. This condition requires treatment by a doctor, and it often lasts throughout the pregnancy.

During one pregnancy, my nausea and vomiting were severe. Thankfully, this wasn't during my whole pregnancy, just the first 12 weeks.

There wasn't much I could do, other than suffer through it. I tried to eat small amounts of food and keep hydrated. I didn't want to take any drugs that could potentially have bad side effects.

What was comforting was knowing that the morning sickness was eventually going to go away! That's the great thing about morning sickness; I just woke up one morning, and it was gone!

—*Barbara Goff, MD, a mom of two and a professor of obstetrics and gynecology and the director of gynecologic oncology at the University of Washington Medical Center in Seattle*

∽◎

During my pregnancy, I had such severe morning sickness that my doctor put me on prescription medication. The vomiting was killing me.

I took an antinausea medication daily 15 minutes before I got out of bed in the morning. Even taking the medication, I still was sick, but at least I was able to function.

Another thing that helped was carrying ginger hard candy in my pocket everywhere I went. It helped settle my stomach. I also packed snacks such as carrots or grapes. I took a variety of snacks to work each day because I never knew ahead of time what food would agree with me. My advice is when you're pregnant, never leave the house without a snack! Morning sickness in pregnancy is caused by high levels of hormones, but it is worsened by hypoglycemia, or low blood sugar. Eating small meals frequently helps to keep your blood sugar levels balanced without overdistending your stomach. Some of the best food selections to consider are from the carbohydrate food group: crackers and breads. Avoid greasy, fatty foods.

Sometimes hot tea helped my nausea, with three teaspoons of sugar. I figured I'd rather throw up liquids than food. Drink whatever tastes good as long as you can keep it down.

—*Aline T. Tanios, MD*

∽◎

During my first pregnancy, I vomited all day long, all over the place, for the better part of eight months. The story that "this is only going to last a few weeks" was not true for me.

I tried everything that anyone suggested—from eating citrus fruit to wearing metallic wrist bands to hypnosis. I would have done anything to stop vomiting, but nothing worked. I didn't stop throwing up until my son was born.

At that time, I was in my residency. When I came into the residents' rooms heading for the bathroom, all of the men would clear out. The women stuck around; it didn't seem to bother them! I knew where every single public toilet was in the hospital, and I probably threw up in every one of them at least once.

How did I cope? I carried a toothbrush and breath mints in my pocket. I could be in the middle of talking with a patient, excuse myself to the bathroom, vomit, brush my teeth, and get right back to talking. You have to keep moving forward, despite the nausea and vomiting.

There are some foods that I learned to avoid because they were so awful to throw up—pineapple, yogurt, and watermelon to name a few. The sight of them makes me sick to this day!

The best news I can give you is that just because you had terrible morning sickness in one pregnancy doesn't mean you'll have it again. During my second pregnancy, I didn't throw up a single time.

—*Carrie Brown, MD, a mom of two and a general pediatrician who treats medically complex children and specializes in palliative care at Arkansas Children's Hospital in Little Rock*

Mommy MD Guide–Recommended Product
Sea-Band Antinausea Bands

One of the many challenges of pregnancy is that you can't take many medications while pregnant. Luckily, there's one simple solution for morning sickness that's completely drug free: acupressure. Pressing on the acupressure points on your wrists, called the nei kuan points, often helps alleviate nausea, whether it's caused by morning sickness or a bumpy car ride.

You'll find several products on the market that stimulate these points, and one is Sea-Band Antinausea Bands. These elastic wrist bands have plastic studs that apply gentle pressure to the acupressure points. You can buy them online at **WWW.SEA-BAND.COM** or in stores.

Chapter 5
Week 5

Your Baby This Week

YOUR BABY'S SIZE
This week, your baby is around 0.05 inch long, about the size of an "l" in this book.

YOUR BABY'S LATEST DEVELOPMENTS
By the beginning of this week, you could see the cluster of cells as a tiny nubbin of tissue on an ultrasound. Although the embryo is still in the shape of a flat disk, your baby's body is starting to form.

Your baby's brain and spinal cord, muscles, and bones are beginning to take shape. A row of dark cells appears down the back of the embryo, and later these cells will fold, close together, and become the neural tube. This is the critical time to be taking folic acid, which is key to your baby's central nervous system development.

The earliest form of your baby's heart is starting to develop. Your baby's heart is the first organ to begin to function. Around the end of this week, your baby's heart will begin to beat. You wouldn't be able to hear it yet, but you might be able to *see* your baby's heart beat on an ultrasound.

YOUR LATEST DEVELOPMENTS
You have probably missed your period. Around a week after your missed period, a home pregnancy test will come back positive.

Morning sickness might well be kicking in. It's so named because it often starts in the morning and abates as the day goes on.

Another common early pregnancy symptom you might be feeling is fatigue. We're not talking about dozing-off-in-front-of-the-TV fatigue. Often the fatigue women feel in pregnancy is more of the hit-by-a-Mack-Truck variety. This is common, and it should pass. If you can manage to get up off of the couch, this is an excellent time to start a gentle workout program, and exercise might actually help you gain more energy. If you already exercise, talk with your doctor or midwife about your routine to see if you should make any adjustments.

You might be noticing changes in your breasts. Often in early pregnancy, women notice a tingling feeling. Your breasts might feel heavy, and they might even look larger. The areolas around your nipples might change in color, and already you might spot veins on the surface of your breasts. These changes are all caused by the high levels of estrogen needed to support your pregnancy.

Throughout your pregnancy, and beginning this week, you might feel a slight tugging or tightness in your lower abdomen. The ligaments that are attached to your uterus are stretching to make room.

Your cervix also begins to swell. You might feel some tenderness from an increase in blood vessels. After intercourse, this might cause some light spotting. That's probably not cause for alarm, unless you also have heavy bleeding and/or cramps along with it. But it's always a good idea to discuss any concerns you have with your doctor or midwife.

JUSTIFICATION FOR A CELEBRATION

By the beginning of this week, the cluster of cells is recognizable as an embryo!

Taking Photos of Your Belly

It's wonderful to start traditions from the very beginning. This week you might want to have someone take some photos of you—especially of your belly. Then you might want to take similar shots each month of your pregnancy.

❧

My husband took photos of my pregnant belly about once a month. It was a fun tradition, and it's neat to look back on the photos of my growing belly.

—*Lezli Braswell, MD, a mom of one daughter and two sons and a family medicine physician currently working in an emergency room fast track in Columbus, GA*

❧

A friend of mine and I were pregnant at the same time, and we took lots of photos of us together.

—*Debra Luftman, MD, a mom of a teenaged daughter and a teenaged son, a board-certified dermatologist in private practice, a coauthor of* The Beauty Prescription, *the developer of the skincare line of products Therapeutix, and a clinical instructor of skin surgery and general dermatology at UCLA*

❧

I had often heard that people don't take as many photos of their second child. I wanted to be sure we had photos and also to ensure that they were special. So I had a photographer come to our home while I was pregnant. She took such beautiful photos of my belly and our whole family.

I also scheduled her to return shortly after we brought our son home from the hospital. I knew that even though we might not have as many candid photos of him, we'd have some very special professional ones.

—*Michelle Paley, MD, PA, a mom of a six-year-old daughter and a two-year-old son and a psychiatrist and psychotherapist in private practice in Miami Beach, FL*

❧

My favorite part of my pregnancy was taking photos of my pregnant belly. It would have been neat to have started this earlier, but I was superstitious and scared to do it too soon, so I wouldn't let my husband take any photos until week 32!

But at week 32, we wrote "32" on my belly in lipstick and took a photo, and then we did the same the next week, and the week after that. After that we started writing messages to our babies in lipstick on my belly before taking the pictures. It was fun!

—*Jennifer Gilbert, DO, a mom of three-month-old twins and an ob-gyn at Paoli Hospital in Pennsylvania*

RALLIE'S TIP

During my first pregnancy, I was so self-conscious about my rapidly ballooning midsection that I wouldn't allow my husband to take photos of my belly. If I had it to do over, I would relax and enjoy my beautiful pregnant belly, and I would have lots of pictures to remind me of my amazing transformation.

Calculating Your Due Date

It's amazing to think that just a decade or so ago, women had to wait to see their doctors or midwives to learn their due dates. Today, you'll find dozens of pregnancy calculators online that can calculate your due date in the blink of an eye. Simply Google "pregnancy due date calculator." Enter the first day of your last menstrual period, and voilà! Your due date will pop up.

But don't get too attached to it! Only about 5 percent of babies arrive on their actual due dates.

When I thought I might be pregnant, I calculated my due date on my own. You can use calculators online, but I simply used a pregnancy wheel that I got on my ob-gyn rotation as a medical student. You just dial in the date of your last period, and it calculates your due date. Then when I got to my first doctor's visit, they confirmed it.

—*Kerri A. Daniels, MD, a mom of one toddler daughter and an instructor in the department of pediatrics at the University of Arkansas for Medical Science in Little Rock*

I have a pregnancy wheel, so I used that to calculate my due date. I also did early ultrasounds on myself to check the measurements and estimate my baby's due date.

—*Diane Connelly, MD, a mom of a six-year old daughter and an ob-gyn in HMO practice in Riverside, CA*

I used an ovulation kit when I was trying to get pregnant, so I knew when I had ovulated. I was able to calculate my due date based upon both my last menstrual period and my ovulation date, which came out to the same due date on the pregnancy wheel.

—*Ashley Roman, MD, MPH, a mom of two daughters, ages three years and six months, and a clinical assistant professor in the department of obstetrics and gynecology at the New York University School of Medicine in New York City*

When I was pregnant, even though I must have been given a due date, I didn't pay any attention to it. I knew better than to get attached to a certain date. To this day, I don't know if my daughters were born close to their arbitrary due dates or not.

—*Stacey Marie Kerr, MD, a mother of two grown daughters, a family physician with strong roots in midwifery, and the author of* Homebirth in the Hospital, *in Santa Rosa, CA*

Fighting Fatigue

If you're tired, you're in good company. Fatigue in early pregnancy is very common. You can blame your soaring progesterone levels. Also, lower blood sugar levels, increased blood production, and lower blood pressure might all be conspiring to make you sleepy.

One thing that's perfectly normal and really common, but not always talked about is overwhelming exhaustion in the first trimester. Even getting up to go to the bathroom is a chore. The fatigue is caused by your rising hormones.

I remember the exhaustion well. I was around five weeks pregnant, and I suspected I was pregnant, but I didn't know for sure yet. I was working as an attending physician at a nursing home, and I was talking to the head nurse. I was supposed to make rounds to see my patients.

> **? When to Call Your Doctor or Midwife**
>
> If your fatigue is so overwhelming that you can't focus on your work or if you're a hazard while driving, contact your doctor or midwife right away.

"I can't get myself up out of this chair," I told the nurse. "I'd rather look at these charts than at the patients."

"Don't worry about it," the nurse said. "You're pregnant!"

I was completely exhausted—so tired I could barely move—for around four weeks. By the second trimester, my energy levels started to rise.

—*Erika Schwartz, MD, a mom of two and the director of www.*
DrErika.com, who's been in private practice for more than 30 years in
New York City, specializing over the past 15 years in women's health,
disease prevention, and bioidentical hormones

I was very tired at some points in my pregnancies. I remember one day during my third pregnancy, I was so tired, I told my kids we were going to sit on the couch and pretend to watch TV. (We didn't have a TV until my kids were 10.) They fell for it for a little while.

—*Nancy Rappaport, MD, a mother of two teenaged daughters and a*
teenaged son, an assistant professor of psychiatry at Harvard Medical
School, an attending child and adolescent psychiatrist in the Cambridge,
MA, public schools, and the author of In Her Wake: A Child
Psychiatrist Explores the Mystery of Her Mother's Suicide

I'm usually on the go, so the biggest thing I noticed about my pregnancy was feeling very tired. I never went to sleep so early and slept in so late as I did during the first trimesters of all of my pregnancies. I tried to stay awake as long as possible, but I'd fall asleep at my desk. So I ended up just going to bed early.

—*Dianna K. Kim, MD, a mom of three and an ob-gyn in private practice*
in Vernon Hills, IL, at the Midwest Center for Women's Healthcare

Especially at the beginning, pregnancy can be exhausting. I think you just have to rest when you need it. When your body tells you to rest, you have to do it. A lot of times we women push ourselves to do more. But pregnancy is not the time to do that. I took naps whenever I was tired in my pregnancies.

—*Kelly Campbell, MD, a mom of three and an ob-gyn in private*
practice at Women's Healthcare Physicians in West Bloomfield, MI

Before I got pregnant, when pregnant women would complain about being tired, I used to think, "Ha, you should walk a day in my shoes." But when I was pregnant with my oldest daughter, I was working 80- to 100-hour work weeks, and I have never been more exhausted in my entire life.

I didn't know how physically exhausted pregnancy makes women. The fatigue is destructive. When I was pregnant, I would put my head down on my desk and fall asleep with mad commotion going on all around me. I'd come home from a 12-hour shift, and I'd fall asleep on the couch. We had a one-bedroom apartment, and I couldn't make it into the bedroom. My husband would carry me into the bedroom, and I'd sleep the entire night in whatever position he put me in. When my alarm went off 12 hours later, I could hardly get out of bed.

I just slept as much as I could in the first trimester until the fatigue eased up in the second.

—*Marra Francis, MD, a mom of three daughters and an ob-gyn who's based in The Woodlands, TX*

When I would get home, I would try to put my feet up and rest. This is much harder when you have another child at home. You're already a mom! You still need to make dinner, get your child ready for bed, make lunches for the next day, and more. I found it much harder to rest during my second pregnancy.

I found that taking just a few minutes, even just five, to sit down made a huge difference in my energy level.

—*Barbara Goff, MD, a mom of two and a professor of obstetrics and gynecology and the director of gynecologic oncology at the University of Washington Medical Center in Seattle*

During the first three months of my first pregnancy, I was so unbelievably fatigued. If someone had told me that they'd shoot me if I didn't get up off of the couch, I would have said, "Just go ahead and get it over with."

I was even more tired during my second pregnancy. It's challenging to find the energy to take care of your older child because you're so drained. What was comforting the second time around was that I knew the fatigue was going to pass. I told myself that if my child had to watch an extra video a day so I could get some rest, it was okay. I'd engage her in activities where she could play and I could sit (or better yet, lie down) next to her. That way she knew I was there, but I could still relax.

I think this is a key time to engage the help of family and friends. It's not a bad favor to ask a family member or friend to watch your children for an extra few hours so you can rest.

—*Lauren Hyman, MD, a mom of two and an ob-gyn at West Hills Hospital and Medical Center in West Hills, CA*

＠ィ＠

When I was pregnant with my first daughter, I was in medical school. For those first few weeks, I was so very tired. I'd tell my husband that I'd be upstairs studying. But when he'd come home from work, he'd find me fast asleep with a book on my face.

I napped when I could and tried to exercise regularly. I tried continuing with running, but that stopped feeling good around 18 weeks, so I got into "aqua-jogging" and swimming, which was great especially at the end of pregnancy when I felt enormous. Being in the water made me feel lighter and allowed me to relax.

I probably didn't do this as well as I should have, but I always tell my patients to drink enough water throughout the day. I remember the first trimester being the worst in terms of fatigue. And I don't remember having too much time to feel tired during my second pregnancy—probably because I had a toddler at home and I was on clinical rotations in the hospital during the day. I did carry water with me during the day (along with snacks) and had a mind-over-matter attitude that I was going to get through my rotations day by day.

—*Janet Lefkowitz, DO, a mother of two girls and an ob-gyn in private practice in Rhode Island*

RALLIE'S TIP

I was in my last year of residency during my third pregnancy. Standing on my feet was simply too exhausting, so I made great use of the rolling stools in our practice. I sat on one every chance I got.

I'd even roll it in the hall between exam rooms instead of walking. Sometimes I'd ask other people to push me! When you're tired, don't walk if you can stand, don't stand if you can sit, don't sit if you can lie down, and sleep whenever you can.

In the first three months of my pregnancies, I couldn't seem to get enough sleep! I felt as if I could curl up and snooze just about anywhere, anytime of the day. I found that if I took a short nap during my lunch hour, I was less likely to doze off unexpectedly. After eating my lunch, I would dim the lights in my office, lean back in a comfy chair with my feet propped up on a stack of books, and set the alarm on my pager to wake me in 20 or 30 minutes. After a short nap, I'd wake up refreshed and re-energized, ready to tackle the rest of the day.

～✑

During my pregnancies, I remember being really tired all of the time. I was so exhausted, I thought I might have chronic mononucleosis. But no, it was just the pregnancy.

For most women, the fatigue goes away after a few months, but unfortunately, for me it didn't. There wasn't anything I could do, just push on.

—Diane Truong, MD, FAAP, a mom of one daughter and one son
and a pediatrician in a multispecialty group practice in Southern California

Coping with Breast Changes

Some breast changes might be welcome, such as their increase in size. Other changes are less welcome, such as tingling, heaviness, and pain. All of them are caused by hormones, and perhaps are partly because your body is preparing to breastfeed your baby in a few months.

Women who have had cosmetic breast implants might be feeling more tender than other women, and your skin might feel especially taut and uncomfortable. That's because your own breast tissue is growing. You might also fear you won't be able to breastfeed your baby. You could talk with your doctor or midwife about it, or discuss it with a lactation consultant.

～✑

My husband and I had our wedding when I was 14 weeks pregnant. I had the most beautiful breasts I've ever had! I wasn't really showing; my breasts were just larger. I looked great in my wedding dress!

—Patricia S. Brown, MD, a mom of two daughters, ages nine and seven,
and a three-year-old son and a psychiatrist at Columbia-New York Child
and Adolescent Telepsychiatry and in private practice in Cresskill, NJ

During pregnancy, in addition to my growing belly, my breasts were growing too. Rather than investing in a lot of maternity clothing, I bought flowing, empire waist dresses. They were loose enough to accommodate my growing belly and breasts.

—*Lezli Braswell, MD*

✺

I had a lot of breast soreness with my second pregnancy. In another pregnancy, it was so bad that I felt like I had been beaten across the chest with a baseball bat. It was very uncomfortable. One thing that made it better was standing in a hot shower with the water flowing over my chest. It also helped to wear a comfortable bra that fit well, although that's challenging when your breasts are a different size every week!

—*Kristie McNealy, MD, a mom of seven- and four-year-old daughters and a two-year-old son, who's pregnant with another son, and a blogger at www.KristieMcNealy.com, in Denver, CO*

✺

My husband and I had been trying to get pregnant for quite a while. Being impatient, I think I tried for six months before I went to see a specialist to find out if there was something wrong. I did six months of infertility treatment and still didn't get pregnant.

At that time, I sort of took a break from trying to get pregnant. I was starting my last year of residency as chief resident, and I decided it was too much stress. I started training for a marathon, running 35 miles each week. I wasn't keeping track of my cycle, and I even stopped taking my prenatal vitamins. One day I ran a half marathon, and I told my running partner, who's also an ob-gyn, that I needed to buy new bras because my breasts hurt. She asked me when my last period was and told me to take a pregnancy test. Turns out, I was pregnant! My first clue was the breast pain.

—*Marra Francis, MD*

Starting a Gentle Pregnancy Exercise Program

As nice as it might be to get a free pass on exercising for nine months, pregnancy isn't going to give you one. Even—perhaps especially— pregnant women should exercise for at least 30 minutes most days. Exercise can help reduce many pesky pregnancy complaints, such as constipation, backache, and swelling. It might help prevent or treat gestational diabetes, the type of diabetes that women can get during pregnancy. Exercise also increases energy and improves mood.

Of course, training for a marathon isn't such a great idea right now, even if you wanted to. Instead, try pregnancy-friendly exercises such as walking and swimming. You'll want to avoid any type of exercise that puts you at risk for falls (such as bicycling and skiing), physical contact (such as ice hockey, soccer, and basketball), and incredible atmospheric pressure (such as scuba diving).

If you've been walking or swimming before your pregnancy, it's safe to continue to do so. But talk with your doctor or midwife before trying a new exercise program. And definitely talk to your doctor or midwife if you have risk factors for preterm labor, vaginal bleeding, or other medical conditions such as high blood pressure.

∼⌒∽

I was active before getting pregnant, and that didn't change after I found out I was pregnant. For example, I always take the stairs, never the elevator. Even in my ninth month, I was still trudging up those stairs!

—*Diane Connelly, MD*

∼⌒∽

I was very physically fit going into my first pregnancy, and I did a Buns of Steel pregnancy workout every day. It's the best pregnancy workout ever.

For my second and third pregnancies, I bought a few new pregnancy workout DVDs because I started to get bored doing the same one over and over. I found one featuring salsa dancing, which was great.

I worked out every single day of all three of my pregnancies. I really think it helped ease my pregnancy symptoms and made my labor go better. Plus I felt good during my pregnancies, and I also felt that I *looked* good.

—*Patricia S. Brown, MD*

∼⌒∽

Walking and running are my favorite workouts. I just put on my shoes and go. For me, having to go to the gym is a barrier to exercise that I don't need.

As great as cardiovascular exercises like walking and running are, don't neglect your upper-body work! A few weeks ago, I was at the orthopedist's office in so much pain I thought I was going to die. I strained my shoulder very badly by carrying around my 26-pound toddler.

—*Stephanie Ring, MD, a mom of two sons, ages six and two, and an ob-gyn at Red Rocks Ob-Gyn in Lakewood, CO*

⁓

I ran the very first Walt Disney World marathon when I was seven weeks pregnant with my first child. I had only found out I was pregnant a few days before. I stopped running at mile 14 because I was having trouble staying warm. I went to a medical tent and explained I was pregnant and cold and wanted a ride to the finish line. The Disney Cast Member looked a little nervous and asked, "Does your doctor know this?"

I exercised throughout my pregnancy, and I think having strong core muscles made my pushing in labor more effective.

—*Melanie Bone, MD, a mom of four "tweens" ages 15 to 12, a gynecologist, the founder of the Cancer Sensibility Foundation, and the author of the syndicated column* Surviving Life *and the book* Cancer, What's Next?, *in West Palm Beach, FL*

⁓

When I was pregnant with my daughter, I was in my residency, so I didn't have time to exercise much. I walked when I could.

Before I got pregnant with my son, I had started running three miles a few times a week. After I got pregnant, I kept that up for a while, but then I realized I was too tired. Plus as my belly got bigger, I didn't feel comfortable running. I started doing the elliptical trainer at the gym and walking on our treadmill.

—*Lezli Braswell, MD*

⁓

I love to run, but I stopped running very early in my pregnancy. I didn't feel comfortable running while pregnant. With my changing body shape and loose joints, I worried about twisting my ankle.

I'm thin and lean, and I usually get too cold in pools, so I rarely swim. But when you're pregnant, you tend to be warmer, so even for those of us who don't like to swim, it's great in pregnancy. Because I didn't feel coordinated, I swam in the handicap lane, although of course I don't think of pregnancy as a handicap. I figured if anyone wanted to kick an eight-month-pregnant woman out of the handicap lane, so be it!

—*Nancy Rappaport, MD*

I swam throughout my pregnancies. Swimming doesn't put any pressure on your back or your legs. When you're buoyant in the water, you can really increase your heart rate, which keeps you fit. But it doesn't stress your body like running can.

—*Debra Luftman, MD*

⤳

I exercised all the way through all of my pregnancies. I walked, and I swam laps—hard. In the water, you're buoyant, and you can get your heart rate up and use all of your muscles without the burden of the extra weight of your belly. Swimming is wonderful!

I credit exercise for the ease of my deliveries and the health of my children. I think that exercise is an invaluable, underrecognized, way to increase your chances of having a healthy pregnancy and a healthy child.

—*Ann Kulze, MD, a mother of four children, ages 20, 19, 18, and 14, a nationally recognized nutrition expert, motivational speaker, physician, and the author of the critically acclaimed book* Dr. Ann's 10-Step Diet: A Simple Plan for Permanent Weight Loss and Lifelong Vitality

⤳

A lot of women think that they can't exercise during pregnancy. I remember working out at the gym and getting odd looks from people. Other people at the gym would see me jogging and ask if it was okay for me to run.

If you're having a normal, healthy pregnancy, there's no reason not to exercise. This isn't the 1960s, when they told pregnant women to sit down and put their feet up. Today, we know that exercise is very important and beneficial during pregnancy. As long as you're healthy, exercise is key to preparing your body for labor and delivery.

Before my pregnancy, I was active. I like to run, but by the time I was around five months pregnant, it was hard for me to run. I wanted to do some sort of exercise, so I took up swimming. I hadn't swam laps since I was a child, but for the last four months or so of my pregnancy, I swam three times a week at the pool at my gym. Even now, I swim once or twice a month.

—*Mary Mason, MD, a mom of a nine-year-old girl and six-year-old boy, an internist, and the chief medical officer for a multi-state managed care company that coordinates care for about 70,000 pregnant Medicaid moms a year*

When I had my two older children, I was living on a farm, and we walked and gardened. We lived a very active life. You cannot eat junk food and sit on your butt the entire pregnancy and expect your baby to just pop out.

When I was pregnant with my younger children, I was no longer living on a farm, but I tried very hard to be physically active. It was during my residency, so I didn't have time for aerobics classes, but I took the stairs every chance I had. I think that staying in shape is vital to having a pleasant pregnancy and a good delivery.

—*Hana R. Solomon, MD, a mom of four, ages 35 to 19, a board-certified pediatrician, the president of BeWell Health, LLC, and the author of* Clearing the Air One Nose at a Time: Caring for Your Personal Filter

∽

I exercised so much before getting pregnant—running, aerobics, weight lifting—that my doctor actually advised me to dial it back a bit when I got pregnant. My doctor's office was on the sixth floor, and one day he fussed at me because I took the steps instead of the elevator.

My doctor urged me to relax, which I tried to do.

—*Kerri A. Daniels, MD*

Chapter 6
Week 6

Your Baby This Week

YOUR BABY'S SIZE

Your baby is growing rapidly. Over the past few weeks, your baby has gone through the greatest size and physical changes of her entire life.

By now, your baby is about the size of a sesame seed, about 0.06 to 0.16 inch long. That's still small, but visible to the naked eye!

YOUR BABY'S LATEST DEVELOPMENTS

Around this time, your baby's neural groove closes. Her brain chambers are already starting to form.

Your baby's eyes are forming. What color will they be?

Also, your baby has started to develop ears. Two slight indentations have formed on the sides of your baby's head, and her ears will eventually come from there. Early facial features are beginning to form. Cells are moving around to form your baby's mouth, chin, and neck.

At this point, your baby still has a tail, but not to worry. The tail will shrink up and then disappear altogether. This week, limb buds appear, which is where your baby's arms and legs will be. Those arms will someday hold you tight, and those little legs will kick with delight.

By this time, the placenta begins to exchange nutrients, oxygen, and waste between you and your baby.

Your baby's lungs, pancreas, and liver are now beginning to form. The thyroid is developing. The first of three sets of kidneys form, although interestingly this set never becomes functional. These are all vital stages in your baby's development.

YOUR LATEST DEVELOPMENTS

Your uterus is already beginning to grow. Just a few weeks ago, it was around the size of a large plum. Already it's as big as an apple! You might have gained a few pounds by now. Perhaps your clothes are even a little snug around your waist. That is unless morning sickness or heartburn is making it hard to eat. But at the same time, you might already be having food cravings, which are very common in pregnancy.

Ironically, moodwise you might be feeling very similar emotions to those you feel before you get your period. You might feel more teary, emotional, irritable, and moody than usual, due to fluctuating hormones.

If your head is pounding, that's not uncommon. Headaches are unfortunately a usual symptom of pregnancy. You might also feel light-headed or dizzy, especially if you jump up too suddenly.

You might have to urinate very frequently for the next few weeks. Your kidneys are in overdrive, processing the extra waste your baby is producing. Plus, your growing uterus is pressing on your bladder.

Your breasts might feel heavier, fuller, and tender. You might notice your areolas darkening.

Tired? You're probably still feeling quite a lot of fatigue. Rest when you can. Never since you were a baby yourself have you had a better excuse for a nap.

JUSTIFICATION FOR A CELEBRATION

This is the one time in your life you'll be happy that your pants feel snug!

Handling Headaches

Many people might be surprised to learn that headaches are very common in pregnancy. Nearly one in five pregnant women has a migraine at some point during pregnancy.

Hormonal changes in pregnancy cause increased blood volume, including around the brain. This in turn can trigger frequent, mild headaches. Headaches can also be caused by cutting back on caffeine, dehydration, fatigue, lack of sleep, low blood sugar, and stress.

The challenging part about headaches in pregnancy is that you can't take strong medications to alleviate them.

∽

During my third pregnancy, I started getting migraine headaches all of a sudden. It was awful. My doctor mentioned that niacin can cause headaches, and we realized it was the extra niacin in the prenatal vitamins that was doing it. The prenatals I was taking contained 200 percent of the recommended Daily Value for niacin. I stopped taking the prenatals, and sure enough, my migraines went away.

—*Patricia S. Brown, MD, a mom of two daughters, ages nine and seven, and a three-year-old son and a psychiatrist at Columbia-New York Child and Adolescent Telepsychiatry and in private practice in Cresskill, NJ*

∽

When I was 13 weeks pregnant, right around the time my morning sickness went away, my migraines started. I'd wake up with a headache each day, and it would get worse as the day went on. It was very hard to cope with the terrible headaches. I found that combining Tylenol and a nap was the best. Thank goodness, the migraines lasted only about three weeks! (Talk with your doctor or midwife before taking this or any medication.)

—*Kristie McNealy, MD, a mom of seven- and four-year-old daughters and a two-year-old son, who's pregnant with another son, and a blogger at www.KristieMcNealy.com, in Denver, CO*

∽

I had a headache every day during my second trimester. I found that taking Tylenol and Sudafed each morning helped. I don't have a history of migraines, so I didn't think they were migraines, just pregnancy-related headaches. (Talk with your doctor or midwife before taking this or any medication.)

I also found that when I was busy, I felt better. Sitting home feeling sorry for myself wasn't the way to go! Working kept my mind off of my headaches.

—Ann LaBarge, MD, a mom of four children, ages 16 to six, and an ob-gyn in private practice at the Midwest Center for Women's Healthcare in Park Ridge, IL

I do get migraines, but fortunately I only had one during my pregnancy. I took Tylenol and a medication called Phenergan that my doctor prescribed for me and gave me the okay to take. It's an anti-nausea medicine, but I have found it really helpful for my migraines. I had suppositories, which are so helpful when you are already feeling sick. Your gut really slows down with a migraine, so oral medications don't work very well. Suppositories aren't the easiest thing, but when you're really suffering, you'll try anything.

Fortunately, the medicine also makes me sleepy. My husband got me a cold washcloth for my head, and I retreated to my bedroom. I was able to sleep and get relief pretty quickly. I was fine after a night of sleep.

During my pregnancy, I also got a few regular headaches. I took Tylenol, and they went away. (Talk with your doctor or midwife before taking this or any medication.)

—Katja Rowell, MD, a mom of a four-year-old daughter, a family practice physician, and a childhood feeding specialist with www. familyfeedingdynamics.com, in St. Paul, MN

? When to Call Your Doctor or Midwife

Headaches are generally harmless during pregnancy. But if you have a migraine or a headache that feels unlike any that you've ever felt before, call your doctor or midwife right away. Also call your medical care provider if your headache is sudden, explosive, occurs after you've fallen or hit your head, or if it's accompanied by fever or a stiff neck, vision changes or slurred speech, or nasal congestion, dental pain, or pain underneath your eyes.

Feeling More Aches and Pains

Around this time, it's common for aches and pains to begin. And they're not going away anytime soon. Your whole body is changing, and your growing breasts and belly throw off your center of gravity. Common places to ache include your back, pelvis, hips, and legs.

∽

Before I got pregnant, I didn't realize the number of aches and pains that are typical of pregnancy. Your body goes through tremendous changes—to your pelvis, lower back, hips, and abdomen. Even my rib cage was achy; it felt like someone was poking me. Sometimes I felt odd, sharp pains out of the blue. These are all normal occurrences of pregnancy, but it's still good to mention these aches and pains to your doctor.

I found that physical therapy was wonderful for aches and pains. I did not have time to go during my first pregnancy, but I highly recommend physical therapy to my patients.

—Jennifer Kim, MD, a mom of three girls, ages eight, five, and four; an ob-gyn in private practice in Evanston, IL, at the Midwest Center for Women's Healthcare; and a clinical assistant professor at the University of Chicago, Pritzker School of Medicine

∽

During my pregnancies I was working as a physician full-time. I thought that the pregnancies were just awful to go through! I hurt in all sorts of places; I was nauseated and hot; I gained a huge amount of weight; and I didn't even look good! I felt huge, and I couldn't stand being pregnant. However, the results—having my babies—were wonderful.

—Sandra Carson, MD, a mom of two grown sons and the director of the Center for Reproduction and Infertility of Women & Infants Hospital in Providence, RI

∽

In both pregnancies, I had uterine cramping. They felt like odd twinges—mildly uncomfortable but

MommyTIME — Take a Bubble Bath

Sometimes aches and pains can be eased by simple stress reduction measures. Try techniques that have eased your stress in the past, such as a bubble bath. Calgon, take me away!

not painful. I think many women don't expect them, but they can be totally normal. As your uterus stretches, you feel a little cramping.

As long as it's just minor cramping, I don't think you need to call your doctor, but if it's combined with bleeding, I'd call a doctor.

—Ashley Roman, MD, MPH, a mom of two daughters, ages three years and six months, and a clinical assistant professor in the department of obstetrics and gynecology at the New York University School of Medicine in New York City

∽

During my pregnancies, I had a lot of aches and pains in my legs and back, but I continued to work right up to the day I delivered. I didn't do anything special for the aches and pains, just suffered through them.

—Melanie Bone, MD, a mom of four "tweens" ages 15 to 12, a gynecologist, the founder of the Cancer Sensibility Foundation, and the author of the syndicated column Surviving Life *and the book* Cancer, What's Next?, *in West Palm Beach, FL*

∽

Before I got pregnant, I was very surprised when my patients complained during their pregnancies. I thought to myself, *You're so lucky to be carrying a healthy child. I don't understand why you'd complain about a few aches and pains.*

I imagined that when I got pregnant, birds would bring me ribbons, and rabbits would dance around my feet. When I got pregnant, I realized how really downright uncomfortable it can be! Even though some women feel it's the best nine months of their lives, the majority of us have extraordinarily valid complaints.

Being pregnant myself gave me an appreciation for how difficult the different periods of those nine months can be. I thought to myself, *This is ridiculous! How do women live through this?* I think I was tested with a little bit of everything. I had a touch of all of the common pregnancy complaints: heartburn, nausea, aches and pains, etc.

In general, my theory is that every pregnant woman gets hit by at least one major complaint. Some women are plagued by acid reflux, others get carpal tunnel syndrome, and still others have pelvic pressure. While you can try to alleviate these complaints, unfortunately you often have to just grin and bear it. And keep in mind how fabulous the reward is at the end!

—*Lauren Hyman, MD, a mom of two and an ob-gyn at West Hills Hospital and Medical Center in West Hills, CA*

Dealing with Dizziness

When you stand up quickly, you might have the panicky sensation that you're about to pass out. Many pregnant women feel "head rushes," sudden bouts of fuzzy vision and light-headedness.

Several factors combine to cause dizziness in pregnancy. They include low blood pressure, low blood sugar, and increased blood volume.

When your blood vessels dilate, it can cause your blood pressure to drop. To combat the low blood pressure, instead of hopping up out of a chair, take your time and hold onto something to steady yourself if need be. Drinking enough water, milk, and juice can help keep you hydrated and also alleviate dizziness.

To keep your blood sugar levels steady, eat several small meals during the day.

Because your blood volume is increasing during pregnancy, your heart must pump faster and harder. Your resting heart rate is much higher now than it was a few short weeks ago. This causes you to become dizzy.

Dizziness can cause you to fall, which can be dangerous for you and for your baby. This is a great time to eliminate tripping hazards around your home, such as throw rugs and items left on staircases. Taking time to do this now will *save* you time later, after your baby is born. You won't want there to be things lying around then, putting you in danger of falling while you're carrying your baby. Be especially careful when getting out of bed first thing in the morning and getting in and out of the bathtub.

~~

The first clue I was pregnant was dizziness. One day at work, I was examining one of the nurses I worked with. All of a sudden, I got really dizzy. The nurse looked at me quizzically.

"Are you pregnant?" she asked.

I thought, *Hmmm. I guess I could be!* And it turns out, I was.

—*Elissa Charbonneau, DO, a mom of an 18-year-old son and a
16-year-old daughter and the medical director of the New England
Rehabilitation Hospital in Portland, ME*

RALLIE'S TIP

*I was in my residency training during my second and third pregnancies. I was
plagued with dizziness, especially whenever I had to stand for long periods of
time or when I smelled strong odors. Working in the hospital, I was on my feet
most of the day, and strong odors were impossible to avoid. Whenever I felt
myself getting dizzy, I just had to stop and drop. I'd sit on a chair if I could
find one, or I'd plop down on the floor if I couldn't. If I didn't sit down and
put my head on my knees, I was sure to faint.*

Dizziness is common in pregnancy. Women who faint easily when they're
not pregnant are even more likely to faint when they are pregnant. When
you're pregnant, higher levels of progesterone cause the veins in your lower
body to dilate. If you're dehydrated, feeling very hot, or standing in one spot
for a long time, you might feel dizzy and/or pass out.

I didn't have a problem with dizziness or fainting, and part of the reason
might have been that I drank a lot to keep hydrated.

—*Gina Dado, MD, a mom of two daughters and an ob-gyn with
Arizona OBGYN Affiliates, Paradise Valley Branch, in Scottsdale, AZ*

I've always tended to get head rushes, caused by low blood pressure. This
was much more pronounced during pregnancy. I'd get up out of bed and
almost black out.

I told my obstetrician about it, and he did a thorough exam and ruled
out any worrisome causes with lab work. Once I knew the dizziness wasn't
dangerous and was normal for me, the most important thing was to anticipate
it. I knew that if I stood up too quickly and stepped right away, I'd feel light-
headed. Instead, when I got out of bed, I'd sit up first and pause at the edge
of my bed for 30 seconds, and *then* I'd stand up. After I stood from a sitting
position, I steadied myself for a minute or two before walking or moving.

—*Katja Rowell, MD*

Peeing All of the Time

It's not your imagination: You have to go to the bathroom *a lot*. Another sign of early pregnancy is frequent urination. You probably feel like you have to go to the bathroom frequently, even sometimes when your bladder is practically empty.

This symptom will come and go throughout pregnancy. Early in pregnancy, you might feel that you have to go to the bathroom more frequently because of the hormone hCG and the fact that your body has more fluid during pregnancy. But in your second trimester, just when you've located all of the bathrooms in all of the stores where you like to shop, you might not have to pee as often. That's because your uterus is growing and rising higher, and it's consequently putting less pressure on your bladder. But you'll get to put your bathroom–location knowledge to good use once again in your third trimester. Toward the end of pregnancy, the baby moves lower in your pelvis to prepare for birth. That increases the pressure on your bladder, causing even more frequent urination.

Cutting back on caffeine, which you are likely doing anyway, might help. Caffeine is a diuretic, which means it makes you have to urinate more often. It's very important to go to the bathroom when you have to. Otherwise, you risk developing a urinary tract infection. (See "Preventing and Treating Urinary Tract Infections" on page 180.)

⌒⌒

I was aware that I might have to urinate often during pregnancy. But it surprised me that I had to awaken eight times a night to go to the bathroom. That became so tiring.

—*Amy J. Derick, MD, a mom of one 15-month-old son who is
17 weeks pregnant with her second son. Dr. Derick is a dermatologist
in private practice at Derick Dermatology in Barrington, IL*

⌒⌒

It was frustrating that early in my pregnancies I had to go to the bathroom all of the time. My husband and I kept long car rides to a minimum, and I really tried to avoid airplanes because they don't let you get out of your seat very often.

You really can't do anything about it. I just tried to focus on the fact that it would go away after a few weeks. I continued drinking and eating well despite having to pee all of the time.

—*Kristie McNealy, MD*

I noticed urinary frequency early in all of my pregnancies. I tend to have a hyperactive bladder anyway, and it progressed as the pregnancies went along. It was pretty horrific in the last two months. I'd feel the urge to urinate every 15 minutes if I was standing up. I sat down whenever I could, and I always knew where the closest bathroom was.

—*Ann Kulze, MD, a mother of four children, ages 20, 19, 18, and 14, a nationally recognized nutrition expert, motivational speaker, physician, and the author of the critically acclaimed book* Dr. Ann's 10-Step Diet: A Simple Plan for Permanent Weight Loss and Lifelong Vitality

Chapter 7
Week 7

Your Baby This Week

YOUR BABY'S SIZE

Your baby will have a tremendous growth spurt this week, more than doubling in size. At the beginning of this week, he is about the size of a BB pellet, 0.16 to 0.2 inch long. But by week's end, he will measure about ½ inch. At this stage, babies are measured crown to rump because their legs are often bent, making it hard to measure them.

YOUR BABY'S LATEST DEVELOPMENTS

Around this time, your baby's eyelids might have closed. They will soon seal shut, and they'll remain that way for several months. Your baby's nose, mouth, and jaw are now visible. Whom will he look like?

Changes are happening quickly in your baby's brain. The cerebral hemispheres are growing. And this week, your baby's brain forms its three main sections, the forebrain, midbrain, and hindbrain. The hypothalamus is formed, which has a very important job. It maintains the body's status quo, keeping blood pressure, body temperature, and fluid balance steady and regulating emotions, hunger, and thirst.

Because your baby's inner ear is now connected to his middle ear, he's getting closer to hearing his first favorite sound—your voice.

Even though your baby's teeth won't erupt until months after he's born, his teeth are developing beneath his gums.

Your baby's heart has now divided into left and right chambers. Your baby's spleen is beginning to develop. The spleen is critical for immunity. It produces antibodies and removes bacteria and worn-out red blood cells from the blood.

Your baby's arms have grown longer, dividing into a hand segment and an arm-shoulder segment. The leg buds now are short fins. Both the hands and feet have digital plates where tiny fingers and toes will develop. This week, your baby's kidneys have started to produce urine.

Even though this huge mystery hasn't been revealed to you yet, your baby's sex was determined at the instant of conception. Now, primitive cells are arriving at your baby's genital area and developing into either female or male structures. Nipples are beginning to form whether your baby is a girl or a boy.

Your baby's lifeline, the umbilical cord, is now well established. It contains a large vein and two arteries that deliver blood and nutrition to your baby. Right now, your baby's intestines are actually inside of the umbilical cord. Once your baby's body is big enough to accommodate the intestines, they will migrate there.

Your latest developments

Your moods right now really might be running amok. Major changes are going on with your hormone levels, and that has a dramatic effect on your mood. Even if your mood swings make you feel out of control, try to keep in mind that this is only temporary—merely a side effect. It probably isn't helping your emotional state that you feel too pooped to pop.

You still might be struggling with morning sickness and heartburn. Even if *you* feel awful, your baby feels fine! You might be feeling some abdominal aches, pains, and twinges due to your growing uterus. By now it's nearly doubled in size! That's also why you have to pee so often. It's putting more and more pressure on your bladder.

In addition to your uterus growing, the actual *cells* in your uterus grow. They increase between 17 and 40 times their nonpregnant size. This is caused by the extra estrogen in your body.

Justification for a celebration

You can't feel it yet, but your baby is testing out his new arms and legs! He's swimming and kicking all around inside the amniotic sac.

Trying On Maternity Clothes Just for Fun!

If you're lucky enough to have a maternity store nearby, such as Japanese Weekend, or even just a department store with a large maternity section, why not check it out? Sometimes they have belly pillows that you can slip on under clothes to approximate what you'll look like as your pregnancy progresses!

While you're there, you might consider buying some pregnancy bras. Your regular bras are likely uncomfortable; they just don't fit quite right anymore. The investment in pregnancy bras will be worth it. Droopy, saggy breasts will only cause you backaches and pain.

Consider soft sports bras. They'll be able to stretch as your breasts grow. Steer clear of underwire bras. At the least, those pesky wires digging into your breasts will be uncomfortable, and they might harm the later development of your milk ducts.

At this time, you might find it comfortable to wear a bra at night.

⁓

I did try on some clothes early in my pregnancy just for the fun of it. I also managed to be a bridesmaid twice while pregnant. It was fun trying on bridesmaid dresses in the first trimester and estimating what I would look like at 30 weeks pregnant, using one of those fake tummy pillows. It was an interesting experience, and it worked out okay. For one wedding, I managed to find a maternity dress that matched everyone else's dresses. For the other wedding, I made the right guess on a bigger size, but unfortunately the alterations to the dress cost about twice as much as the dress itself.

—*Kristie McNealy, MD, a mom of seven- and four-year-old daughters and a two-year-old son, who's pregnant with another son, and a blogger at www.KristieMcNealy.com, in Denver, CO*

⁓

I think that women should show off and really celebrate their pregnancies. That wasn't the case when I was pregnant.

My oldest daughter is 18, and when I was pregnant and a doctor in training, we hid our pregnancies! I certainly didn't tell anyone I was pregnant, and I wore a large blouse with a big scarf hanging over it so no one would know I was pregnant. When my colleagues and I got pregnant, we tried to convince everyone that "I'm a doctor. Everything is fine. Nothing will be different. Don't look at me that way."

Fortunately the world has changed. Today, people know that pregnancy is beautiful; pregnant women are beautiful. I'm sorry that I missed that. Today, pregnant women know that they look gorgeous and spectacular. Pregnancy is powerful. I think that women should relish in the changes their bodies go through. You can show off and feel proud. It's great that our culture has changed in such a short time.

—*Eva Ritvo, MD, a mom of two teenaged daughters, an associate professor and vice chairman at the Miller School of Medicine of the University of Miami, and a coauthor of* The Beauty Prescription

Sure try on some clothes, but spread out the fun. Don't do everything for the baby in the first trimester. Save as much as you can for the end. (It will be hard!) The first two trimesters are exciting on their own—ultrasounds, a growing baby, milestones, and morning sickness. I found that the last trimester is just l-o-n-g. I saved those weeks for clothes shopping, baby showers, decorating, name picking, and daydreaming about those sweet little baby cheeks.

—*Tyeese Gaines Reid, DO, a mom of one, an emergency medicine resident physician at Yale New Haven Hospital in Connecticut, and the author of a time management book,* The Get a Life Campaign

Feeling More Emotional

If Kleenex commercials make you cry and your partner is driving you nuts, you're not alone. Blame it on changes in both your hormone and neurotransmitter levels, which are substances that allow nerve cells to communicate with each other. You might find it helpful to talk with a friend or family member, or even a counselor.

When I was pregnant, I was so much more emotional. I'd cry even watching the news! My husband and I would laugh afterward, realizing it was just my hormones from the pregnancy causing it.

—*Gina Dado, MD, a mom of two daughters and an ob-gyn with Arizona OBGYN Affiliates, Paradise Valley Branch, in Scottsdale, AZ*

During my pregnancies, commercials made me cry at the drop of a hat. As a blogger, I enjoy reading people's blogs, and both happy stories and tragedies make me cry.

—*Kristie McNealy, MD*

❧

I don't remember feeling overly emotional or sensitive, but if you ask my husband, he might have a different answer for you!

During my pregnancy, I was very sensitive to smells, especially the smell of steak. The first time I came home from work and had a meltdown because my husband had cooked steak, he became more sensitive to my changes in mood.

—*Ashley Roman, MD, MPH, a mom of two daughters, ages three years and six months, and a clinical assistant professor in the department of obstetrics and gynecology at the New York University School of Medicine in New York City*

RALLIE'S TIP

I was a little more emotional than usual during pregnancy, and it usually embarrassed me, especially when I got all weepy and teary-eyed for no apparent reason. But sometimes, my pregnancy-induced sensitivity emboldened me. Toward the end of my third pregnancy, I was working with a male surgeon who had the habit of calling all the women he worked with "Missy." After about two weeks, I just couldn't take it anymore, and I told him so in a very forthright manner. He was shocked that a young female resident had the audacity to confront him, and I was almost as shocked as he was! If my emotions hadn't been fueled by pregnancy hormones, I don't think I would have ever had the courage to speak my mind.

❧

I remember one time during my pregnancies when I was really emotional. I had a huge argument with my husband. He was planting foxgloves in our garden, which can be poisonous. I asked him how he could be so thoughtless planting them in my garden. I thought he must be intent on poisoning our child! It was completely illogical: If you're a little kid, you can off yourself in any number of ways. Plus, the baby wasn't even born yet! It would be years before he would be able to grab those flowers.

But at that time, I felt more vulnerable than usual. My body was changing, and my balance was changing, yet I felt very protected at the same time.

—Nancy Rappaport, MD, a mother of two teenaged daughters and a teenaged son, an assistant professor of psychiatry at Harvard Medical School, an attending child and adolescent psychiatrist in the Cambridge, MA, public schools, and the author of In Her Wake: A Child Psychiatrist Explores the Mystery of Her Mother's Suicide

I probably was more sensitive during my pregnancies, but I fought it. I was raised by a Navy captain, and in our home emotions were not valued. I learned early on to control my emotions because they didn't get me anything.

When I was pregnant, I tried not to be too vulnerable. But I was scared—terrified actually—of the change that this was going to bring to my life. I knew that becoming a mother would make me more vulnerable in my relationship with my partner. I tried not to show my vulnerability and emotions though. That might have partly been why I was so sick throughout my pregnancy. I think stress might have added to that. But I just lived each day and dealt with what I had.

—Stacey Marie Kerr, MD, a mother of two grown daughters, a family physician with strong roots in midwifery, and the author of Homebirth in the Hospital, *in Santa Rosa, CA*

Delegating Pet Care

If you have pets, you might want to delegate their care to someone else during your pregnancy. Dogs aren't much of a danger, except for them jumping on you or causing you to fall.

Cats, on the other hand, may carry a parasite called Toxoplasma gondii that can cause a condition called toxoplasmosis, which can be dangerous to your baby. If a mother is infected between weeks 10 and 24, it puts the baby at a small risk (around 5 percent) of premature birth, low birth weight, fever, jaundice, and other problems. Later in your pregnancy, the risk of damage to your baby is decreased because most of his organs have already developed. If you're infected, an antibiotic can reduce the likelihood that your baby will be infected.

Around 15 percent of women in the United States are immune to toxoplasmosis, which protects their babies as well. But there's no practical way to be sure that you're one of them. You're more likely to be immune if you've owned cats for a long time because you might have already had the infection and overcome it. Because the parasite is excreted in cat feces, cats can track it all over the house on their paws. (Eeew.) In addition to asking your partner to clean out the litter box, he should also vacuum and mop frequently. (Is that a cheer we hear?)

Other pets, such as hamsters and reptiles, also carry dangerous pathogens, such as salmonella bacteria, which can be harmful to you and your baby. If you have these pets, keep them in their cages and don't handle them during your pregnancy.

If you have birds, as long as they're healthy, they shouldn't pose any problems to you or your growing baby.

⁓

When I found out that I was pregnant, I asked my husband to change the cat litter box for me. Cat feces can contain a parasite called *Toxoplasma gondii*. The parasites multiply in cats' intestines and are shed in their waste. When people handle cat feces, they can contract the parasite and get an infection called toxoplasmosis, which can threaten the health of an unborn child.

My husband is a surgeon, and when he was on call or out of town, I'd use a disposable cat litter box. You pull off the wrapper and throw the whole box away when it's full. That way I never had to handle the litter.

—*Mary Mason, MD, a mom of a nine-year-old girl and six-year-old boy, an internist, and the chief medical officer for a multi-state managed care company that coordinates care for about 70,000 pregnant Medicaid moms a year*

⁓

When I was pregnant with my daughter and older son, we had a cat. My husband was in his surgery residency and was away a lot, and he didn't like that cat one bit. So I did change the litter box. But I didn't inhale. Everything was fine.

—*Lezli Braswell, MD, a mom of one daughter and two sons and a family medicine physician currently working in an emergency room fast track in Columbus, GA*

I didn't have any pets when I was pregnant, but even if I had, I would have cared for them myself. If I had a cat, I wouldn't have minded changing its litter box. In my 20 years of practice, I have never seen a case of toxoplasmosis, and I don't believe it is a real concern for most pregnant women in urban and suburban areas.

I'm very laid back. I ask patients why they would treat themselves differently when they are pregnant. Do they think it's okay to care for a pet or eat sushi when they aren't pregnant but not when they are? Seems a little silly to me.

—*Melanie Bone, MD, a mom of four "tweens" ages 15 to 12, a gynecologist, the founder of the Cancer Sensibility Foundation, and the author of the syndicated column* Surviving Life *and the book* Cancer, What's Next?, *in West Palm Beach, FL*

When I was pregnant, we had a hamster. They carry a disease that can be dangerous for pregnant women. So I relinquished my hamster care duties to my husband. He didn't think it was so great.

—*Sonia Ng, MD, a mom of seven-year-old and one-year-old sons and a pediatrician and expert in sedation at Children's Hospital of Philadelphia Pediatric Care at Princeton Health Care System in Princeton, NJ*

RALLIE'S TIP

I actually didn't delegate my pets' care. My dogs kept me active during my pregnancy. After a long, hard day of work, I usually just wanted to go home and collapse on the couch, but I couldn't deny my dogs their exercise. Taking a brisk walk in the fresh air with my two happy dogs always energized me and lifted my spirits.

During my first pregnancy, we had two large dogs that were absolutely glued to me. One was a yellow lab that we raised from a puppy, and the other was a Great Dane we rescued while I was pregnant. He weighed 120 pounds! He would just stand and press his big head against my belly, as if trying to protect me from everyone. He circled the wagons and didn't want anyone near me.

While I was pregnant, I left cleaning up the yard to my husband. Pretty early on I stopped walking the dogs too. Between the two of them, there was almost 200 pounds of dog, and I didn't want to be dragged across the park if they got excited about something.

—*Kristie McNealy, MD*

Cooling the (Heart)burn

Even women whose only prior experience with heartburn is those ubiquitous TV commercials (How do you spell relief? R–O–L–A–I–D–S) might experience heartburn themselves during pregnancy. Nearly a quarter of pregnant women get heartburn during their first trimesters. At least *half* of women will have it sometime during pregnancy. Heartburn can begin at any point in pregnancy, and it sometimes becomes more severe toward the end of pregnancy.

Heartburn is very aptly named: It feels like a burning sensation in the middle of your chest. You might also have an acid or bitter taste in your mouth.

There are several reasons why you might be feeling the burn. First, even though you're eating for two, ironically, higher levels of the hormone progesterone during pregnancy slow down digestion. Plus, your uterus is crowding other organs in your abdomen. As your pregnancy goes along, your baby presses on your digestive tract. Also, your esophagus slackens during pregnancy.

As these factors combine, stomach fluids containing acid and digestive enzymes splash backward through the valve-like sphincter that separates the stomach from the esophagus, exposing the sensitive lining of the esophagus to acid and causing you pain.

❧

During my first pregnancy, I had heartburn in my first trimester. In my second and third pregnancies, I had much worse heartburn, but only in the third trimester. In addition to eating smaller, more frequent meals, I found that drinking milk soothed it.

—*Patricia S. Brown, MD, a mom of two daughters, ages nine and seven, and a three-year-old son and a psychiatrist at Columbia-New York Child and Adolescent Telepsychiatry and in private practice in Cresskill, NJ*

During one pregnancy, I had really bad heartburn. Lying with my upper body propped up on pillows helped. Drinking ice water also eased the heartburn.

—*Elissa Charbonneau, DO, a mom of an 18-year-old son and a 16-year-old daughter and the medical director of the New England Rehabilitation Hospital in Portland, ME*

During my second pregnancy, I had a lot of heartburn. All I could eat was white foods, such as potatoes, toast, and eggs. Because I had so much heartburn, everyone said the baby would have tons of hair. Turns out when she was born, she had about two strands on her head.

—*Erika Schwartz, MD, a mom of two and the director of www. DrErika.com, who's been in private practice for more than 30 years in New York City, specializing over the past 15 years in women's health, disease prevention, and bioidentical hormones*

During my pregnancy, I had a lot of nausea and heartburn. I believe that nausea that occurs after the first trimester is often associated with acid reflux.

I found it helped if I didn't eat too much at once. Also, I tried not to *drink* too much at once because too much liquid in my stomach made me nauseated. I usually love pasta with tomato sauce, but I had to avoid it when I was pregnant. Finally around week 19, the nausea and heartburn went away, and I was able to eat and drink more normally.

—*Jennifer Kim, MD, a mom of three girls, ages eight, five, and four; an ob-gyn in private practice in Evanston, IL, at the Midwest Center for Women's Healthcare; and a clinical assistant professor at the University of Chicago, Pritzker School of Medicine*

During my first pregnancy, I had heartburn, but I could manage it by changing position and sleeping more upright. Sometimes simply turning to my right side would make it better.

But when I was pregnant with triplets, I had terrible, unrelenting heartburn. Each night, it would wake me around 1 am, even if I last ate at 7 pm.

The heartburn was so bad that I talked with my doctor, and he suggested I take over-the-counter Pepcid. (Talk with your doctor or midwife before taking this or any medication.) I also discovered that eating ice cream and sipping a little milk helped. So I coated that heartburn with some ice cream! The combo of medicine and ice cream eased the heartburn enough that it wasn't waking me up anymore. Of course, by then I was waking up for a zillion other reasons.

—Sadaf T. Bhutta, MBBS, a mom of a three-year-old daughter and 18-month-old triplets and an assistant professor and the fellowship director of pediatric radiology at the University of Arkansas for Medical Sciences and Arkansas Children's Hospital, both in Little Rock

I had horrific acid reflux when I was pregnant with my twins. I had to take medication because otherwise I couldn't eat enough to gain weight.

If I lay down flat in bed the last trimester, the heartburn was worse. So I slept in a chair.

—Susan Wilder, MD, a mom of an older daughter and twin girls, a primary care physician, and CEO and founder of Lifescape Medical Associates in Scottsdale, AZ

I've had heartburn on and off with this pregnancy. With my first baby, I had a horrible stomach flu, and after I got over that flu, I had the worst heartburn. Nothing helped. I think it was connected to the stomach

Mommy MD Guide-Recommended Product
Tums

"Toward the end of my pregnancies, I had terrible heartburn," said Karen Heald, MD, a mom of four boys and a board-certified family physician in private practice outside Atlanta, GA. "I sat up in bed at night and couldn't sleep very well. I took quite a lot of Tums, rather than other over-the-counter medicines, because I figured the Tums also gave me calcium."

You can buy Tums at drugstores, grocery stores, and mass merchandisers and online.

bug because the heartburn kicked in right afterward. Perhaps the heartburn was caused by my vomiting so much. The heartburn was vicious. I tried eating small meals and cutting out acidic foods, but it didn't really help. The best news I can give is that it all went away when the baby came!

—*Kristie McNealy, MD*

? When to Call Your Doctor or Midwife

If your heartburn is so severe that you can't eat or sleep, call your doctor or midwife the next business day. You might need to control it with medication.

My worst pregnancy symptom from the second month till my delivery was horrible heartburn. I'm prone to it anyway, and pregnancy made it worse. I didn't gain much weight during the last month of my pregnancy because if I ate anything after noon, I couldn't lie down at night.

Don't be afraid to take medication if that's what your doctor recommends. During my first pregnancy, all I could take was over-the-counter Mylanta. I took so much of it, I bought three bottles at a time at Target. My husband remembers me shaking the bottle at 3 am many nights. During my second pregnancy a few years later, it was okay to take Zantac. When I hesitated, my doctor said, "Don't you remember how miserable you were last time?" So I took it, and it helped a lot.

—*Sharonne N. Hayes, MD, a mom of two and the director of the Women's Heart Clinic at Mayo Clinic in Rochester, MN*

RALLIE'S TIP

I never had heartburn in my life until I was pregnant. I tried to control it with dietary changes, but that was difficult because I was starving all of the time. Eating a huge amount of food made the heartburn worse, pushing the food and acids back up into my esophagus, which causes burning and pain. I still ate a lot, but I made myself eat smaller meals, even breaking up one meal into three mini-meals. I certainly wasn't denying myself any calories!

I discovered that drinking soft drinks helped my nausea, but it made my heartburn worse. Anything with bubbles seemed to stir things up, and at one point, I had to swear off even clear sodas like ginger ale.

Chapter 8
Week 8

Your Baby This Week

YOUR BABY'S SIZE

Your baby grows so quickly at this point that if she continued to grow this fast, she would be a 15-foot-tall one-month-old. This week, your baby is about the size of a marble, measuring ½ to ¾ inch long.

YOUR BABY'S LATEST DEVELOPMENTS

Your baby's nose now has a tiny tip. Her ears continue to form. Inside her mouth, her tongue has formed as well as 20 buds for her baby, or milk, teeth. Your baby is likely to be born with smooth gums, unless she's one of a very few born with one or two neonatal teeth.

Your baby's arms are longer now, and her elbows bend. Her arms are curved slightly over her heart, as if in an embrace.

Speaking of your baby's heart, her aortic and pulmonary valves are now present.

This week will bring a lot of lung development. By the end of this week, your baby's lungs will have their basic structure. They look like a miniature version of your own lungs.

Your baby's hands and feet now have digital rays that will become fingers and toes.

Prior to this, your baby's body was curved into a C. But now she's starting to uncurl. Your baby's embryonic tail continues to shrink.

Around this time, the placenta begins to produce human placental lactogen. This pregnancy hormone helps your baby to grow. It also stimulates milk production in your breasts.

Amazingly, your baby can now make reflexive movements in response to outside stimuli. For example, if your partner talks at your belly or presses on your pelvis, your baby will wriggle and "dance" in response.

YOUR LATEST DEVELOPMENTS

Although your waist is expanding, you probably still fit into most of your clothes. Enjoy them—for now. Already, your uterus is the size of a grapefruit. All of this growth might be causing you mild cramps and twinges of pain.

Around this time, you might begin to have problems with gas and bloating. Squeezing yourself into too-small clothes isn't going to help, so you'll want to gravitate toward looser, elastic waistbands.

Heartburn might begin this week. It's also very common during pregnancy to be sensitive to tastes and smells. This is probably not helping morning sickness if you're still dealing with it.

You might already be having some Braxton Hicks contractions, which are also sometimes called "false" contractions. But you won't feel them yet.

Although you can't see it, you might be interested to know that your cervix might have a blue tint. This is caused by the increased blood flow. It also continues to soften, and it's now sealed off by a mucus plug, which was created by your body secretions.

As early as this week, you might notice increased white or light yellow vaginal discharge. Get used to it, because you'll probably have it during most of your pregnancy. It's aptly called leukorrhea, a not-too-pleasant name for a not-too-pleasant symptom.

JUSTIFICATION FOR A CELEBRATION

Your "skinny" jeans no longer fit! (When else in life would you want to celebrate that?!)

Going to Your First Prenatal Visit

Most of the time, most of us don't look forward to going to the doctor. But your first prenatal visit is one appointment you're probably anxiously awaiting.

When you find out that you're pregnant, it's a good idea to schedule this first appointment. Practitioners vary widely on when this first visit is scheduled. It could be as early as eight weeks, or as late as 13!

In the meantime, while waiting for the day to arrive, it's a good idea to jot down some notes and questions. Write down the first date of your last menstrual period. Your doctor or midwife will ask you that to calculate your due date, using a pregnancy wheel. (It'll be interesting to compare that with the date you found online.) Your doctor or midwife might also ask how many days are in your typical cycle. Then he or she will aim to adjust your estimated due date accordingly.

Your first appointment will probably be long. You might be asked about your health history, your partner's health history, and that of your families. Your doctor or midwife will likely talk with you about prenatal vitamins and medications.

Get ready to kick off your shoes, because at this and every visit, they're likely to check your weight. Your doctor or midwife will note your height, and some doctors and midwives make note of a woman's shoe size as well, although neither measurement is a very good indicator of pelvis size.

At this first appointment, you might be given several tests. Very likely, your blood pressure will be checked at this and every visit. You might have to pee in a cup, and your urine will be tested for proteins and sugar. You might also be checked for sexually transmitted diseases, cervical cancer with a Pap smear, and HIV/AIDS.

At some point, your doctor or midwife will likely order a complete blood count. They'll draw some blood and check your iron levels and white blood cell count for infection. (Low iron levels indicate anemia. See "Preventing and Treating Anemia" on page 257.) Also, you'll have a rubella titer to see if you have immunity against German measles, which is also known as rubella.

Perhaps at your first visit, your doctor or midwife will draw more blood to determine your blood type and Rh factor. Everyone's blood is one of four types: A, B, AB, or O. It's important to know your blood type in case you need to receive blood. The Rh factor is one of several proteins that are present on the surface of red blood cells. If your blood has this protein, you're Rh positive. If your blood lacks the protein, you're Rh negative. More than 85 percent of people are Rh positive, leaving only 15 percent of us to be Rh negative. If you're Rh negative, but your partner is Rh positive, your baby could be Rh positive. This disconnect between you and your baby can cause problems in pregnancy. You could develop antibodies to your baby. And then if a small amount of your baby's blood mixes with your blood, your body might respond as if you're allergic to the baby, which can be dangerous for your baby. But not to worry, all of this can be easily prevented with an injection of Rh immunoglobulin, which is a blood product that prevents sensitization.

That's a lot of testing! But there's one test you might want to request: a thyroid test. Women with higher-than-normal levels of thyroid-stimulating hormone (TSH) have four times the chance of miscarriage than women with normal levels, according to one study. If your TSH levels are high, your thyroid function will be closely minitored.

Be sure to bring your date book along to your visit. On your way out, some doctors and midwives schedule a bunch of prenatal appointments at a time, which is handy.

During this visit, you'll learn a lot about your doctor or midwife, and his or her staff. You will be going to many, many appointments over the next months. If you don't have a good feeling about this visit, don't be afraid to find another practitioner.

⌒

For both of my pregnancies, I went to a midwife instead of an obstetrician. The midwife has an office that in many respects looks like any obstetrician's office. The visits were longer than most ob visits, however, lasting around a half hour each. I really felt that my needs were being met and that I was being heard.

—*Lauren Feder, MD, a mom of two sons, a nationally recognized physician who specializes in homeopathic medicine, and the author of* Natural Baby and Childcare *and* The Parents' Concise Guide to Childhood Vaccinations, *in Los Angeles*

I was living in France with my husband when I was pregnant. I had a very nice doctor, and my appointments were very friendly.

At the time, my French wasn't that good, and my doctor didn't speak Spanish, so we spoke English at my doctor visits. What really saved our conversations, though, was that so much of them were medical in nature. We both understood that perfectly well!

—*Lilian Morales, MD, a mom of an 11-year-old daughter and a physician in Bogotá, Colombia*

RALLIE'S TIP

Although I'm a physician myself, I had lots of questions for my obstetrician during my pregnancy. I wanted to make sure that the signs and symptoms I was experiencing during pregnancy were normal. Because I had trouble remembering my questions during the excitement of my visits, I began to jot them down on a piece of paper. After misplacing my list several times, I began writing my questions in my date book. If my next appointment was on the first of November, I'd write my questions on the "November 1" page. Because I kept my date book with me at all times, I could write down my questions whenever they occurred to me, and I didn't have any trouble finding them when I met with my doctor.

◌

I think it's so important to get—and keep—your husband involved. When men go to the doctor's office for these appointments, they feel that they're not really a part of it. The doctor tends to be looking at everything from the woman's perspective; she's the patient after all. The guys often fall by the wayside.

I think we women have to try to understand that and include them. I tried very hard to be supportive of my husband and include him in everything from the very beginning. He came with me to appointments and tests. Often the doctor would talk directly to me, and so I was careful to bring my husband into the conversations.

—*Jennifer Gilbert, DO, a mom of three-month-old twins and an ob-gyn at Paoli Hospital in Pennsylvania*

Having an Early Ultrasound

Getting a glimpse at your baby via ultrasound is very exciting. Many doctors and midwives send moms-to-be for ultrasounds around this time to confirm a due date or to check for problems.

An ultrasound uses high-frequency sound waves to create a picture. The machine transforms echoes into black-and-white images that you can see on a monitor. Early in your pregnancy, a probe might be inserted into your vagina for an "internal ultrasound." (It might feel a little odd, but it's not painful.) Later in your pregnancy, a wand is used on the *outside* of your belly.

Generally, moms-to-be are given some printed-out ultrasound images. These printouts are wonderful keepsakes, but they're really quite fragile. They can deteriorate quickly. Most ultrasound images are printed on thermal imaging paper. They can turn brown when exposed to light for even a short time. They're also sensitive to heat and pressure.

To preserve your baby's first "pictures," put them into specially designed keepsake frames and hang them out of direct sunlight. Or place them into an acid-free photo album. You could also scan them on a computer. Then you'll have a digital copy saved on your computer and to e-mail to your friends and family.

❧

Early in my pregnancies, my obstetrician did quick ultrasounds in her office to confirm the baby's due date and to see the heart beating. They were fun, and my ob always gave me pictures to take home.

—*Lezli Braswell, MD, a mom of one daughter and two sons and a family medicine physician currently working in an emergency room fast track in Columbus, GA*

❧

I had already had an early ultrasound, but I tricked my friend into giving me another one. She's an obstetrician as well and had been really supportive of me while my husband and I were trying to get pregnant.

After I found out I was pregnant, I wanted to surprise her with the news, so I went to her office and acted like I was having abdominal pain. I asked her to do an ultrasound to find out what was "wrong." When she did the ultrasound, she saw the gestational sac right away. It was wonderful to share my good news with her.

—*Diane Connelly, MD, a mom of a six-year-old daughter and an ob-gyn in HMO practice in Riverside, CA*

You'd think that having ultrasound machines right in my office, I'd have been doing ultrasounds every minute of every day during my pregnancy to check on the baby.

But actually, I was pretty mellow when it came to checking on the baby. I only had the ultrasounds that my doctor recommended.

—*Ashley Roman, MD, MPH, a mom of two daughters, ages three years and six months, and a clinical assistant professor in the department of obstetrics and gynecology at the New York University School of Medicine in New York City*

I have ultrasound machines in my office, and during my pregnancies I could scan myself as often as I liked. During my first pregnancy, I scanned myself a lot because I just wanted to watch what the baby was doing.

But by the time I was pregnant with my fourth baby, the novelty had worn off, and I wasn't that interested in doing it anymore.

—*Melanie Bone, MD, a mom of four "tweens" ages 15 to 12, a gynecologist, the founder of the Cancer Sensibility Foundation, and the author of the syndicated column* Surviving Life *and the book* Cancer, What's Next?, *in West Palm Beach, FL*

During my last pregnancy, I had a nuchal fold scan, which is an early ultrasound that's done when you're between 11 and 14 weeks pregnant to check for Down syndrome, some other chromosomal abnormalities, and major congenital heart problems.

During the test, the technician measures the clear space in the tissue at the back of the baby's neck. If the space is larger than average, it might mean that more fluid has accumulated there, which could indicate a disorder such as Down syndrome.

The technician found that my baby's space was in the very high, but still normal, range. I was concerned, but fortunately the blood test to complete the first trimester screen revealed a low risk for Down syndrome, Trisomy 13, and Trisomy 18 (chromosomal disorders).

—*Dianna K. Kim, MD, a mom of three and an ob-gyn in private practice in Vernon Hills, IL, at the Midwest Center for Women's Healthcare*

Noticing Odd Tastes and Smells

On the TV show *Psych*, one of the main characters, Gus, jokes about his "super sniffer." Likely, right about now, you're noticing you have a super sniffer too. Your sense of smell is more acute, and it's also more sensitive. This is due to the extra estrogen circulating in your body. Even tastes and smells that you normally like might make you feel nauseated.

❧

In both of my pregnancies, I've had a heavy metallic taste in my mouth. This taste was the first symptom I had, and with my second son it was how I knew I was pregnant.

Perhaps because of the extra blood flow to my mouth, I taste the iron in the blood. I really don't know the cause. I have never found a way to remove the taste, but I get used to it. I hardly notice it anymore.

—*Amy J. Derick, MD, a mom of one 15-month-old son who is 17 weeks pregnant with her second son. Dr. Derick is a dermatologist in private practice at Derick Dermatology in Barrington, IL*

❧

Some women have such a profound sense of smell during their pregnancies that certain odors will make them vomit. I carried a cut lemon with me, and when an odor triggered my nausea, I'd sniff the lemon to ease the feeling.

—*Gina Dado, MD, a mom of two daughters and an ob-gyn with Arizona OBGYN Affiliates, Paradise Valley Branch, in Scottsdale, AZ*

❧

During my pregnancy, I was very sensitive to smells. They really bothered me. I remember the smell of eggs in the morning would make me sick immediately, and I'd have to go outside to get away from it. Living communally, I had less control over the smells in the kitchen. I was sick a lot.

—*Stacey Marie Kerr, MD, a mother of two grown daughters, a family physician with strong roots in midwifery, and the author of* Homebirth in the Hospital, *in Santa Rosa, CA*

❧

For around the first month of my pregnancy, certain smells made me nauseated. The one I remember in particular is mayonnaise! I couldn't stand it. If I smelled mayo, I quickly tried to smell something different instead.

—*Lilian Morales, MD*

During my pregnancies, smells really bothered me. The smell of coffee was disgusting to me.

I also had an aversion to red meat. I couldn't stand the smell of steak, and I usually love steak. During my pregnancy, the smell of steak was so offensive to me that if I came home from a 24- or 36-hour shift at the hospital and my husband had cooked steak the night before, I could tell! My sense of smell was that acute.

My husband thought he was in the clear if he cooked it while I was at the hospital. But when I came home, the smell was still overwhelming. I had to ask him not to do it anymore.

—*Ashley Roman, MD, MPH*

&

During my pregnancy, there were some smells I couldn't stand. Actually, the smell of anything cooking made me ill. My husband cooked his food outside on the grill for months. I didn't eat a whole lot, but I wasn't skinny to begin with. I joked that my baby was living off the fat of the land. Because I couldn't stand the smell of the hospital cafeteria, the other residents would ask me what I thought I could eat and bring it back for me.

—*Carrie Brown, MD, a mom of two and a general pediatrician*
who treats medically complex children and specializes in palliative
care at Arkansas Children's Hospital in Little Rock

&

During my pregnancy, I was very sensitive to certain smells. I usually love the smell of coffee, but during pregnancy it made me sick. Also the smell of pine needles made me want to vomit. Some evergreen trees grew next to our driveway, and I had to run from the driveway into my house. Just the smell of those trees made me sick.

Another smell that really bothered me during my pregnancies was artificial orange. I remember we gave our dog an orange-scented flea dip, and it had a very strong orange smell. To this day, even though my son is 18 years old, that artificial orange smell still makes me nauseated.

—*Elissa Charbonneau, DO, a mom of an 18-year-old son and a*
16-year-old daughter and the medical director of the New England
Rehabilitation Hospital in Portland, ME

RALLIE'S TIP

During my pregnancy, I wasn't sensitive to many smells at home, but the minute I stepped into the hospital, I would begin to feel queasy. I was especially sensitive to chemical smells, including the industrial cleaning solutions, air fresheners, and antiseptic soaps and lotions.

To counteract the unpleasant, nausea-inducing smells, I carried a small tube of eucalyptus ointment in my pocket, and I dabbed a bit under my nose whenever the need arose. I found the smell of the eucalyptus blocked the unpleasant odors around me, quelled my nausea, and had a calming effect on me. As a backup, I carried a pack of ginger candy in my pocket, which helped alleviate my nausea.

∽

In the beginning of my second pregnancy, for some reason, the smell of other kids' diapers made me sick. I work in the sedation unit, and we ask parents to change their kids' diapers before letting us put them to sleep. If they peed during the imaging and leaked, they would require more medication for sedation.

If I smelled a dirty diaper, I would practically run out of the room gagging. It was hard to look the parents in the eye sometimes. I explained to the parents what was happening, and they were very understanding. Having their doctor gag in order to avoid giving their kids more medication was a good trade-off. Lots of the mothers said that smells bothered them during their pregnancies too.

I was so grateful that my other son was older and long out of diapers. I don't know how I would have changed his diapers if he was still wearing them!

—*Sonia Ng, MD, a mom of seven-year-old and one-year-old sons and a pediatrician and expert in sedation at Children's Hospital of Philadelphia Pediatric Care at Princeton Health Care System in Princeton, NJ*

Worrying Constructively

It's perfectly normal to worry during your pregnancy. We won't mention all of the things you could be worried about, in case you haven't thought of them yet!

Try to use all of this nervous energy for good, and come up with ways to ease your anxiety when you can. Some women find that deep breathing is calming. You can learn many different techniques online, but you could try simply closing your eyes and breathing in and out slowly for a few counts: one, two, three.

Talking worries over with a friend or your partner can help. A worry shared is a burden lifted.

∽◌◠

Physicians see so many things that our imaginations can run wild. We've seen the worst-case scenarios. I think we have to be especially disciplined at staying positive. It is key to remind ourselves that statistics are on our side, and we are far more likely to have a healthy baby than an unhealthy baby.

—*Nancy Rappaport, MD, a mother of two teenaged daughters and a teenaged son, an assistant professor of psychiatry at Harvard Medical School, an attending child and adolescent psychiatrist in the Cambridge, MA, public schools, and the author of* In Her Wake: A Child Psychiatrist Explores the Mystery of Her Mother's Suicide

∽◌◠

Sometimes doctors become worriers during their pregnancies because we see the worst outcomes. For example, during my first pregnancy, I was working in the neonatal intensive care unit, where all the babies were premature or sick.

But I kept reminding myself that most of the time during most pregnancies, nothing bad happens. Most of the time you feel well, you have a normal delivery, and you have a healthy baby. The outcome for most of us is really great!

I had three lovely pregnancies. I really had nothing special going on— very easy pregnancies.

—*Ayala Laufer-Cahana, MD, a pediatrician, mother, artist, serious home cook, and the founder of Herbal Water Inc., in Wynnewood, PA*

∽◌◠

Early on in our training, physicians have to deal with the reality that the things you see happen to your patients could happen to your family. We develop mechanisms to handle the uncertainty and the reality of what could happen in life. During my pregnancy, I tried to keep the perspective that just

MomMy TIME Try Breathing Exercises

It's amazing that something as simple as breathing can calm you down and ease your worries. But it's true: Regular, mindful breathing can help reduce stress and paradoxically give you energy. Here's one breathing technique that you can use twice a day, or even just when you find your mind dwelling on upsetting thoughts.

Sit in a comfortable chair. Place your right hand on your chest and your left hand on your abdomen. Take a deep breath in through your nose. You should notice that your hand on your abdomen is rising higher than your hand on your chest. Slowly exhale through your mouth.

Next, take a slow, deep breath in through your nose. Hold it for a count of seven. Slowly exhale through your mouth for a count of eight. Gently contract your ab muscles to completely get all of the air out of your lungs. This is the key to this exercise: Exhaling all of the air out of your body. Repeat the cycle four more times.

Once you have this pattern down, you might want to add words to make it work even better. For example, when you inhale, you could say to yourself the feeling that you want to have, such as "relaxation," and when you exhale, you could say to yourself the feeling that you want to get rid of, such as "stress."

because something happened to someone else didn't mean it was going to happen to me.

—*Ruth D. Williams, MD, a mom of twins—a boy and a girl—and another boy, and an ophthalmologist in private practice at the Wheaton Eye Clinic in Wheaton, IL, who specializes in the diagnosis and treatment of glaucoma*

During pregnancy, women have all kinds of symptoms and all kinds of worries. And both the symptoms and the worries are likely to change throughout pregnancy. This is perfectly normal, and in a strange way, this is preparation for being a parent.

Parenting is a constantly moving target. Just when you get good at something, the demands change. For example, once my daughter and I got to be really good at nursing, she didn't want to do it anymore. I was crushed. *What am I going to do with all of this milk I'm producing?* I wondered. Just when you figure out how to do something, your kids need something else. It's extraordinarily challenging, but in a good way.

Becoming a parent matures you more than anything else. I've been through medical school, marriage, divorce, illnesses, and the death of loved ones. But nothing has matured me as much as becoming a mother.

—*Eva Ritvo, MD, a mom of two teenaged daughters, an associate professor and vice chairman at the Miller School of Medicine of the University of Miami, and a coauthor of* The Beauty Prescription

Coping with Food Aversions

It's very common for women to have aversions to food during pregnancy, even to foods they usually like. These aversions can be caused by hormonal changes. Meat, for some reason, is a common food aversion. If you can't stand the sight or smell of meat, make sure to get protein from other sources, such as beans, eggs, and nuts.

∽

During my pregnancy with my daughter, I had an aversion to water! It made me nauseated. I used to love to drink water, but when I was pregnant, I could only drink flavored water, juice, or Gatorade.

—*Dianna K. Kim, MD*

Mommy MD Guide-Recommended Product
Humco Cola Syrup
Cola Syrup is all old-fashioned remedy for nausea that you might find helpful. It's Coca-Cola syrup without the carbonation. It does contain caffeine, though.

You can buy Humco Cola Syrup at drugstores or online for around $3 for a four-ounce bottle.

During my pregnancy, I couldn't stand the taste of coffee. I also suddenly developed aversions to foods I normally love: Brussels sprouts and broccoli. They just didn't appeal to me when I was pregnant.

—*Ann Kulze, MD, a mother of four children, ages 20, 19, 18, and 14, a nationally recognized nutrition expert, motivational speaker, physician, and the author of the critically acclaimed book* Dr. Ann's 10-Step Diet: A Simple Plan for Permanent Weight Loss and Lifelong Vitality

I like to eat. I'm definitely a live-to-eat person! During my first pregnancy, my husband was working as a chef. He cooks with a lot of garlic and pepper. Generally I like that too. But when I was pregnant, I couldn't stomach the smell of cooking garlic and pepper.

I made my husband change out of the clothes that he wore to the restaurant on the porch before coming inside. He would remove his clothes in the middle of a Maine winter night and then run into our apartment and throw the clothes into the washing machine. He was such a good sport!

—*Janet Lefkowitz, DO, a mother of two girls and an ob-gyn in private practice in Rhode Island*

When I was pregnant, I couldn't even hear the word "ham" without getting nauseated. I just couldn't hear that word. I never particularly liked or disliked ham, but if I even thought about how it looked or smelled, I would get sick. My husband used to tease me about it, joking, "Don't say what?"

—*Marra Francis, MD, a mom of three daughters and an ob-gyn who's based in The Woodlands, TX*

Chapter 9
Week 9

Your Baby This Week

YOUR BABY'S SIZE
Your baby measures around 1 to 1¼ inches long, about the size of a Ping-Pong ball.

YOUR BABY'S LATEST DEVELOPMENTS
With each passing day, your baby looks more and more like himself. His features will continue to sharpen and take shape. His external ears are now well formed, and he even has earlobes. Your baby's tongue is developing.

By now your baby has developed muscles and nerves throughout his entire body. All of your baby's organs have formed. From now on, they will mature. His intestines have begun moving into his abdominal cavity from the umbilical cord. Because your baby is larger and stronger, if he's in the right place at the right time, you'll be able to hear his heartbeat on a handheld Doppler.

This week, your baby's arms and legs are longer. Your baby's fingers and toes are formed. (Someday soon, you'll be able to count them!) Your baby can open and close his hands and grab his nose or umbilical cord. He might even begin sucking his thumb. Right now, your baby's fingertips are slightly enlarged because his touch pads are developing. This week, the tiny swirls are forming on his fingertips. (And in a few short years, those fingertips will leave sticky juice prints all over your home!)

Even though your baby's sex organs are forming, male and female organs appear very similar at this point. So if you had an ultrasound, you probably couldn't tell if your baby is a boy or a girl yet.

Your baby is cushioned and protected by the amniotic fluid that surrounds him. Right now, there's only about 1 teaspoon of fluid, but that amount will continue to increase. Around this time, when your baby opens his mouth, he even gulps some fluid in, which is perfectly fine. Your baby can't drown in the amniotic fluid because he doesn't use his lungs to breathe. He gets his oxygen via the umbilical cord—from you.

YOUR LATEST DEVELOPMENTS

Your blood volume continues to increase. You don't feel this extra blood, but you feel plenty of its effects, such as frequent urination and dizziness. You're also still likely very fatigued. Having more blood in your system protects you and your baby from harm when you lie down or stand up during your pregnancy. And it also is a safeguard during labor and delivery, when you'll lose some blood.

You might be noticing more breast changes. The sweat glands in your areolas, which are called Montgomery's tubercles or Montgomery glands, have enlarged. They look like little pimples. They also start to secrete a fluid to lubricate the nipples, to help to protect them from drying and cracking during breastfeeding. Interestingly, after your first pregnancy, they never shrink back completely. An outer ring of lighter-colored tissue starts to appear on the breasts, called the secondary areola. It's probably an old wives' tale, but perhaps that's to make your nipples more visible for the baby to find later on when breastfeeding.

The skin in your genital area also will start to darken, and that mucus-like vaginal discharge might have increased.

Did someone turn up the heat? In pregnancy, many women feel warmer than usual. Because of the increased estrogen, metabolic rate, and blood flow, your body is producing more heat. Feeling hot like this might not be helping your mood either. Dressing in layers can help.

JUSTIFICATION FOR A CELEBRATION

This week your baby's embryonic tail has disappeared!

Telling Family and Close Friends the Good News

Choosing when to tell your family and close friends that you're pregnant is a very personal decision. Some women tell their families and close friends right away, while others wait until they see or hear the baby's heartbeat, or even until after they're out of their first trimesters. Of course, if your family and friends guess, that's out of your control!

∽

I took a home pregnancy test around seven days after I suspected I might have gotten pregnant. I hadn't even missed a period yet.

I was so excited that the test was positive that I called my mom right away. Back when my mom got pregnant, the rabbit had to die to let you know you were expecting. My mom had no conception of quick pregnancy tests. When I told her that I was pregnant, she asked, "What are you talking about?"

"Mom," I said, "in this day, you can pee on a stick a few days after you conceive and find out." She was blown away by the news.

—*JJ Levenstein, MD, FAAP, a mom of one son in college and a pediatrician in private practice in Southern California*

∽

My husband and I waited to tell anyone I was pregnant until we confirmed at my first doctor's visit that everything looked okay. Then we called both of our moms and let them know. Both of our moms already have lots of grandkids, and I was touched at how excited they were to hear about *our* baby.

I was excited to tell my friends that I was pregnant, but I didn't want to hurt anyone's feelings if they weren't told first. So I got everyone onto the same conference call, and I told them all at once. They were all especially excited because I was the first in our circle of friends to get pregnant.

—*Kerri A. Daniels, MD, a mom of one toddler daughter and an instructor in the department of pediatrics at the University of Arkansas for Medical Science in Little Rock*

∽

My husband and I didn't tell our family we were expecting until after I had an amniocentesis and the results came back okay. I was around 18 weeks along, and we told everyone when we went to visit my family for my nephew's wedding.

I told my sister that I was pregnant when she came out to meet us at the car. After that, the news spread like wildfire.

—*Susan Wilder, MD, a mom of an older daughter and twin girls, a primary care physician, and CEO and founder of Lifescape Medical Associates in Scottsdale, AZ*

⁓

My husband and I had been trying to get pregnant for a couple of years, so it was definitely a blessing when we found out I was pregnant. But as an older mom, I was nervous about telling people until we were sure everything was going well.

I didn't even tell my mom until I was around five months pregnant. She lives out of state, which made it much easier to keep it a secret! One day when she was visiting, we went out to breakfast. I showed her an ultrasound photo and said, "I have one of these!" My mom realized right away what I was saying, and her face broke into a huge smile.

—*Monica Lee-Griffith, MD, a mom of one, an ob-gyn, and senior staff, Henry Ford Health System in metropolitan Detroit*

⁓

My husband and I were cautious about telling people that I was pregnant at first because the miscarriage rate is fairly high. We waited until I was around 10 or 12 weeks pregnant to tell our family. By that time, I was reassured because I had seen the baby's heart beating.

To tell my parents, we put some ultrasound photos in with my dad's birthday card. To tell my in-laws, we gave my father-in-law a Father's Day card and told him he would get a grandfather card next year. It took him a little while to get it!

—*Diane Connelly, MD, a mom of a six-year-old daughter and an ob-gyn in HMO practice in Riverside, CA*

⁓

My husband and I agreed not to tell anyone—not even our parents—that I was pregnant until I was past my 12th week. I know that women miscarry most commonly within those first 12 weeks, so after that I figured there would be a better chance that everything would be okay. Plus, by then we had seen the baby's heart beating on an ultrasound, which was very reassuring.

My husband and I were fortunate that our parents lived near each other. We invited my husband's parents to my parents' home, and we told everyone at the same time. They were all very surprised! The news of our second pregnancy slipped out much sooner, but I was less concerned about anybody knowing.

—*Janet Lefkowitz, DO, a mother of two girls and an ob-gyn in private practice in Rhode Island*

෴

My husband and I had been married for 10 years before I got pregnant with our daughter. Our family had long given up on us having children.

When I got pregnant, we were building a new home. At the time, it was framed, so you could see where each room was. My in-laws came to visit one day and see the house in progress. My husband and I took them through the house, room by room. When we got to the last bedroom, I said, "This is the nursery." They kindly said, "Maybe someday." And I said, "Yes, in January!" They were so happy and surprised that they started to cry.

—*Kelly Campbell, MD, a mom of three and an ob-gyn in private practice at Women's Healthcare Physicians in West Bloomfield, MI*

Watching Out for Bleeding

Vaginal bleeding can occur in the first trimester and not be a sign of problems. In fact, anywhere from 20 to 30 percent of women experience some bleeding in early pregnancy. Bleeding during the second or third trimesters is more worrisome.

Bleeding can be a sign of a miscarriage, but about half of pregnant women who bleed do not have miscarriages. Very early bleeding, around 6 to 14 days after conception, could be implantation bleeding. Bleeding can also be caused by some pelvic or urinary tract infections or by having sex. Other conditions during later pregnancy can cause bleeding, such as placenta previa, which is when the placenta lies low in the uterus and partly or completely covers the cervix, or placenta abruption, a condition in which the placenta detaches from the uterine wall.

෴

I had some bleeding in my second pregnancy around five weeks. It was significant, and I was scared. It lasted for a few days, and I tried to take it easy.

I tried to think positive thoughts, and I hoped that everything would work out. My doctor did an ultrasound, which was concerning with a slow heartbeat, but my repeat ultrasound a few days later showed that everything was fine.

—Jennifer Kim, MD, a mom of three girls, ages eight, five, and four; an ob-gyn in private practice in Evanston, IL, at the Midwest Center for Women's Healthcare; and a clinical assistant professor at the University of Chicago, Prtizker School of Medicine

Early in my pregnancy, I had bleeding. It turned out there was a bruise behind the placenta called a subchorionic hematoma. It's a common reason for women to have bleeding in the first trimester. I tried to rest when I could, although I couldn't take a lot of time off. It was a good reason for me to see one of the higher-risk obstetricians. The bleeding stopped after my first trimester.

—Ellen Kruger, MD, a mom of two teenagers and an ob-gyn in an academic and clinical practice in New Orleans, LA, with Ochsner Health System

When to Call Your Doctor or Midwife

If you have bleeding, call your doctor or midwife right away. Don't wear a tampon, douche, or have sexual intercourse. Wear a pad or panty liner so you can monitor how much you're bleeding and what type of bleeding it is.

Bleeding early in the first trimester can be a sign of an ectopic pregnancy. This means the egg has implanted outside of the uterus, usually in the fallopian tube. Other symptoms of an ectopic pregnancy include cramps, tenderness in the lower abdomen, shoulder pain, nausea, and lower back pain. Call your doctor or midwife right away if you experience these symptoms.

Later in pregnancy, bleeding can signal a problem, especially in the second and third trimesters.

Having Genetic Testing or Counseling

Around this time, you might have the option to see a genetic counselor. Some doctors and midwives recommend them, especially for women older than age 35 or people with a family history of a genetic illness.

If you see a genetic counselor, you'll be asked lots of questions about your health, your partner's health, and your families' health histories. You might give blood and tissue samples that will be tested for genes that carry diseases, such as Tay-Sachs, sickle cell anemia, and cystic fibrosis.

If you have these genes, but not the condition itself, you're called a "carrier." But if both you and your partner carry the genes for one of these three conditions, it can be passed along to your baby.

∽

I had a cystic fibrosis carrier screening done years ago when I was an egg donor, at my recipient's request. It was helpful because now I know I'm not a carrier.

Cystic fibrosis is an inherited chronic lung condition that causes a thick, sticky mucus to accumulate in the lungs and digestive tract. Two of my three kids have had respiratory issues, and it was nice to know it wasn't cystic fibrosis right off the bat.

—*Kristie McNealy, MD, MPH, a mom of seven- and four-year-old daughters and a two-year-old son, who's pregnant with another son, and a blogger at www.KristieMcNealy.com, in Denver, CO*

∽

I had genetic testing done while I was pregnant, but I had a very positive outlook and a strong conviction that my babies would be healthy.

Since then, I've also trained to be a geneticist. I'm very glad that I had my kids before that! As an obstetrician, you see a lot of routine cases and deliver a lot of healthy babies, and only occasionally do you have to deliver bad news. On the other hand, as a geneticist, I deal with the rare and the unusual so frequently that the rare and the unusual become the norm. I'm grateful that I had my kids before I learned a lot of specialty genetics because it might have made my pregnancies much more stressful.

—*Siobhan Dolan, MD, MPH, a mom of three, a consultant to the March of Dimes, and an associate professor of obstetrics and gynecology and women's health at Albert Einstein College of Medicine/Montefiore Medical Center in the Bronx, NY*

∽

I had amnios with each of my pregnancies, except for my first because I was just shy of 35 then. It was no big deal. But I remember my doctors insisted that I have genetic counseling before my amnios. I found the counseling to be very enlightening because genetic counselors like to tell people a whole lot more than they need to know. I think they might scare people unnecessarily! I've seen many women leave genetic counselors with their heads spinning with numbers and fears. Even I left worrying that my chances of having a problem were pretty high. But everything turned out just fine.

—*Melanie Bone, MD, a mom of four "tweens" ages 15 to 12, a gynecologist, the founder of the Cancer Sensibility Foundation, and the author of the syndicated column* Surviving Life *and the book* Cancer, What's Next?, *in West Palm Beach, FL*

Avoiding Scary Baby Stories and Reality TV

It's tempting to watch reality TV shows about labor and delivery. As you flip through the channels, they're sure to grab your attention. But most labors and deliveries shown on TV are exciting and dramatic. Watching that could make you anxious and worried about your *own* labor and delivery. And it really doesn't offer much help for you to imagine the most dramatic scenarios of what your labor and delivery could be like. There's no way to know how it will go until it happens.

Like no other time in life, when you're pregnant, people want to tell you scary stories. People would come up to me and talk about their labors, or their friend or family member's labor, and all of the things that went terribly wrong.

The truth is most pregnancies and labors are uneventful. But no one's going to tell you that because it's not a good story. The deliveries with high drama are the ones that people talk about. "Happy, healthy woman delivers happy, healthy baby" does not sell newspapers. Ignore the stories as best you can.

—*Ellen Kruger, MD*

When I was pregnant with my triplets, I was put on bed rest early on. I worked from home, but I also watched TV to pass the time. I'd flip through the channels, and I was truly fascinated by all of the baby-related reality TV shows. I watched *A Baby Story*, *Adoption Stories*, you name it. I was actually inspired at the time by early episodes of *Jon and Kate Plus 8*. If Kate could

? When to Call Your Doctor or Midwife

If your worries are interfering with your day-to-day life, in other words preventing you from doing the things that you love, or if you feel depressed or down for more than two weeks, talk with your doctor or midwife about it.

handle life with sextuplets, I figured that I can make it with triplets!

Even the scary baby reality TV shows didn't frighten me. I had enough faith in God that with the help of my ob and especially my mom (who stayed with us for several weeks to help me around the house), I would have a good outcome.

—*Sadaf T. Bhutta, MBBS, a mom of a three-year-old daughter and 18-month-old triplets and an assistant professor and the fellowship director of pediatric radiology at the University of Arkansas for Medical Sciences and Arkansas Children's Hospital, both in Little Rock*

I didn't have to watch reality TV to hear scary stories. Because I was an older mom, I went to a high-risk obstetrician. They call this "advanced maternal age." I hated that because I felt so young and healthy.

They seemed to focus on and worry so much about bad outcomes that they scared me every time I went in. Their approach was very frightening to me. I don't mind taking things seriously, but I'm very optimistic by nature, so I always tried to look at the more positive side of things.

—*Ruth D. Williams, MD, a mom of twins—a boy and a girl—and another boy, and an ophthalmologist in private practice at the Wheaton Eye Clinic in Wheaton, IL, who specializes in the diagnosis and treatment of glaucoma*

As a medical student, I had a bit of "med student syndrome," which is when you're convinced that you have the medical ailment that you're learning about.

One of the required trainings for pediatric residency was a six-week rotation through the neonatal intensive care unit (NICU). Because I was pregnant during this time, I asked my chief residents not to put me in the NICU so I wouldn't have to worry that my baby would have everything I'd see on rounds. They were very accommodating of my request. I guess they didn't want a crazy woman on their hands!

Diane Truong, MD, FAAP, a mom of one daughter and one son and a pediatrician in a multispecialty group practice in Southern California

I remember just before my second baby was born, I was out eating dinner, and a woman started to tell me in graphic detail about her horrific pregnancy! I turned to her and said, "I cannot listen to these stories anymore."

Sometimes people feel the need to say all sorts of things. It could be that they have anxiety, or they might feel the need to relive an experience that was difficult for them. They forget that you are in transition, and you don't want your mind to be filled with horror stories.

I think that all you have to do is gently explain that you don't wish to hear any more. You're preparing for a healthy pregnancy and a healthy baby, and you want to focus on that.

—Nancy Rappaport, MD, a mother of two teenaged daughters and a teenaged son, an assistant professor of psychiatry at Harvard Medical School, an attending child and adolescent psychiatrist in the Cambridge, MA, public schools, and the author of In Her Wake: A Child Psychiatrist Explores the Mystery of Her Mother's Suicide

Feeling Overheated and Sweating

If you live in Minnesota, feeling warm might be a welcome change. If you live in Florida, it might be sending you over the edge. Either way, it's very common to feel warm and overheated in pregnancy.

During your pregnancy, you might even have hot flashes. Between 50 and 70 percent of pregnant women do. The hot flashes often happen at night, and they can make you really thirsty in addition to feeling very, very hot. It might help to sleep in lighter clothing and place a cup of water on your nightstand.

Feeling warm is due partly to your expanding circulatory system and increased metabolic rate. The blood supply to your skin has increased. Because your veins are more dilated, your body is better able to eliminate heat from your skin. This helps cool you, but it's not always enough.

Here's one benefit to feeling warm: It might not matter if you can't zip up your winter coat because your belly is in the way.

Speaking of warm, it's a good idea to avoid hot tubs, saunas, and electric blankets during pregnancy. After around 15 minutes in a 102°F hot tub, your body temperature can reach 102°F. Studies suggest that temperature might cause problems in your baby.

⁓

I tend to be cold. So when I was finally warm in my pregnancy, it was actually very pleasant.

—*Diane Connelly, MD*

⁓

I'm cold all of the time. During my pregnancies, I was uncomfortably hot, but there wasn't much I could do about it.

I was very lucky that I had a wonderful obstetrician who encouraged me and told me that being so hot was normal. I just focused on looking forward to having healthy babies.

—*Sandra Carson, MD, a mom of two grown sons and the director of the Center for Reproduction and Infertility of Women & Infants Hospital in Providence, RI*

⁓

I remember one point in my pregnancy, I was seeing a young man who had cancer. The exam room door was closed, and I got really hot and felt like I was going to pass out. I opened the door to let in more air, and I sat down. After that, I was fine.

—*Debra Luftman, MD, a mom of a teenaged daughter and a teenaged son, a board-certified dermatologist in private practice, a coauthor of* The Beauty Prescription, *the developer of the skincare line of products Therapeutix, and a clinical instructor of skin surgery and general dermatology at UCLA*

⁓

I was pregnant during the summer in Texas, and I was warm all of the time. At night, I set the air-conditioning to 65, but still I was sprawled out on the bed. My husband slept in flannel pajamas under a goose-down comforter. If he rolled over and touched me, I screamed, "Stop touching me! It's too hot!" I was so miserable.

—*Marra Francis, MD, a mom of three daughters and an ob-gyn who's based in The Woodlands, TX*

I was pregnant during the summer, and it was very hot. I carried a battery-operated fan everywhere—even into meetings. I also carried a bottle of water all of the time, and I drank as much as I could to stay hydrated.

I wore layers. I often had just a sundress or a cotton top with spaghetti straps under my white coat!

—*Katja Rowell, MD, a mom of a four-year-old daughter, a family practice physician, and a childhood feeding specialist with www. familyfeedingdynamics.com, in St. Paul, MN*

Chapter 10
Week 10

Your Baby This Week

YOUR BABY'S SIZE
This week, your baby is around the size of a golf ball. She measures about 1¼ to 2 inches, crown to rump.

YOUR BABY'S LATEST DEVELOPMENTS
Because most congenital malformations occur before the end of this week, your baby will soon have a very critical part of her development safely behind her.

This week, your baby's brain will grow dramatically, producing around 250,000 neurons every single minute. Your baby's eyes are nearly formed, complete with irises and pigmentation. Your baby's ears are starting to move up her head. Her head is becoming more rounded now.

Your baby's nails and hair begin to be visible this week.

Your baby's teeny stomach has begun producing stomach acids. Her kidneys are also producing urine. Her liver is producing red blood cells.

If you haven't been able to hear your baby's heart beat yet, this week you should be able to hear it via Doppler at your doctor's or midwife's office. What a reassuring, wonderful sound that is!

If your baby is a boy, his testes have started to produce testosterone. If your baby is a girl, her clitoris has begun to form from the same cells that would have developed into a penis if he were a boy.

Your baby's legs are developed. In the coming weeks, they'll only continue to grow.

Your baby's spine continues to elongate. Also, her skeleton is replacing the cartilage with bone. Your baby's skin might soon be covered with lanugo. This is a fine hair that insulates your baby until she has enough fat to keep her warm.

YOUR LATEST DEVELOPMENTS

It might be harder and harder to keep your pregnancy a secret. Besides your excitement showing, your belly is starting to protrude. Your nipples also might be sticking out more than usual. You might develop dark, blotchy areas of skin, called melasma or pregnancy mask. Almost three out of four pregnant women get this, on the upper lip, cheekbones, and brow.

You could see a dramatic increase in fatigue this week. Your emotions might still be very sensitive.

This week, you might have some vision changes. Your vision might be blurred, you might see floaters, and your contact lenses might not fit right. These symptoms are caused by the pressure increasing behind your eyes as your body takes on more fluid and blood and because your cornea becomes around 3 percent thicker than it was pre-pregnancy.

Even if you don't normally get nosebleeds, you might have them in pregnancy. They're common, caused by increased levels of the hormones estrogen and progesterone. Your nose might also be increasingly stuffy.

You might notice that your hands and feet have sprouted bulging veins. Your veins are stretching to make room for the extra blood coursing through them. Don't worry: The veins will shrink back and be less visible after your baby is born.

All of a sudden, you might find yourself more clumsy than before. Glasses and plates might seem to leap out of your hands and crash on the floor. It's not your imagination. A hormone called relaxin is loosening up your ligaments and joints in preparation for birth. Unfortunately, relaxin doesn't discriminate: It loosens the joints and ligaments in your hands as well as the ones in your pelvis.

JUSTIFICATION FOR A CELEBRATION

At the end of this week, your baby graduates from being an embryo to being a fetus!

Hearing or Seeing Your Baby's Heart Beating

As early as five or six weeks into your pregnancy, you might be able to see your baby's heart beating on an ultrasound. Each time you go to your doctor or midwife, he or she is likely to listen to your baby's heartbeat using a handheld instrument called a Doppler. This is an amazing, reassuring sound, and most moms-to-be never get tired of hearing it.

⤜⤏

The first time I heard my baby's heartbeat, I was at work. I had one of the sonographers I work with check me to make sure everything was okay. It was very fun!

—Ashley Roman, MD, MPH, a mom of two daughters, ages three years and six months, and a clinical assistant professor in the department of obstetrics and gynecology at the New York University School of Medicine in New York City

⤜⤏

I'm an ob-gyn, and I work in an office where I could do an ultrasound of my babies anytime I wanted to. That was a real advantage because I was so afraid for them. I either listened to their heartbeats or looked at them each and every day of my pregnancies.

I have a policy in my practice that if a mom-to-be calls and she is worried and needs to hear her baby's heartbeat, I have her come in. I never tell them no. I understand how that anxiety feels.

—Kelly Campbell, MD, a mom of three and an ob-gyn in private practice at Women's Healthcare Physicians in West Bloomfield, MI

⤜⤏

I listened to my baby's heartbeat often during my pregnancy. It's always reassuring in pregnancy to hear that. The fetal heartbeat should be regular and between 110 and 160 beats per minute. Of course, it can be higher or lower, depending on if the baby is moving. Their heart rates go up when they move, just like ours do.

I even got to let my family hear my baby's heartbeat. I live in California, and my family lives in Atlanta. I called my parents and put the fetal Doppler on my belly so that they could hear my baby's heartbeat over the phone.

—Diane Connelly, MD, a mom of a six-year-old daughter and an ob-gyn in HMO practice in Riverside, CA

When I saw my baby's heart beating, I felt so reassured. I didn't want to tell anyone that I was pregnant until I saw the baby's heart beating at eight weeks. I didn't want to get all excited and tell my friends and family and then, if something happened, have to go through telling everyone the bad news.

—*Gina Dado, MD, a mom of two daughters and an ob-gyn with Arizona OBGYN Affiliates, Paradise Valley Branch, in Scottsdale, AZ*

Discovering You're Having Twins, Triplets, or More

According to *Twins* magazine, the incidence of fraternal twins varies by race. In parents of African descent, twins occur in 1 birth per 70; of Caucasian descent, in 1 birth per 88; of Japanese descent, in 1 birth per 150; and of Chinese descent, in 1 birth of 300. Genetic factors don't affect the incidence of identical twins; they're simply a special occurance.

Often, twins are discovered at an ultrasound around 12 weeks. Sometimes, however, two tiny sacs are spotted as early as six weeks. At 12 weeks, the sonographer can tell if the twins are fraternal or identical.

In any event, discovering you're having twins, triplets, or more is bound to be a moment you'll remember forever.

When I found out I was pregnant, I went for an ultrasound. I looked at the monitor, and I thought I was looking at a split screen! I saw two sacs! The ultrasound tech smiled and said, "Oh no, there are two!"

—*Susan Wilder, MD, a mom of an older daughter and twin girls, a primary care physician, and CEO and founder of Lifescape Medical Associates in Scottsdale, AZ*

I didn't find out I had a twin pregnancy until I went in for my ultrasound around 21 weeks. It was the most exciting moment of my life. At that same time, I found out that I was having a boy and a girl. It was the perfect dream come true.

—*Ruth D. Williams, MD, a mom of twins—a boy and a girl—and another boy, and an ophthalmologist in private practice at the Wheaton Eye Clinic in Wheaton, IL, who specializes in the diagnosis and treatment of glaucoma*

With my first pregnancy, my husband and I were nervous to tell anyone we were pregnant too soon. But a few years later, when we tried to get pregnant again, we were much more up-front with our family that we were doing in vitro fertilization. It was nice to have their support every step of the way.

When we found out we were having twins, I remember showing my mother-in-law the ultrasound pictures of the embryos. She saw her grandsons at the 16-cell stage! That's something most people don't get to do.

—*Kelly Campbell, MD*

❧

When my husband and I were at an early ultrasound, we found out that we were having twins! You could clearly see the two sacs, and the sonographer said, "It's two!" I could cry just thinking about it.

Somehow I always knew it would be twins, though. But my first thought was: *I'm so glad we aren't having triplets!* I was thrilled—but also scared. I wondered, *How am I going to carry a twin pregnancy?* And then, *How am I going to continue to have a professional career with twins?*

—*Jennifer Gilbert, DO, a mom of three-month-old twins and an ob-gyn at Paoli Hospital in Pennsylvania*

❧

I had in vitro fertilization to become pregnant with all of my kids. When my firstborn turned one, I was 34 years old. All of the literature says that after 35, even a healthy woman's fertility nose-dives. I have polycystic ovarian syndrome, so I knew that my fertility would be even lower.

I went through one more IVF cycle, and as I had with my daughter, I had three embryos transferred. Although two of the three embryos had died in the first trimester during my first pregnancy, by week 12 of my second pregnancy, they all looked great! My ob-gyn said, "I think this time you're going to have all three babies!"

For the first few months, my husband and I were in denial. This isn't happening to us! My husband was especially in denial about needing a minivan. He checked into every type of SUV, but of course none of them could accommodate four babies. (Our daughter would only be 20 months old when the triplets were born.) And so we bought a minivan.

—*Sadaf T. Bhutta, MBBS, a mom of a three-year-old daughter and 18-month-old triplets and an assistant professor and the fellowship director of pediatric radiology at the University of Arkansas for Medical Sciences and Arkansas Children's Hospital, both in Little Rock*

Enjoying Sex during Pregnancy (No Kidding!)

If you're having a normal, low-risk pregnancy, sex is safe. In fact, it might help reduce your stress and increase your intimacy with your partner.

After having sex, you might have a little spotting or some cramping in your lower back and abdomen. As long as it's not severe pain or heavy bleeding, it should be just fine.

❦

Before I got pregnant, my husband and I had a healthy sex life. We had a lot of sex while I was pregnant too. In fact, we had sex the morning my water broke. We just found ways to make it happen. Sex was relaxing for me and lovely for him. It's good to bank up a lot of "credit," because after the baby comes, you won't be able to have sex for a while.

—*JJ Levenstein, MD, FAAP, a mom of one son in college and a pediatrician in private practice in Southern California*

❦

I think many husbands fear that they could hurt the baby during sex. But that's not something to worry about. You're not going to poke the baby in the eye! It's perfectly safe to have sex right up until you deliver as long as everything's going normally.

For me, I really needed that closeness with my husband. I felt so huge, and my husband was very supportive. Just having him close, hugging, holding hands, etc., helped me to feel better.

—*Gina Dado, MD*

❦

Sex during pregnancy was fabulous. It's "perma" lube! I felt incredibly sexy when I was pregnant—the sexiest I ever felt. Of course postpartum, the Dolly Parton look wasn't harmful either. I think that my husband and I have the best sex in the universe. This continues to strengthen the relationship throughout the marriage, despite

When to Call Your Doctor or Midwife

If you experience heavy bleeding or severe cramping in your lower back or abdomen after having sex, call your doctor or midwife right away.

the sleepless nights, the terrible twos, and the teen years. Your relationship with your partner will get you through all the difficult times—and we all have them!

I think some women turn inward during pregnancy, and they don't share with their partners. My husband and I worked through whatever issues we had to in order to maintain our relationship.

I believe that if you don't continue to explore your sexuality with your partner, the relationship will end. Sex is necessary to make a relationship lifelong. You have to have that rebonding on a fairly frequent basis.

—Hana R. Solomon, MD, a mom of four, ages 35 to 19, a board-certified pediatrician, the president of BeWell Health, LLC, and the author of Clearing the Air One Nose at a Time: Caring for Your Personal Filter

Watching Out for Vision Changes and Dry Eyes

Some women experience changes with their vision and eyes during pregnancy, such as blurry vision, floaters, and problems with contact lens fit. The good news is that all of these symptoms should pass a few weeks after your baby is born. After your fluid levels return to normal, by around six weeks after delivery, your eyes should too.

During my pregnancy, I saw occasional floaters in my vision. It might be due to more fluid being retained in your body.

My floaters just came and went, and after my baby was born, they went away entirely. Floaters can be a normal occurrence in pregnancy, but they might indicate other complications of pregnancy.

—Jennifer Kim, MD, a mom of three girls, ages eight, five, and four; an ob-gyn in private practice in Evanston, IL, at the Midwest Center for Women's Healthcare; and a clinical assistant professor at the University of Chicago, Pritzker School of Medicine

During my pregnancy, I briefly went blind. Well, okay maybe not totally blind, but my vision got so blurry for a few minutes that I couldn't see.

It was very scary. I could see fuzzy shadows, and I could distinguish dark from light, but that was it. I was walking to my office in the city, and I had to run my hand against a wall to guide me.

It only lasted around 10 minutes, but I went to a neurologist to find out what had happened. He said it was a migraine headache.

—Joanna Dolgoff, MD, a mom of a seven-year-old son and a four-year-old daughter, a board-certified pediatrician/child obesity expert with practices in Manhattan and Roslyn Heights, NY, creator of an online child weight loss program (www. DrDolgoff.com), and author of the book Red Light, Green Light, Eat Right

I don't recall having any eye changes during my pregnancy. But it's true that the moisture content of the cornea can change during pregnancy. Some women might have problems with contact lens fit during pregnancy, and women with diabetes can experience progression of diabetic retinopathy. It's really important to maintain strict control of your blood sugar and see your doctor for an eye exam while you're pregnant.

—Ruth D. Williams, MD

Staunching Nosebleeds

During pregnancy, your blood volume increases by up to 50 percent. Your circulatory system is expanding to allow for this increase in blood volume. This can cause occasional nosebleeds. Also, the extra progesterone and estrogen in your body causes your mucous membranes to swell. Your nose might start to bleed all of a sudden, without warning and for no apparent reason.

> **? When to Call Your Doctor or Midwife**
>
> Because women with diabetes can experience progression of diabetic retinopathy during pregnancy, it's really important to carefully control your blood sugar and see your doctor for an eye exam.
>
> Vision problems, such as blurry vision, can be a symptom of preeclampsia, which is a cluster of symptoms that includes swelling and high blood pressure. Call your doctor or midwife right away if your vision problems are accompanied by swelling, headaches, and/or flulike aches and pains.

Drinking plenty of water and other noncaffeinated beverages such as milk and juice can help to prevent nosebleeds. To treat a nosebleed, hold a cold washcloth on the bridge of your nose, applying gentle pressure.

RALLIE'S TIP

I had several nosebleeds during my pregnancies, especially during the winter months when the indoor air was warm and very dry. I found the best way to stop a nosebleed was to sit upright in a chair and simply pinch my nostrils firmly together for three to five minutes. I learned the hard way that tilting my head back wasn't such a great idea. The taste of blood at the back of my throat made me gag, which caused my nose to bleed even more.

Mommy MD Guide-Recommended Product
Systane Lubricating Eye Drops

"My job is very computer-based, and pregnancy made my eyes more tired than usual," says Sonia Ng, MD, a mom of seven-year-old and one-year-old sons and a pediatrician and expert in sedation at Children's Hospital of Philadelphia Pediatric Care at Princeton Health Care System in Princeton, NJ. "Looking at the computer screen also gave me dry eyes.

"What helped was using preservative-free Systane Lubricating eye drops in my eyes," Dr. Ng adds. "I use the preservative-free drops because I'm allergic to the preservatives. The one time I used drops with preservatives, my eyes turned really red like I had pinkeye. When you work in a hospital and your eyes are red, swollen, and gunky, people really don't want you to touch their children.

"During my pregnancy, I put the drops in my eyes as needed. I kept a bottle in each of my bags, so I would always have one with me."

You can buy Systane Lubricating eye drops in drugstores and online for around $10.

Women often get nosebleeds during pregnancy because the blood vessels in their nasal passages dilate

I personally didn't get any nosebleeds, but I slept with a humidifier and do recommend Ocean Nasal Spray (a saline spray you can buy at drugstores) to keep your nasal passages moist. (See "Mommy MD Guide-Recommended Product: Ocean Spray" on page 147.)

—*Gina Dado, MD*

? When to Call Your Doctor or Midwife

If you have frequent nosebleeds, tell your doctor or midwife at your next appointment. If you have a gushing nosebleed, or one that you can't stop, go to the emergency department.

Chapter 11
Week 11

Your Baby This Week

YOUR BABY'S SIZE

This week, your baby is around 1½ to 2½ inches long, about the size of a billiard ball. He's entering a period of rapid growth. His length will double in the next three weeks, and over the next few weeks, his weight will increase five-fold.

YOUR BABY'S LATEST DEVELOPMENTS

Even though you can't feel it, your baby is in almost constant motion. The teeny gymnast has plenty of room to flip all around, doing somersaults in the amniotic fluid.

Hair follicles are appearing on your baby's scalp. With the exception of your baby's lungs and brain, his organs will all start to regularly perform their tasks this week. Your baby's brain and lungs will continue to develop throughout your pregnancy.

Your baby's genitals are beginning to show distinguishing features. By the end of this week, the sex organs should be visible on an ultrasound. A penis is easier to detect than a clitoris.

Around this week, the placenta begins to give your ovaries a break and produce more hormones.

YOUR LATEST DEVELOPMENTS

Your uterus is almost big enough to fill your pelvis now. Your doctor or midwife might be able to feel the uterus through your abdomen just above the pubic bone. If not now, soon. Looser, more comfy clothing is certainly in order. All of this growth might be giving you some round ligament pains. As your uterus expands, the ligaments attached to it are forced to stretch. Ouch! Hopping up quickly can make the pain worse, so try to move slowly.

With any luck, your skin looks more glowing and shiny now.

Your breasts might have gone up a cup size, or two or more. Don't panic! This growth should stop soon. If the skin stretching is causing you to itch, cocoa butter might help. The good news is the soreness might have decreased by now.

Your gums might be swelling, causing them to bleed. They're also more vulnerable to bacteria, plaque, gingivitis, and even periodontitis. If you don't already have an appointment to see your dentist, it's a good idea to make one soon in your pregnancy.

Pregnancy is such a different experience for everyone. Some women find that their hair and nails grow faster and thicker. Other women lose some of their hair, and their fingernails break like eggshells. These changes might be due to pregnancy hormones or the increased blood in your body.

At this point, you might certainly still be experiencing nausea and fatigue. You're more likely to be having heartburn now than earlier in your pregnancy.

Many women start to feel breathless at around this stage, even when they're not exerting themselves. Your organs are all working very hard, demanding more oxygen than usual. During pregnancy, your oxygen requirements rise by up to 20 percent.

Here's a welcome change: Your mood might be leveling out. However, it's at this point in pregnancy that the reality often sets in for a woman's partner. So he might just be beginning to panic . . .

JUSTIFICATION FOR A CELEBRATION

Your baby's face is filling out now, making him look more and more like an infant, and more and more like himself.

Having a Pregnancy Massage

As long as you find a massage therapist with the experience and equipment to give prenatal massage, it can be a wonderful, relaxing experience.

∽◌∽

I highly recommend having a pregnancy massage. It really helped me relax. I had a few massages during my pregnancies, and they were wonderful. I get achy because of my job, and the massages helped to relieve that.

—*Jennifer Kim, MD, a mom of three girls, ages eight, five, and four; an ob-gyn in private practice in Evanston, IL, at the Midwest Center for Women's Healthcare; and a clinical assistant professor at the University of Chicago, Pritzker School of Medicine*

∽◌∽

MomMy TIME — Buy Yourself Some New Luxurious Toiletries

Now would be a great time to treat yourself to some soothing new bath products. Lavender is very relaxing. Or perhaps choose vanilla, which will come in handy after your baby is born. A 2005 *Developmental and Behavioral Pediatrics* study found that babies are comforted by the scent of vanilla.

You'll find a wonderful selection of skin- and bathcare products at terrific prices at Bath & Body Works, which are in malls across the country, or online at **www. BathAndBodyWorks.com.**

During my pregnancy, I got massages every two weeks. Massage therapists use special massage tables with holes in them to accommodate pregnant women's bellies. The massages helped relax my muscles and me. It's important to relax as much as you can during pregnancy to avoid muscle cramps. I didn't have many muscle cramps during my pregnancy, and I think it was because I was so proactive about getting massages.

—*Debra Luftman, MD, a mom of a teenaged daughter and a teenaged son, a board-certified dermatologist in private practice, a coauthor of* The Beauty Prescription, *the developer of the skincare line of products Therapeutix, and a clinical instructor of skin surgery and general dermatology at UCLA*

I had a couple of massages before I got pregnant, and I had a few while I was pregnant. I went to a massage therapist who was specially trained in working with pregnant women,

At the time, I had sciatica—pain in my lower back that ran down my leg. There's not much you can do for sciatica when you're pregnant because many of the traditional medications are not safe to take in pregnancy. The massage helped a bit temporarily. The best part of it was the hour of relaxing and being pampered.

—*Lezli Braswell, MD, a mom of one daughter and two sons and a family medicine physician currently working in an emergency room fast track in Columbus, GA*

During my third trimester, I had sacroileitis, which caused a stabbing pain in my right gluteus muscle. Stretching and pregnancy massage were wonderful. Even though the pain was still there until after I delivered, massage gave me an hour of relief and relaxation.

—*Gina Dado, MD, a mom of two daughters and an ob-gyn with Arizona OBGYN Affiliates, Paradise Valley Branch, in Scottsdale, AZ*

Getting the First Trimester Screening

There's a very important reason why this is called a *screening*: The results of this test do not *diagnose* a problem. They merely estimate what a person's *chances* are of having a problem. The results help your doctor or midwife to decide whether further testing might be warranted, such as a chorionic villus sampling or amniocentesis. (See "Having a Chorionic Villus Sampling" on page 150 and "Having an Amniocentesis" on page 203.)

This screening is usually done between weeks 11 and 14. A study published in the *New England Journal of Medicine* a few years ago found that this test is the most accurate, noninvasive screening available for chromosomal abnormalities.

The first trimester screening is actually two tests in one: a blood screening test and an ultrasound. It's used to identify risks for chromosomal abnormalities, such as Down syndrome, and heart defects. The blood test measures two key pregnancy hormones: human chorionic gonadotropin (hCG) and pregnancy-associated plasma protein A (PAPP-A). If these levels are abnormally high or low, it might indicate a problem.

During the ultrasound part of this screening, the technician measures nuchal translucency, which is the thickness at the back of the baby's neck. An increase in this space could suggest a chromosomal abnormality, such as Down syndrome, or a heart defect. However, the test cannot identify neural tube defects.

The results of these two tests are then combined with other information, such as the mother's age, to determine the risk to the baby.

This test often replaces other tests, including the triple screen or quad screen. Those tests are performed later, in the second trimester, and they are less accurate than the first trimester screening.

If you elect to have the first trimester screening, you'll usually have your results back within a week. However, because this test doesn't actually *diagnose* anything, instead merely predicting risks, many women elect not to take this test at all.

～

I had the triple screen test with each of my pregnancies. During my last pregnancy, I was 35, what they call "advanced maternal age," so I was slightly concerned. My husband and I hoped for the best, and fortunately the test didn't indicate any problems.
  —*Dianna K. Kim, MD, a mom of three and an ob-gyn in private practice in Vernon Hills, IL, at the Midwest Center for Women's Healthcare*

～

I had a triple screen test, which is also sometimes called a triple test or a multiple marker screening. The test is usually done between weeks 15 and 20 of pregnancy. They drew a bit of blood and tested it for three substances that they then use to estimate a baby's chance of having an abnormality or genetic disorder.

The test was optional, but I was glad that I had it. Even though I wouldn't have done anything if the test suggested there might have been a problem, I thought it would be best to prepare myself.
  —*Rebecca Kazin, MD, a mom of three girls and the medical director of the Johns Hopkins Dermatology and Cosmetic Center at Green Spring Station in Lutherville, MD*

I had screening tests for Down syndrome during both of my pregnancies. During my second pregnancy, my test came back abnormal, which was very stressful. Ironically, I received the results when I was across the country at a national Maternal Fetal Medicine meeting, but I had to wait until my return home five days later to have amniocentesis performed. Those were the longest five days. Fortunately, everything came back fine.

—*Ashley Roman, MD, MPH, a mom of two daughters, ages three years and six months, and a clinical assistant professor in the department of obstetrics and gynecology at the New York University School of Medicine in New York City*

During all three of my pregnancies, my husband and I decided not to do the triple screen test. We decided that even if we had a baby with health problems, it wouldn't change how we would have behaved.

—*Lezli Braswell, MD*

Feeling Hungry and Eating Well

It's not unusual for women to feel an intense, gnawing hunger in pregnancy. Make the best of this and eat the healthy foods you and your baby need.

During my pregnancies, I ate the best that I ever have in my entire life. I was so conscious that everything I put into my mouth was going to the baby.

—*Patricia S. Brown, MD, a mom of two daughters, ages nine and seven, and a three-year-old son and a psychiatrist at Columbia–New York Child and Adolescent Telepsychiatry and in private practice in Cresskill, NJ*

When I was pregnant with my two sons, I was ravenously hungry. I had true hunger pains; my stomach hurt.

I'm usually very lean, especially prior to pregnancy, and I think it was nature's way of getting me to put a little fat on. I listened to my body and ate when it told me to, though it wasn't always telling me to eat the best things!

—*Ann Kulze, MD, a mother of four children, ages 20, 19, 18, and 14, a nationally recognized nutrition expert, motivational speaker, physician, and the author of the critically acclaimed book* Dr. Ann's 10-Step Diet: A Simple Plan for Permanent Weight Loss and Lifelong Vitality

In my first pregnancy, I ate nonstop. I had 20 meals a day. This was before we knew what was good for you, so I ate a bagel in the morning before work. Then I'd eat breakfast in the hospital cafeteria. Lunch at work was a blur, but I'd stop for pizza and McDonald's on my way home! I never worried about gaining weight, and in the end I had no problem losing it anyway.

—*Erika Schwartz, MD, a mom of two and the director of www. DrErika.com, who's been in private practice for more than 30 years in New York City, specializing over the past 15 years in women's health, disease prevention, and bioidentical hormones*

As a doctor and also a mother, I believe that nothing in the world matters more than health—not money, not your appearance, and not your job.

So when I was pregnant, I was fanatical about my health. For example, I haven't had a sip of soda since I found out I was pregnant with our first daughter! My husband and I decided that we didn't want to do anything to neglect my health—and therefore the health of our baby—because if anything went wrong, we would blame ourselves.

In hindsight, it's ironic that I was so fanatical about my health because my oldest daughter has cerebral palsy. But it did give me comfort to know that I was as healthy as I could possibly be during my pregnancy.

I think it's important to give your children the best start for their health from the very beginning, and that is pregnancy. It's a tremendous responsibility to have a baby growing inside of you. That baby is 100 million percent depending upon you. You owe it to your baby to create the healthiest environment that you can by eating right—and also by exercising and avoiding stress as much as possible.

—*Eva Ritvo, MD, a mom of two teenaged daughters, an associate professor and vice chairman at the Miller School of Medicine of the University of Miami, and a coauthor of* The Beauty Prescription

Clearing Up Skin Changes

Your skin is certainly not immune to changes during pregnancy. Acne and pregnancy mask are a few skin changes you might encounter. On the flip side, all of the extra blood in your veins might be giving you a lovely, rosy complexion, and the extra hormones might make your skin smooth and shiny.

A few lucky pregnant women have less acne during pregnancy. If you usually break out before your period, you're more likely to break out while you're pregnant too. Often in pregnancy, women are more acne prone or their skin is drier than usual. As your hormone levels change, it can trigger increased oil production. Pesky pimples can appear on your face, and also on your neck, shoulders, and back. Drinking water might help to flush oil and bacteria from your pores and prevent pimples.

Pregnancy mask affects almost three-quarters of all pregnant women, but for some reason a lot of women haven't heard of it. Its medical name is melasma, and it's caused by increased levels of a hormone called melanin. That's the same hormone that causes your skin to darken in the sun. In pregnancy, you might notice dark, blotchy areas of skin, especially on your brow, cheekbones, and upper lip. Exposure to the sun will make it worse, so it's helpful to stay out of the sun and wear sunscreen. During pregnancy,

Mommy MD Guide-Recommended Product
Eminence Organic Skin Care

"I had pregnancy acne," said Gina Dado, MD, a mom of two daughters and an ob-gyn with Arizona OBGYN Affiliates, Paradise Valley Branch, in Scottsdale, AZ. "This was very difficult because when you're pregnant, you're supposed to be glowing and beautiful. I was not glowing, and I didn't feel beautiful. I had acne all around my jawline. It was devastating.

"When you're pregnant, you want to avoid products containing glycolic acid, retin A, and salicylic acid. I used products from organic skincare lines such as Eminence Organic Skin Care. You can use benzoyl peroxide and some other more natural skincare products. And of course, there's always concealer to cover it up."

You can buy Eminence Organic Skin Care in fine salons and spas worldwide. Visit WWW.EMINENCEORGANICS.COM for details.

your skin might be more sensitive to certain ingredients in sunscreen, so test it on a small area of skin before slathering it all over.

~

During my first trimester of pregnancy, I had a lot of acne. I wasn't expecting that at all. Thankfully, I was able to cover it with makeup.

—*Patricia S. Brown, MD*

~

During my pregnancy, I had a little acne. I used over-the-counter benzoyl peroxide, and that seemed to clear it up after only a few treatments. Because continued use seemed to dry out my skin, I'd stop using it for a while until the acne flared up again.

—*Lezli Braswell, MD*

~

I didn't have a problem with acne during my pregnancies. But my skin seems a little bit wrinkly! After my first son was born, my skin returned to normal. One of my patients observed that I looked younger.

"Yes," I explained. "That's because for nine months I hadn't used Botox."

—*Amy J. Derick, MD, a mom of one 15-month-old son who is 17 weeks pregnant with her second son. Dr. Derick is a dermatologist in private practice at Derick Dermatology in Barrington, IL*

? When to Call Your Doctor or Midwife

Do not take any prescription medications while pregnant, including those for acne, without the approval of your doctor or midwife. Accutane (isotretinoin) in particular is very dangerous in pregnancy.

Because your skin is an organ and anything you put on it is absorbed into your body, you must be very careful about what you put on your skin during pregnancy. Products containing retinol are especially worrisome, and their safety during pregnancy is suspect.

If you're having problems with your skin, talk with your doctor or midwife at your next appointment.

RALLIE'S TIP

I'll never forget how horrified I was when I first noticed a brown discoloration on my upper lip. I thought I was growing a mustache! On closer inspection, I realized that it wasn't facial hair, but rather a change in skin pigment. I had never heard of "pregnancy mask," so I had no idea what it was or how long it would last. Fortunately, it was easily disguised with makeup, and it went away a few months after my delivery.

∽

One unusual symptom I had during pregnancy is that all of the hair on my legs fell out. I'm not sure if it was due to hormonal changes or because my legs were so swollen. But I didn't care what the cause was; I was thrilled! Six months after my baby was born, though, all of the hair grew back.

Just as perplexing, during my pregnancy I grew hair on my boobs and stomach. It looked sort of like the hair Jeff Goldblum had in *The Fly*. It really freaked me out. *What next?*

I plucked out the thick ones on my boobs. But I was afraid to wax the ones on my belly for fear it would cause stretch marks. Thankfully, it all fell out after my baby was born.

—*Sonia Ng, MD, a mom of seven-year-old and one-year-old sons and a pediatrician and expert in sedation at Children's Hospital of Philadelphia Pediatric Care at Princeton Health Care System in Princeton, NJ*

Chapter 12
Week 12

Your Baby This Week

YOUR BABY'S SIZE
Your baby measures around 2½ inches now, from crown to rump. She's about the size of a tennis ball.

YOUR BABY'S LATEST DEVELOPMENTS
Your baby might begin to hiccup. Some women feel their babies' hiccups before they feel kicks. You can tell hiccups from kicks because hiccups are rhythmic.

All of your baby's structures are formed, and they're continuing to develop and grow. Your baby's pituitary gland, at the base of her brain, is now starting to make hormones. These hormones are responsible for growth and blood pressure regulation.

This week, your baby's voice box, or larynx, is developing. Even though your baby isn't able to cry in utero, she'll cry the minute she's born when her throat and mouth are cleared of fluid. It will be one of the best sounds that you have ever heard.

Your baby's digestive tract continues to mature. Around this week, her pancreas begins to produce the hormone insulin, which will help to digest sugars.

Your baby's skeleton is beginning to develop hard bone centers in the cartilage of her fetal bones. This process is called ossification. Inside your baby's tiny bones, the marrow is beginning to produce white blood cells, which are her first weapons against infections.

Around this time, your baby's small intestine can now produce contractions in preparation to later push food through her bowels.

Your baby's tiny fingernails and toenails are growing. You might have to cut them soon after she's born.

YOUR LATEST DEVELOPMENTS

Your uterus is growing quickly. For these first few months of pregnancy, this growth is caused by estrogen and progesterone. But later, your uterus also grows because it's stretched by the growth of the baby and placenta. You might also be noticing weight gain in your breasts, hips, and legs. By now you've probably gained around two to four pounds, perhaps more if you were underweight prior to getting pregnant. This is justification for a shopping trip for some looser clothing— or for raiding your partner's closet.

With any luck, your nausea and fatigue are beginning to abate. You might notice an increase in your appetite.

You might already be feeling back pain and strain. Practicing good posture and stretching can help prevent it.

Because your uterus is moving higher in your pelvic region, it's putting less pressure on your bladder, so you might not have to urinate as often.

An increase in vaginal secretions plus greater blood flow to genital organs might make sex better than ever. Some couples find that not having to worry about birth control helps too. You might feel closer to your partner than ever, because of the baby you have created together. But on the other hand, a loss of libido is perfectly normal too. Your breasts might still be sensitive, you might still feel too tired, your weight might make you uncomfortable, and you just might not feel like it.

Although varicose veins are more common later in pregnancy, it's not unusual to have them already.

During pregnancy, your immune system dials down. Because of this, you're more likely to catch colds and other illnesses.

JUSTIFICATION FOR A CELEBRATION

Your baby has developed the sucking and rooting reflexes, which will help her to find your breast or a bottle after she's born.

Buying (or Borrowing) Some Looser Clothing

If it hasn't happened already, someday soon your underwear, pants, and skirts won't fit. Besides gaining weight in your belly, you might also be gaining weight in your hips and legs. Some looser clothing will definitely make you more comfortable.

~

Early in my pregnancy, I bought a lot of stretch pants and other forgiving clothes that could "grow" with me.

—Elissa Charbonneau, DO, a mom of an 18-year-old son and a 16-year-old daughter and the medical director of the New England Rehabilitation Hospital in Portland, ME

~

A few months into my first pregnancy, I bought a few pairs of new pants that were a size bigger than what I normally wore. Even though it cost a bit, I knew that I was going to have more children. Plus I knew I'd wear the pants

Mommy MD Guide-Recommended Product
BellaBand

"Because I had such severe morning sickness for about half of both of my pregnancies, I actually *lost* weight at first," said Ashley Roman, MD, MPH, a mom of two daughters, ages three years and six months, and a clinical assistant professor in the department of obstetrics and gynecology at the New York University School of Medicine in New York City. "I was able to get away without wearing maternity clothes for most of my pregnancies.

"When I found that I could no longer zip up my pants, I purchased BellaBands, which are the best gift for any pregnant woman," Dr. Roman said. "With a BellaBand, I could wear my regular pants, unbuttoned and unzipped, and the BellaBand would hold them up. Then I simply put one of my larger sweaters over them. I saved a whole lot of money on maternity clothes!"

You can buy BellaBands for around $26 online. Or find a store near you using the "store locator" on **WWW.INGRIDANDISABEL.COM**.

again after the baby was born while my body returned to pre-pregnancy size. They were a great investment!

> —*Lezli Braswell, MD, a mom of one daughter and two sons and a family medicine physician currently working in an emergency room fast track in Columbus, GA*

RALLIE'S TIP

When I first started showing, I couldn't wait to go shopping for maternity clothes. What I didn't know with my first pregnancy is that I would be wearing maternity clothes for what seemed like forever—not just during the pregnancy but also for a few months after the delivery while I was trying to lose my pregnancy weight.

In the early stages of my second pregnancy, I bought regular shirts and pants in bigger sizes instead of maternity clothes that emphasized my pregnancy. I was comfortable wearing them while my belly was growing during my pregnancy and then again while my belly was shrinking after the delivery.

Monitoring Your Weight

During pregnancy, your weight might be the topic of much debate. Some practitioners monitor weight very carefully; others have a more laissez-faire attitude. You'll probably kick off each and every prenatal appointment by kicking off your shoes and stepping on the scale.

If you've started out your pregnancy at a healthy weight, most experts recommend that women eat an additional 300 calories each day, about the number in a cup of yogurt and a piece of fruit, to gain between 25 and 35 pounds. Generally, women gain two to four pounds in their first trimesters and then about a pound each week in the second and third.

If you were underweight before pregnancy, you should probably gain a little more, as much as 40 pounds. If you were overweight, you should gain only 15 to 25 pounds. If you were obese before getting pregnant, you should gain only 11 to 20 pounds. If you're carrying twins, you should probably gain 37 to 54 pounds, if you began at a healthy weight.

As with many things in life, slow and steady wins the race. Keeping your weight gain steady and gradual is helpful for many reasons. For one, it might help to minimize stretch marks.

I'm 5 feet tall and before I got pregnant, I weighed 108 pounds. I gained between 25 and 33 pounds in each pregnancy, and I was terribly uncomfortable. I topped out at 141. I didn't pig out during my pregnancies, but I ate what I felt like I needed to eat. I didn't worry about my weight because I knew I could lose it after the babies were born.

—Melanie Bone, MD, a mom of four "tweens" ages 15 to 12, a gynecologist, the founder of the Cancer Sensibility Foundation, and the author of the syndicated column Surviving Life *and the book* Cancer, What's Next?, *in West Palm Beach, FL*

I normally wear a size 2 or 4. I decided that during my pregnancy, I wasn't going to overly restrict my caloric intake. So I gained 45 pounds my first pregnancy. I'm pregnant again now, and I'm unfortunately above my desired weight, so I'm going to cut back just a little.

—Amy J. Derick, MD, a mom of one 15-month-old son who is 17 weeks pregnant with her second son. Dr. Derick is a dermatologist in private practice at Derick Dermatology in Barrington, IL

With my first baby, I gained around 25 pounds, and with my second I gained 20 pounds. It was hard not to gain more. I really tried to avoid empty calories like soda and chips. I ate a lot of low-fat dairy, which is important for extra calcium. I also snacked on nuts, which offer both carbs and protein.

Mommy MD Guide-Recommended Product
Digital Scale

Digital scales are handy, easy to use, and inexpensive. You could buy a basic scale for less than $20 at a discount store, or you could spend several times that.

Try before you buy. Make sure you can see the scale's readout clearly. Confirm that it uses the units you want, which is likely pounds. You might want a scale that reads to tenths of a pound, so you can more closely monitor your weight going up now, and in a few months going back down.

The extra weight puts a tremendous amount of stress on your frame, and if you're carrying around more than the ideal number of pounds, you'll feel it even more. I had a lot of aches and pains, especially backache.

—*Stephanie Ring, MD, a mom of two sons, ages six and two, and an ob-gyn at Red Rocks Ob-Gyn in Lakewood, CO*

I'm generally thin, and I found if I watched what I was eating, I gained a healthy amount of weight. I gained 26 pounds with each pregnancy. The interesting thing is I gained exactly the same amount of weight with each pregnancy, even though my babies were totally different weights: 8 pounds, 11 ounces; 6 pounds, 14 ounces; and 7 pounds, 8 ounces.

—*Dianna K. Kim, MD, a mom of three and an ob-gyn in private practice in Vernon Hills, IL, at the Midwest Center for Women's Healthcare*

I gained 39 pounds with both of my pregnancies. It probably wasn't the best thing, but I did let myself indulge in foods a little more than usual. During pregnancy was the first time I felt at peace in my body. I believed that it wasn't about what I looked like; it was about what I felt like inside. Plus, it was hard to feel badly about myself when I was getting so much positive attention, like my husband staring and rubbing my belly.

—*Joanna Dolgoff, MD, a mom of a seven-year-old son and a four-year-old daughter, a board-certified pediatrician/child obesity expert with practices in Manhattan and Roslyn Heights, NY, creator of an online child weight loss program (www.DrDolgoff.com), and author of the book* Red Light, Green Light, Eat Right

I gained 50 pounds with my first baby, which I would not recommend to anybody. One thing that contributed to my weight gain was the fact that I had a lot of morning sickness. I felt nauseated and hungry at the same time, and eating made me feel better. The most comforting foods to me were salty, bready things. I lived in Philadelphia at the time, and I ate loads of soft pretzels. Another thing that contributed to my weight gain was that I had a lot of swelling. I think a lot of the weight was water.

During my second pregnancy, I gained only 30 pounds. I was more careful about what I ate. Also, I was no longer living in the soft-pretzel capital of the world! And I didn't have as much swelling during my second pregnancy.

—*Elissa Charbonneau, DO*

In my first pregnancy, I went to an obstetrician I knew in New York City, and he told me I shouldn't gain more than 10 to 15 pounds. That was the last time I went to see him.

During that pregnancy, I gained 50 pounds, and I gained 40 pounds during my second pregnancy. (My daughter was born five weeks early, and she already weighed six pounds, so we would have both been quite large if she had gone to term.) That was the most weight I've ever gained in my entire life. Otherwise my weight has only fluctuated five pounds.

I believe that as long as your health is good and you're feeling good, your weight will balance out. It's a fallacy that if you gain a lot of weight during pregnancy, you won't be able to lose it.

—*Erika Schwartz, MD, a mom of two and the director of www. DrErika.com, who's been in private practice for more than 30 years in New York City, specializing over the past 15 years in women's health, disease prevention, and bioidentical hormones*

It can be awfully shocking when you step on a scale during pregnancy. I think I was told to gain 10 pounds the first 20 weeks and then 15 to 20 pounds the second 20 weeks. In my first pregnancy, I was so excited to be pregnant. It was hard not to think that I could eat all this great stuff. Ten pounds comes on very quickly.

But when it comes down to it, you should eat only around 300 extra calories a day to gain the recommended amount of weight during pregnancy. Sometimes people think that's a bowl of ice cream, but actually it's only a serving of yogurt and a piece of fruit. Despite what you see on TV and in the movies, pregnancy isn't a license to eat whatever you want.

I gained about 35 pounds during each of my pregnancies. It was always shocking to see the number on the scale.

—*Mary Mason, MD, a mom of a nine-year-old girl and six-year-old boy, an internist, and the chief medical officer for a multi-state managed care company that coordinates care for about 70,000 pregnant Medicaid moms a year*

I'm 5 feet 2, and my baseline weight is around 120 pounds. When I found out I was having triplets, my doctor told me that I should gain 20 pounds per baby—60 pounds total! This was surprisingly difficult to do because I only had 25 weeks to do it in, the time remaining in my pregnancy.

"Are you kidding me?" I asked him. "That's not going to happen by any healthy means!"

I tried to eat as well as I could, but that's a lot of weight to gain in a short amount of time. I did enjoy eating lots of ice cream and natural 100 percent juices. My mom was staying with us for the last three months of my pregnancy, and she cooked all of my favorite things.

But it was actually challenging to gain all of that weight. Even when you're carrying one baby, your stomach gets full quickly. But with three babies in there, my stomach was really small, and I got full really quickly. I ate small, frequent meals each day instead of three large ones. I also drank as many of my calories as I could. Liquids would slide right through my gastrointestinal system rather than sitting there in my stomach and causing heartburn.

Even though 60 pounds was a lot of weight to gain, I was confident I could lose it all. And I did; I lost every single pound within a few weeks of delivery.

—*Sadaf T. Bhutta, MBBS, a mom of a three-year-old daughter and 18-month-old triplets and an assistant professor and the fellowship director of pediatric radiology at the University of Arkansas for Medical Sciences and Arkansas Children's Hospital, both in Little Rock*

? When to Call Your Doctor or Midwife

If you notice any sudden changes in your weight, such as several pounds up or down in a few days, call your doctor or midwife right away.

Dramatic weight loss might be caused by severe morning sickness. And dramatic weight gain can be a symptom of preeclampsia, which is a cluster of symptoms that includes swelling and high blood pressure. According to the Preeclampsia Foundation, a gain of more than two pounds in a week or six pounds in a month could be cause for concern. Both of these conditions require medical attention.

Preventing and Treating Colds and Flu

Pregnancy has plenty of discomforts. Adding a cold or flu to the mix can really put you down for the count. Yet because your immune system is weakened during pregnancy, so that your body doesn't reject your baby, you're likely to get sick more.

Prevention is the best policy during pregnancy. Wash your hands frequently, keep your distance from people who are sick, rest as much as you can, try to avoid stress as much as you possibly can, and eat plenty of vitamin-rich fruits and vegetables.

Additionally, the Centers for Disease Control and Prevention recommends that pregnant women get flu shots. Because the flu shot doesn't contain any live virus, it's safe during pregnancy. The flu vaccine isn't a wonder shot; it can't protect you against every possible strain of the virus. But it does decrease your odds of catching the flu.

If, despite your best efforts, you do get sick, don't take any over-the-counter cough or cold medications without talking to your doctor or midwife. Home remedies are your best bet. A teaspoon of honey can ease a cough, gargling with salt water soothes a sore throat, and a squirt of saline spray unstuffs stuffy noses.

༄

I was pregnant during cold and flu season. If I was going to be examining a patient who had a cold or sore throat, I wore a mask. Also I washed my hands like crazy!

—*Katja Rowell, MD, a mom of a four-year-old daughter, a family practice physician, and a childhood feeding specialist with www. familyfeedingdynamics.com, in St. Paul, MN*

༄

During my pregnancies I caught a few colds. I found it helped to take a hot, steamy shower to open up my nasal passages. And I sucked on throat lozenges, drank lots of water, and ate good old homemade chicken soup.

You can also take any of the over-the-counter Tylenol products. (Talk with your doctor or midwife before taking this or any medication.)

—*Gina Dado, MD, a mom of two daughters and an ob-gyn with Arizona OBGYN Affiliates, Paradise Valley Branch, in Scottsdale, AZ*

When I was pregnant with my baby, my older daughter was two, and I was constantly getting sick. Last winter, I had five colds in six weeks. You do what you have to do to make it through. Sleep was my best remedy. I slept as much as I could.

—*Ashley Roman, MD, MPH*

During my pregnancies, I had a few colds. I took cold medication. I had read the studies and felt that it was okay. (Talk with your doctor or midwife before taking this or any medication.)

—*Joanna Dolgoff, MD*

I caught a cold at the beginning of my pregnancy, even before I realized I was pregnant. It's not uncommon for women to catch colds and then find out a few days later they're pregnant. A lot of women are more susceptible to colds in their pregnancies because their immune systems are suppressed.

In one pregnancy, I developed a sinus infection. I remember taking Sudafed and Benadryl so I could breathe at night. Once it persisted past a week, I went to my doctor and was prescribed antibiotics, and then it cleared up. (Talk with your doctor or midwife before taking any medications during pregnancy.)

Something that I've heard other people find to be helpful, though I've

? When to Call Your Doctor or Midwife

If you catch a cold or even the flu, the best thing to do is let it run its course. However, if you develop symptoms of a secondary bacterial infection, such as a persistent cough or symptoms that don't go away after 10 days or so, call your doctor or midwife. Also call your doctor or midwife if you develop a fever.

If you're unlucky enough to get a stomach bug with diarrhea, you can self-treat with milk of magnesia for a day. Call your doctor or midwife if you have diarrhea for more than 24 hours however.

never tried them myself, are neti pots.

—Jennifer Kim, MD, a mom of three girls, ages eight, five, and four; an ob-gyn in private practice in Evanston, IL, at the Midwest Center for Women's Healthcare; and a clinical assistant professor at the University of Chicago, Pritzker School of Medicine

During each of my pregnancies, I caught a couple of colds. One time I got strep throat, which completely knocked me down flat. That was awful.

It's practically a rite of passage to catch a cold during pregnancy. I took Tylenol, Sudafed, and Robitussin DM. That combo will pretty much get you through anything! (Talk with your doctor or midwife before taking this or any medication.)

—Ann LaBarge, MD, a mom of four children, ages 16 to six, and an ob-gyn in private practice at the Midwest Center for Women's Healthcare in Park Ridge, IL

When I get colds in pregnancy, I try to get as much rest as possible. If my kids are sick at the same time, I make them join me for naps. I also drink plenty of fluids.

Especially when someone is sick, I keep our home meticulously clean. About six weeks ago, two of my kids and my husband had the flu. I managed to take care of them without getting sick myself! I washed my hands very frequently, placed bottles of hand sanitizer strategically all over the house, and doled out tissues right away to keep my kids from wiping their noses with their hands and arms. Several times a day, I went around the house with a can of Lysol, spraying the doorknobs, light switches, and bathroom surfaces.

I was also very vigilant about not touching my nose and eyes unless I had just washed my hands. This is really hard. If you tell yourself not to rub your eyes, you want to do it all day long!

—*Kristie McNealy, MD, a mom of seven- and four-year-old daughters and a two-year-old son, who's pregnant with another son, and a blogger at www.KristieMcNealy.com, in Denver, CO*

During my second pregnancy, I was having triplets. I was already not feeling so great with morning sickness, and then around six weeks, I caught a terrible gastrointestinal bug. I had diarrhea for weeks.

I was careful to talk this over with my husband, who's also a doctor, because an illness like that, which prevented me from gaining much weight, can be dangerous in pregnancy. I had some electrolyte imbalances for a short time, which got corrected quickly with the right diet. He monitored my blood work and diet carefully, and thank goodness it went away.

—*Sadaf T. Bhutta, MBBS*

Dealing with Gas and Bloating

During pregnancy, it's very common for women to have lots of gas and bloating. Most pregnant women do. Gas can cause abdominal discomfort, and even pain.

The reason why you might have more gas and bloating is that pregnancy hormones relax the muscles in your digestive tract. This slows your digestion, and it can cause gas to build up.

You might find that eating some foods—such as pasta, potatoes, beans, cabbage, and dairy products—makes gas worse. You could try cutting back on these foods, but be sure to make up for their nutrients with other foods. It might help to eat more slowly and chew your food thoroughly. Or eat several small meals each day instead of three larger ones. Avoid drinking from a bottle or straw, chewing gum, and sucking on hard candy.

The good news is, this should all pass a bit after your baby is born.

With this baby, I definitely have a lot of gas and bloating. My doctors tell me he's measuring small, but he's already taking up every square inch of me. For hours after I eat, I feel that if I move too much, everything is going to come right back up.

I try to eat very small meals and stop eating before I feel full. I also prop myself up on pillows, which helps with the feeling that the baby is pushing on my stomach.

—*Kristie McNealy, MD*

RALLIE'S TIP

I did have a little extra gas with my pregnancies. Fortunately, I had a very flatulent Boston Terrier who loved to curl up on the couch next to me and my husband in the evenings. Whenever the need arose, I just blamed everything on that little dog!

Having a Chorionic Villus Sampling

This test, also called a CVS, might be performed between 11 and 13 weeks. This gives it an advantage over amniocentesis, which can be done only later in pregnancy. (See "Having an Amniocentesis" on page 203.) It detects chromosomal abnormalities, such as Down syndrome, and genetic disorders, such as cystic fibrosis, which is an inherited disease that causes thick, sticky mucus to build up in the lungs and digestive tract.

CVSs are highly accurate—98 to 99 percent. Results are available in about a week. More than 95 percent of moms-to-be who have the CVS test learn that their babies do *not* have the conditions that they were tested for. Although the test results will identify any problems, they cannot measure the severity of the conditions.

During a CVS, a doctor places an instrument either through your cervix or abdomen and then removes a sample of tissue from your placenta. That tiny sample is tested for abnormalities.

The test carries a 1 to 2 percent risk of miscarriage. If you have a CVS and are Rh negative, you should receive an injection of Rho-GAM afterward.

~∽~

I had a CVS. It's an invasive test, not used very commonly. It's an early diagnostic test for Down syndrome and other chromosomal disorders. I decided to do it because of my age; I was 39 when my second child was born.

The CVS is a placental biopsy for chromosomes. It's similar to an amniocentesis, but its advantage over amnio is that it can be done earlier.

I won't mince words; it was painful. It can cause a lot of cramping and discomfort. Imagine a needle going into your uterus. I had planned to take the whole day off after my CVS, which was a good idea.

—*Stephanie Ring, MD*

RALLIE'S TIP

I believe there is tremendous value in having a CVS in some circumstances, but my husband and I opted not to have it during my pregnancies. We discussed having this test with our second and third pregnancies, because I was in my mid-thirties, but in the end, we decided against it. We felt that we would love our babies no matter how they came out. Because that was the case, we felt that having the test wasn't really necessary for us, and besides, it could pose a tiny measure of risk for our baby. Once we made our decision, we felt really good about it.

Chapter 13
Week 13

Your Baby This Week

YOUR BABY'S SIZE
Your baby is about the size of a hockey puck, 2½ to 3 inches from crown to rump.

YOUR BABY'S LATEST DEVELOPMENTS
An interesting shift takes place around now. Before this, your baby's head was quite large in comparison to his body. But now his body growth accelerates as his head growth slows. You might say your baby is "growing into" his head.

Your baby's eyes are moving closer together on his face. His ears are in their normal position—the better to hear you now.

Your baby's vocal cords are now formed. He can't cry out loud, though, because sound doesn't travel through fluid—not even amniotic fluid, which is pretty amazing stuff.

This week, your baby's intestines continue to move to their location inside of his abdomen, which is now large enough to accommodate them. Around this time, your baby's liver will start to produce bile, which aids in the digestion of fats.

If your baby is a girl, her ovaries now contain around six to seven million eggs, although many of them degenerate, leaving about one to two million at birth. That's all that she will ever have, and some of them someday could become your grandchildren.

Your baby's placenta continues to grow along with him and develop.

YOUR LATEST DEVELOPMENTS

You're probably starting to show. Your uterus feels like a soft, smooth ball. It's around the size of a small melon. You can probably feel its upper edge about four inches below your belly button.

Around now, at your doctor or midwife appointments, your practitioner will measure the distance between the top of your uterus, which is called the fundus, and your pubic bone, also known as the symphysis pubis. It's always measured in centimeters, and the number of centimeters often corresponds to the number of weeks you are along. For example, at 14 weeks, you'll measure around 14 centimeters.

These next few weeks, dizziness is common. Your rising progesterone level is to blame. It's sending more blood to your baby and placenta, and because less blood returns to your brain, your blood pressure drops, making you feel dizzy and light-headed. Try to move more slowly and deliberately to prevent falls. Drinking a lot of water can help ease the light-headedness.

If you have any birthmarks, freckles, or moles, they might have darkened. This is because the extra estrogen in your body stimulates cells in your skin called melanocytes to make pigment that darkens the skin. They'll probably fade after your baby is born.

Also because of the extra estrogen, right around now, you might spot a line down the middle of your abdomen. (It looks oddly like the seam in a teddy bear!) This is called the linea nigra. The skin down the middle of your abdomen becomes darker or pigments with a brown-black color.

You might find that by now, many of the common first trimester complaints, such as nausea and fatigue, have given way to second trimester symptoms, including a stuffy nose and bleeding gums. Both of these are caused by increased blood flow.

Your breasts might already have started to produce colostrum, the fluid that (if you choose to breastfeed) feeds your baby for the first few days after his birth. If you find that the colostrum is making your shirt damp, you can buy nursing pads to put into your bra.

JUSTIFICATION FOR A CELEBRATION

This is the last week of your first trimester!

Signing Up for Freebies

One of the many perks of pregnancy is free stuff! You'll receive lots of free magazines, booklets, samples, and coupons galore.

‿

When you're pregnant, you receive all sorts of free samples, information, and coupons. I looked through everything. I found lots of helpful information and coupons. One thing that was particularly good was the information on formula. I also found lots of coupons for diapers that came in handy.

—*Dianna K. Kim, MD, a mom of three and an ob-gyn in private practice in Vernon Hills, IL, at the Midwest Center for Women's Healthcare*

‿

American Baby, Babytalk, and a few other magazines give free subscriptions to moms-to-be. Sign up for them. I found that they are easy reading, help pass the time, and have the new and improved baby products in them. You can sign up online at their websites. I also signed up at pampers.com, huggies.com, similac.com, enfamil.com, and similar sites for their free weekly e-mails and to receive their samples in the mail.

—*Tyeese Gaines Reid, DO, a mom of one, an emergency medicine resident physician at Yale New Haven Hospital in Connecticut, and the author of a time management book,* The Get a Life Campaign

Telling Your Boss and Coworkers the Good News

In a perfect world, your boss and coworkers would be every bit as delighted as your friends and family to hear that you're pregnant. But sadly, that's not always the case.

Because of an amendment to Title VII of the Civil Rights Act of 1964, you cannot be fired for pregnancy-related reasons. If your pregnancy limits your activities, your employer is required to accommodate them, just as he or she would if you had any other temporary disability.

Visit the Equal Employment Opportunity Commission's website, www.eeoc.gov, for more information on your rights and pregnancy discrimination.

During my first pregnancy, I was a resident in dermatology. I was so excited that I was pregnant, I could have yelled it from the rooftop.

With my second and third pregnancies, I had to tell my boss and coworkers pretty early on because at my job you have to block off time off and let people know ahead of time. I told as few people as possible and asked them not to tell anyone. I told them I was taking a sabbatical, which is rather funny because not many 35-year-olds take sabbaticals.

> —*Rebecca Kazin, MD, a mom of three girls and the medical director of the Johns Hopkins Dermatology and Cosmetic Center at Green Spring Station in Lutherville, MD*

During my pregnancy, I was in my third year of residency. It was doable, but not the best timing. I was lucky that I was in a large residency group. Early in my pregnancy, I told my classmates that I was pregnant, and I asked if I could do the harder rotations first. That way, as I got heavier and more tired as my pregnancy went along, I wouldn't have to stay up all night on rotations. My colleagues were very helpful in coordinating our schedules.

> —*Diane Truong, MD, FAAP, a mom of one daughter and one son and a pediatrician in a multispecialty group practice in Southern California*

I was shocked to discover that I was pregnant in the spring of my senior year of medical school, just months before I would begin what was going to be the most demanding part of my career—my internship. I thought, *My gosh, what if I can't do this?*

Before I could even tell my husband I was pregnant, I told the head of the department of internal medicine I was going to intern with. The department head encouraged me to persevere, and he promised that they would work with me and that I could get my training under my belt and have time off when the baby was born. And so I forged ahead.

> —*Ann Kulze, MD, a mother of four children, ages 20, 19, 18, and 14, a nationally recognized nutrition expert, motivational speaker, physician, and the author of the critically acclaimed book* Dr. Ann's 10-Step Diet: A Simple Plan for Permanent Weight Loss and Lifelong Vitality

I found out that I was pregnant during my residency. At the time, I was the only person who had dared to get pregnant in the middle of residency training! I was very scared to tell the chairman of my department that I was pregnant, but he was actually very nice about it.

I didn't have to tell my peers that I was pregnant. They guessed. Early on, they started looking at me funny and asking if I was pregnant. I fessed up pretty quickly. They were very supportive of me. A lot of the male residents' wives were having babies at that time, and so they were understanding of what I was going through.

—*Elissa Charbonneau, DO, a mom of an 18-year-old son and a 16-year-old daughter and the medical director of the New England Rehabilitation Hospital in Portland, ME*

Preventing and Treating Constipation

Constipation is very common in pregnancy, and about half of all pregnant women experience it. It can be caused by several factors. First, your uterus is putting pressure on your intestines.

Also, you might not be drinking enough fluid and eating enough fiber. Fluid keeps your stool softer, and fiber makes it bulkier, both of which make it easier to pass. Strive to drink 10 cups of water each day. Because your blood volume is increased, you need to drink more fluid to keep up. Try to eat 25 to 30 grams of fiber each day. Fiber-rich foods include fruits, vegetables, whole grain breads, and breakfast cereals—though not the ones with the word "frosted" in the name!

Another factor contributing to constipation is an increase in progesterone. This causes food to move more slowly through your intestines, which can cause constipation.

Mommy MD Guide–Recommended Product
Metamucil Wafers
These apple-and-cinnamon flavored cookies taste good, and two of them offer six grams of fiber, which is key to warding off constipation. A box of 24 costs around $5 at grocery stores and drugstores.

During my pregnancies, I had some difficulties with constipation. I took an over-the-counter medication my doctor recommended called Colace. (Talk with your doctor or midwife before taking this or any medications.) It's a stool softener, and I took it twice a day starting in my second trimester when I really started to notice the constipation. It's important to keep the stool soft so you don't have to strain.

> ## ? When to Call Your Doctor or Midwife
>
> Constipation isn't usually serious, but occasionally it can be a symptom of another problem. If you have severe constipation, or if it's accompanied by abdominal pain, alternates with diarrhea, or if you pass mucus or blood, call your doctor or midwife immediately.

—*Lezli Braswell, MD, a mom of one daughter and two sons and a family medicine physician currently working in an emergency room fast track in Columbus, GA*

Throughout my first pregnancy, I was really constipated. During my second pregnancy, my doctor recommended a brand of prenatal vitamins that also has a stool softener in it. I thought that it was helping, and I was sure of it one morning when I forgot to take my prenatal vitamin. I took a regular vitamin instead, and all day long I felt like I couldn't poop. That convinced me!

—*Sonia Ng, MD, a mom of seven-year-old and one-year-old sons and a pediatrician and expert in sedation at Children's Hospital of Philadelphia Pediatric Care at Princeton Health Care System in Princeton, NJ*

I tried to eat a lot of fiber during my pregnancy, such as fruits and vegetables, to aid in normal digestion. Also I drank plenty of liquid to prevent constipation. This is very important after you have the baby because if it hurts to go to the bathroom, you'll try to avoid going, which will make your stools harder and more difficult to pass.

Even with all of my efforts, I got an anal tear, which was very painful. It is important to know what we can do to prevent "normal issues" that can occur during the pregnancy and after delivery. The two nutritional points are: Get adequate hydration and use what nature provides us—fruits and vegetables. When you combine them with exercise, you should be feeling your best.

—Aline T. Tanios, MD, a mom of three and a general pediatrician and hospitalist who treats medically complex children at Arkansas Children's Hospital in Little Rock

Visiting the Dentist and Caring for Your Teeth and Gums

Don't imagine for a second that your teeth and gums are immune to pregnancy changes! Your gums become softened and swollen by pregnancy hormones, which makes them more likely to bleed and even to become infected. Also, your gums are more vulnerable during pregnancy to bacteria, gingivitis (inflammation of the gums), periodontitis (inflammation of the structures that support the teeth), and even plaque. More than half of pregnant women get gingivitis. Periodontitis in particular can lead to low birth weight or even premature delivery. Experts think that the same bacteria that cause gum disease can enter your bloodstream and travel to other parts of your body, causing infection.

Regular flossing and brushing are very important during pregnancy. If brushing and flossing make you gag, try a different toothpaste.

Plus, be sure to make and keep your dentist appointments. Your dentist will try to avoid taking x-rays during your pregnancy. But the chance of a single X-ray harming your baby is very low because X-rays are very specific, and your teeth are a long way from your belly. But it's best to avoid having X-rays if at all possible during pregnancy.

If you have the misfortune of needing a dental procedure, don't worry. Local anesthetic should be perfectly safe.

⌒

During my pregnancies, I went in for my regular dentist checkups. I was also very good at flossing while I was pregnant. But that went right out the window after my baby was born.

—Sonia Ng, MD

⌒

During my pregnancy, I had a little gum bleeding. I made sure to keep my regular dental appointments. It's very important to go to the dentist when you're pregnant—even more important than usual. Problems develop and worsen more quickly during pregnancy because your immune system is suppressed. Anything you've got going on in your mouth is going to get worse, faster.

—*Ann LaBarge, MD, a mom of four children, ages 16 to six, and an ob-gyn in private practice at the Midwest Center for Women's Healthcare in Park Ridge, IL*

I went to the dentist early on in my pregnancy. I had found out a few weeks prior that I was pregnant, so they didn't do any X-rays. In fact, I had a filling that was falling out, but they just told me to brush and floss really well and then come to get it fixed after the baby was born.

It's important to see a dentist during pregnancy because pregnancy can wreak havoc on your dental health.

—*Kerri A. Daniels, MD, a mom of one toddler daughter and an instructor in the department of pediatrics at the University of Arkansas for Medical Science in Little Rock*

During my pregnancy, my gag reflex was really strong. Brushing my teeth was especially challenging. I remember dry heaving while brushing my teeth, with my husband giggling about it in the bedroom.

I had to brush my teeth bending over because that helped. To this day, I can only brush my teeth leaning over the sink. If I stand up or if my toothbrush touches the back of my throat, I gag.

—*Marra Francis, MD, a mom of three daughters and an ob-gyn who's based in The Woodlands, TX*

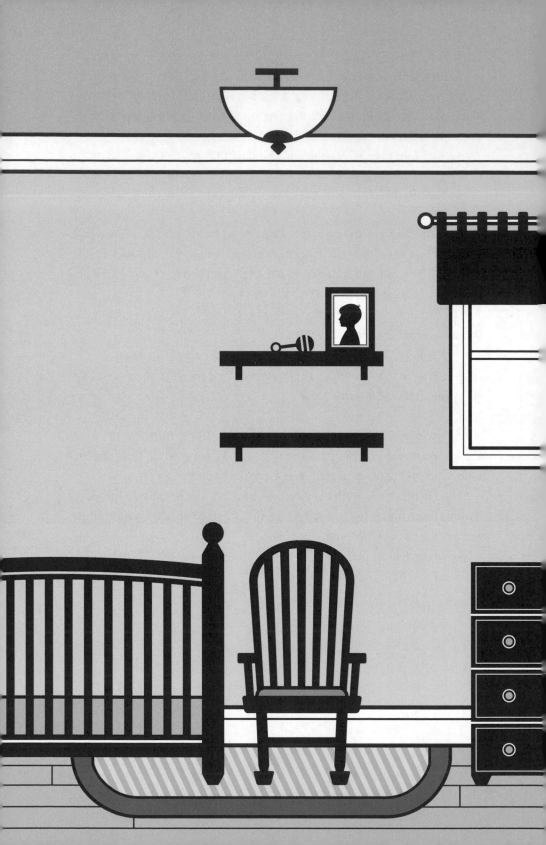

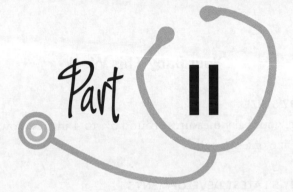

Part II

YOUR SECOND TRIMESTER

Chapter 14
Week 14

Your Baby This Week

YOUR BABY'S SIZE

This week, your baby measures around 3¼ to 4 inches crown to rump, about the size of a soft ball.

YOUR BABY'S LATEST DEVELOPMENTS

Your baby's neck continues to lengthen, and her chin no longer is resting on her chest. There's now a clear separation between your baby's head and shoulders.

Your baby is starting to use her facial muscles—squinting, smiling, and frowning. Taste buds are forming on your baby's tongue. She doesn't have her set of 10,000 yet, but she will.

Around this week, your baby's thyroid gland begins to function. The thyroid gland is located in the front of the neck, just below the voice box, and it produces hormones that regulate metabolism.

Each week, it becomes easier to tell if your baby is a boy or a girl because the external genitalia are increasingly developed. If your baby is a girl, her ovaries are moving down into her pelvis. If your baby is a boy, his prostate gland is starting to develop.

Your baby still has plenty of room, and she's in near constant motion. She's often in synch with your sleeping and waking patterns, sleeping when you sleep. Here's hoping that this continues after she's born!

YOUR LATEST DEVELOPMENTS

You might be starting to show this week. Your uterus is pushing up and out, forcing your belly to stick out.

Your get-up-and-go might have gotten up and gone again. Your circulatory system continues to expand, and its plasma production outpaces your body's ability to produce red blood cells. If you're tired, ask your doctor or midwife about anemia. (See "Preventing and Treating Anemia" on page 257.)

Around this time, you might start to feel short of breath, for two good reasons. First, your lungs are breathing for two, taking in enough oxygen for you *and* your baby. Second, the upward movement of your uterus is putting pressure on organs near your diaphragm.

Your baby's now-functioning thyroid gland needs iodine to work, so eat iodine-rich foods, such as yogurt, milk, mozzarella cheese, and eggs. Table salt has plenty of iodine, but too much of that will raise your blood pressure and worsen swelling.

Around this time, while some moms-to-be have *stuffy* noses, paradoxically others develop *runny* noses. Your ears might suddenly feel clogged too. That's all because of the fluid that your body is producing to help to keep bacteria and viruses out.

Even if you didn't have moles or small growths of skin called skin tags before pregnancy, you might develop them during pregnancy. Existing moles and skin tags might grow. Point out any changing moles to your doctor.

Although you're still probably only seeing your doctor or midwife once a month, it's a great idea to weigh yourself at home weekly. This will help you to monitor your weight gain.

You might feel your baby move soon! Quickening can be felt as early as 14 weeks, although it's more commonly felt after week 16.

JUSTIFICATION FOR A CELEBRATION

Your baby's hearing is probably developed well enough that she can hear you. Why not tell her a story, sing her a song, or read her a book?

Feeling Your Baby Move

Quickening: What an interesting word for such an amazing feeling. You might not have felt your baby move yet, but sometime in the next few weeks, your baby will be strong enough and able to move vigorously enough that you can feel it. *Contact!*

Although some moms-to-be feel their babies move around week 14, others don't feel their babies move until 18 weeks, 20 weeks, or even later. You might feel your baby move sooner if this is your second pregnancy.

Early on, your baby's movements might feel like butterflies fluttering around or ginger ale bubbles rising in a glass. Later, they'll feel more like kicks or jabs.

When I was 16 weeks pregnant, my husband and I took a trip to Alaska. That's where I first felt my baby move! I remember being in the lodge and thinking, *Oh my gosh!* I remember it like it was yesterday.

—*Gina Dado, MD, a mom of two daughters and an ob-gyn with Arizona OBGYN Affiliates, Paradise Valley Branch, in Scottsdale, AZ*

My son was a big mover. He also got the hiccups a lot, which was kind of fun. I could tell the difference between his movements and hiccups because the hiccups were rhythmic.

—*Ellen Kruger, MD, a mom of two teenagers and an ob-gyn in an academic and clinical practice in New Orleans, LA, with Ochsner Health System*

Feeling my baby's movements inside of me was wonderful. I thoroughly enjoyed it. Generally, my baby's movements were subtle. But this is different for everyone. Some of my patients feel like they have little soccer stars in there. At night, when things were calm, I remember lying in bed with my husband and being so excited about feeling my baby move.

—*Diane Connelly, MD, a mom of a six-year-old daughter and an ob-gyn in HMO practice in Riverside, CA*

With a twin pregnancy, you can feel the babies move earlier. Your uterus is growing so quickly, and the top of it is pressing up against your abdomen so much earlier. I felt my twins by 12 weeks!

Feeling your baby move is a very strange thing. I've heard that to some women, it feels like soda bubbles rising. Not to me! To me it felt like there was a person in there. But in a good way. Not like it was an alien or anything—like it was a tiny little person.

—*Kelly Campbell, MD, a mom of three and an ob-gyn in private practice at Women's Healthcare Physicians in West Bloomfield, MI*

When I first felt my triplets moving around week 15, they were moving around a lot. But by around week 20, they were running out of room, and I didn't feel them as much as one might think. I could feel their arms and legs moving and poking me, but I didn't feel them tumbling around anymore. They simply didn't have that much space.

Interestingly, once they settled into position, they stayed there. One of my sons was on my upper left, my other son was on my upper right, and my daughter was in my pelvis. I could clearly tell who was sleeping and who was awake. They are fraternal triplets, and so they each had their own sac, fluid, and placenta.

—*Sadaf T. Bhutta, MBBS, a mom of a three-year-old daughter and 18-month-old triplets and an assistant professor and the fellowship director of pediatric radiology at the University of Arkansas for Medical Sciences and Arkansas Children's Hospital, both in Little Rock*

I didn't feel my baby move until about 20 weeks of pregnancy. This might have made me nervous, but I was taking part in a major research study and having regular ultrasounds. It was great because I was able to see my baby, which was very wonderful and reassuring.

—*Monica Lee-Griffith, MD, a mom of one, an ob-gyn, and senior staff, Henry Ford Health System in metropolitan Detroit*

Taking a Vacation with Your Partner

Your second trimester is a great time to travel. Most of the first trimester discomforts, such as morning sickness, have hopefully passed, and you don't yet have the third trimester discomforts, such as a big belly, to contend with.

It's a good idea to discuss your travel plans with your doctor or midwife first. Pack anything and everything you think you might need to stay comfortable—as long as you're not the person who has to carry the bag! When you're in the car, plane, or train, get up periodically and move around to prevent fluid from pooling in your ankles and feet. Drink plenty of water to stay hydrated as well.

Bon voyage!

❦

I had a really great pregnancy, and I felt good throughout. My husband and I went on vacation to Park City to the snow. I didn't get to ski, but we took wonderful long walks.

—*Debra Luftman, MD, a mom of a teenaged daughter and a teenaged son, a board-certified dermatologist in private practice, a coauthor of* The Beauty Prescription, *the developer of the skincare line of products Therapeutix, and a clinical instructor of skin surgery and general dermatology at UCLA*

❦

During my second pregnancy, we were living in Germany. It was fantastic! Because of Germany's central location, we could take day trips to four different countries. We even went to Paris for two weekends. We enjoyed lots of wonderful food.

—*Ann Kulze, MD, a mother of four children, ages 20, 19, 18, and 14, a nationally recognized nutrition expert, motivational speaker, physician, and the author of the critically acclaimed book* Dr. Ann's 10-Step Diet: A Simple Plan for Permanent Weight Loss and Lifelong Vitality

❦

I really encourage women to take a vacation with their spouses either before they get pregnant or in the first or second trimester. What you don't want to do is take a crazy trip to some exotic country when you're 24 weeks pregnant. If you have a complication, you want to be close to home.

When I was 16 weeks pregnant, my husband and I went to Alaska. To this day, we look back at that trip as one of our favorite vacations.

—*Gina Dado, MD*

❦

My ex-husband, the father of my children, is a travel aficionado. He loves trips. He was not particularly thrilled that I got pregnant. He decided that we had to take a trip every single month of my pregnancy to feel that we did everything we possibly could before the baby was born. We went skiing in Whistler and sight-seeing in Paris, to name a few trips. It was very tiring, but fortunately I'm a high-energy person, even during my pregnancies.

—*Melanie Bone, MD, a mom of four "tweens" ages 15 to 12, a gynecologist, the founder of the Cancer Sensibility Foundation, and the author of the syndicated column* Surviving Life *and the book* Cancer, What's Next?, *in West Palm Beach, FL*

I was nervous during my pregnancy because it was my first, and we had tried for a while before I got pregnant. Generally, my husband and I take a lot of trips, but I was afraid to fly during my pregnancy.

We did go to a small vacation town in Northern Michigan for a wonderful weekend with friends when I was 32 weeks pregnant.

—*Monica Lee-Griffith, MD*

I was pregnant during the last stages of medical school, but my husband and I went out as much as we could to keep our social life going. We even took trips as often as possible. I remember floating in a pool like a beached whale three weeks before I delivered. Those trips helped to keep our relationship strong.

—*JJ Levenstein, MD, FAAP, a mom of one son in college and a pediatrician in private practice in Southern California*

Because I was in the Army when my husband and I got married, we didn't get to take a honeymoon. But when I was 22 weeks pregnant, we went to Costa Rica. It was so cool because I was showing. We got so much wonderful attention everywhere we went.

It was my first pregnancy, and I was naïve. I didn't really pack anything special for my pregnancy. One thing I remember being grateful for, though, is Chap Stick. My lips were always dry. Another thing I took was bottled water. I figured who knew if the water would be safe for a pregnant woman. Of course, that was pre-911 when we were still allowed to bring liquids on planes.

—*Patricia S. Brown, MD, a mom of two daughters, ages nine and seven, and a three-year-old son and a psychiatrist at Columbia-New York Child and Adolescent Telepsychiatry and in private practice in Cresskill, NJ*

During my first pregnancy, when I was 19 weeks pregnant, my husband and I went to Costa Rica. It was a fun trip! I did some things in hindsight I probably shouldn't have, such as going on zip lines! It was great! I overdid it, and I started cramping after that. But I rested, and all was fine.

One thing to remember when traveling is to take along yeast infection medication, especially if you're going to be in the water. Pregnant women are prone to yeast infections. I took some over-the-counter yeast infection medicine along just in case. Who knows where, or even if, they sell Monistat in Costa Rica!

—*Jennifer Kim, MD, a mom of three girls, ages eight, five, and four; an ob-gyn in private practice in Evanston, IL, at the Midwest Center for Women's Healthcare; and a clinical assistant professor at the University of Chicago, Pritzker School of Medicine*

We didn't get to take any special trips during my pregnancies. We were busy working!

—*Elizabeth Berger, MD, a mom of two, a child psychiatrist, and the author of* Raising Kids with Character

Telling Your Other Children the Good News

Moms-to-be vary greatly on when they tell their other children that they're expecting. A lot of it depends on how old the child is. But this could certainly prove to be a very interesting conversation.

I actually told my older son that he was going to have a baby brother before I told my husband. My son asked, "When will we be able to play basketball together?"

"Not for a long time," I explained gently.

Then we went to the store together to buy a card to give to my husband to tell him the news. In the card, my son wrote, "Now that I'm going to be a big brother, can I get a dog?" My husband looked quite confused at first, but then he got it and smiled.

—*Sonia Ng, MD, a mom of seven-year-old and one-year-old sons and a pediatrician and expert in sedation at Children's Hospital of Philadelphia Pediatric Care at Princeton Health Care System in Princeton, NJ*

My first two children are 20 months apart, so our daughter was very young when I was pregnant with our older son. My husband and I bought our daughter a board book about being a big sister, and we read that to her often.

I also got her a doll. I remember after my son was born, she would walk around and hold her doll to her chest like she was nursing.

—*Lezli Braswell, MD, a mom of one daughter and two sons and a family medicine physician currently working in an emergency room fast track in Columbus, GA*

One day during my pregnancy with twins, my older daughter came home from preschool. Her friend's mom had a baby, and my daughter announced, "Mommy, you're supposed to give me a baby 'brudder' and a baby 'sitser.'" I was in shock.

"I am probably going to give you two babies, but I don't know if they'll be boys or girls," I told her.

My daughter appeared satisfied that I would fulfill her demands.

—*Susan Wilder, MD, a mom of an older daughter and twin girls, a primary care physician, and CEO and founder of Lifescape Medical Associates in Scottsdale, AZ*

I had a child every year: My first daughter was 11 months old when I had my second baby. There was no telling her anything! Then my daughter and older son were two years and one year old respectively when my second daughter was born. It wasn't until my last baby was born that they could really understand that a sibling was coming, but even at three years old, it really didn't matter much to my children. They don't remember life without their siblings.

—*Melanie Bone, MD*

My first two daughters are only a year and a half apart, but I waited three years to get pregnant with my third. I wasn't sure how my daughters, who were then ages five and three, would react to the news that I was pregnant, so I tried to wait until I was 12 weeks along to tell them.

But my oldest daughter figured it out before that. In hindsight, it's easy to see how: You show quickly with the third baby, and her line of sight was right at my belly. One day, she asked me, "Mommy, do you have a baby in your belly?" It caught me off guard, and I said, "I ate too much for dinner." But she and her sister kept asking, and so I admitted it pretty soon after that.

I was glad I did because my daughters were so excited that it was extra fun for me too. They talked to their baby sister through my belly button. For a long time after the baby was born, they'd lift up my shirt to talk to the baby. I'd say, "The baby's over there! Stop lifting up Mommy's shirt!"

I had feared that once my daughters knew I was pregnant, they would keep asking day after day when the baby was coming. But they understood that it took nine months, and they waited patiently.

My girls did ask a lot of questions, though. How did the baby get in there? How's the baby going to get out? I answered the questions as clearly and honestly as I could.

—*Rebecca Kazin, MD, a mom of three girls and the medical director of the Johns Hopkins Dermatology and Cosmetic Center at Green Spring Station in Lutherville, MD*

Handling Unsolicited Advice

Everyone has an opinion about everything, especially when you're expecting. Because your emotions might be close to the surface and because pregnancy is so personal, it might be harder than usual to cope with all of the advice coming your way.

During my pregnancy, people tried to give me lots of advice. Everyone has their own ideas and plenty of advice to share. I found it best to listen, say "thank you," and then do what I felt was best. If you try to follow everyone else's advice, it can make you crazy.

—*Michelle Paley, MD, PA, a mom of a six-year-old daughter and a two-year-old son and a psychiatrist and psychotherapist in private practice in Miami Beach, FL*

I'm sometimes saddened and other times amused by the stories my patients tell me about the unsolicited advice they get from people, such as "You need to gain weight; you're too small" or "You need to stop eating; you're too big." I wish people would give advice like that gently—or better yet, not at all! It's very concerning, especially for first-time moms.

I didn't get too much of that because I'm an obstetrician. What questionable advice I did get, I simply ignored.

—*Diane Connelly, MD*

One of my pet peeves is that people with no knowledge or training think that they're parenting experts just because they've reproduced. When you're pregnant, these folks delight in telling you what's wrong with you.

One of my patients, a trial attorney no less, came to my office in tears because an old lady told her she was carrying her baby too low. I asked, "Where did this woman get her medical degree?"

This happens to everyone, even doctors. My mom told me not to raise my hands above my head because the baby would strangle. I laughed, "Mom, I've had my hands in there, and it's not attached. It's okay."

When people give you unsolicited advice, feel free to blurt out the rudest thing you can think of. Then blame it on the pregnancy hormones.

—*Ellen Kruger, MD*

Chapter 15
Week 15

Your Baby This Week

YOUR BABY'S SIZE

This week, your baby measures 4 to 4½ inches long. He's about the size of a bocci ball.

YOUR BABY'S LATEST DEVELOPMENTS

Your baby is still growing quickly. The size of his body is starting to catch up with his head.

At this point, your baby's eyes are still widely separated, but they are now at the front of his face. Your baby's eyelids are still squeezed shut. His external ears are now fully formed. Your baby's inner ear bones are still developing, though. They are beginning to harden, which will help your baby to hear you better and better as your pregnancy continues.

The roof of your baby's mouth has formed by now, and the taste buds on the roof of his mouth have developed.

Your baby's hands are developing more and more. He can suck his thumb and make a fist.

Your baby's muscles are becoming more substantial. His movements are becoming less mechanical and more smooth, like a newborn baby's. Your baby's skin is still so thin that you can practically see through it.

Your baby's sex organs are formed well enough that it's possible to tell by ultrasound if you're having a boy or a girl. But there's still a large margin of error, so you might not want to paint that nursery pink or blue just yet!

Your baby's placenta is fully functioning now. It's producing most of the progesterone needed to support the pregnancy.

YOUR LATEST DEVELOPMENTS

Because your belly is starting to grow, it's probably beginning to make you uncomfortable when you sleep on your stomach. Lying on your back might not feel good either because it could be harder to breathe. Many experts caution that as your uterus gets larger, lying on your back can put your uterus on top of important blood vessels that lie in the back of your abdomen. This can decrease circulation to your baby and parts of you. Try sleeping on your side instead. Propping yourself up with pillows, or your partner, behind you can help. (See "Mommy MD Guide–Recommended Product: Body Pillow" on page 342.)

Your partner might also be having a hard time sleeping. Even if you've never snored before, you might snore now. Pregnancy causes congestion, which in turn causes snoring. Spraying some saline in your nose before bed might help. The good news is, you should stop snoring again after your baby is born.

Your baby's bones are continuing to ossify, which means they need lots of calcium. Get plenty of calcium, such as from low-fat dairy foods, or else that calcium for your baby will come out of *your* bones.

Because of an increase in pregnancy hormones, the glands inside your breasts that will produce milk expand around this time. Your breasts might feel full and heavy. They also might look a bit like a Rand McNally road atlas. Around now most women can see a pattern of dilated veins crisscrossing under the skin of their breasts.

You might still feel nauseated now and again, but most cases of morning sickness ease by now. It might have been replaced by heartburn, which is common in the second and third trimesters.

Right around now, it's common for back pain to begin, caused by the extra weight you're carrying and the added pressure on your tailbone.

JUSTIFICATION FOR A CELEBRATION

Because your baby's bones are getting harder and ossifying rapidly, his skeleton would be visible on an ultrasound.

Choosing the Location for Your Nursery

Where your baby will sleep is a very personal decision. Some parents feel strongly that their babies should sleep in their own cribs, in their own rooms, from day one. Other parents feel just as strongly that babies should co-sleep with their parents, as babies did generations ago and as many babies in other countries still do. Still other parents strike a compromise and place their babies in bassinets in the parents' room.

The American Academy of Pediatrics does not recommend that babies sleep in bed with their parents. However, the AAP encourages babies sleeping in a crib that's in their parents' bedroom, because this has been associated with a reduction in sudden infant death syndrome risk.

Not only didn't we have a nursery for our second baby as my due date approached, we didn't even have a house! When I was pregnant with my second daughter, my husband was racing to build us a one-room cabin in the woods. We moved in on Thursday, hung a few curtains on Friday, rested up on Saturday, and our baby was born on Sunday.

—*Stacey Marie Kerr, MD, a mother of two grown daughters, a family physician with strong roots in midwifery, and the author of* Homebirth in the Hospital, *in Santa Rosa, CA*

Our baby slept in a bassinet in our room for the first few months. You don't use a bassinet for long, so we decided to share one with another friend who had a baby not too long before we did, and then pass it along.

—*Dianna K. Kim, MD, a mom of three and an ob-gyn in private practice in Vernon Hills, IL, at the Midwest Center for Women's Healthcare*

My husband and I didn't have to give much thought to where to put our daughter's nursery. We lived in a one-bedroom apartment at the time! We set up her crib in a corner of our bedroom and dressed it with a pastel-colored bedding set gifted to us from our dear friends.

It worked out fine. You do what you must to accommodate your lifestyle. We lived in that apartment until our daughter was a year old.

—*Diane Truong, MD, FAAP, a mom of one daughter and one son and a pediatrician in a multispecialty group practice in Southern California*

My husband and I decided to put our daughter into her crib in her room right away. She didn't sleep in our room and certainly not in our bed. (Well okay, maybe for one night . . .)

Sleeping is really important. It's like breathing! If you don't take care of yourself, you can't take care of your kids.

—*Michelle Paley, MD, PA, a mom of a six-year-old daughter and a two-year-old son and a psychiatrist and psychotherapist in private practice in Miami Beach, FL*

Even though my husband and I found out early in my pregnancy that we were having twins, we set the babies up in the same room. In hindsight, I don't know if we should have done that because I think they wake each other up. My husband and I considered moving one baby into another room, but the crib had been assembled in the nursery, and we couldn't get it out the door!

—*Jennifer Gilbert, DO, a mom of three-month-old twins and an ob-gyn at Paoli Hospital in Pennsylvania*

When my husband and I found out we were having twins, we decided to have them share a nursery. In fact, we decided to have them share a crib. This worked well for a long time, until my son started climbing out. For a little while he slept in a playpen next to the crib. Then he was bodysurfing on the edge of the playpen and knocked it over. That's when we moved him into a bed.

—*Ruth D. Williams, MD, a mom of twins—a boy and a girl—and another boy, and an ophthalmologist in private practice at the Wheaton Eye Clinic in Wheaton, IL, who specializes in the diagnosis and treatment of glaucoma*

When I became pregnant with my second baby, my husband and I decided to keep the same room as the nursery, and move our older daughter to a new room. This worked out well because I could use the same nursery theme, which was sheep and lambs, so it worked well for a girl and a boy. I had also stenciled "The Lord is my shepherd" on the wall.

Right before our son was born, we simply moved our daughter to her "big girl bed" in her "big girl room." It worked out just fine, and we repeated the process when our second son was born.

—*Lezli Braswell, MD, a mom of one daughter and two sons and a family medicine physician currently working in an emergency room fast track in Columbus, GA*

When my younger daughter's due date approached, we had a tricky situation. Our older daughter was only 23 months old and still sleeping in the crib. My husband and I didn't want to go out and buy another crib. We figured for the first few months after the baby was born, she'd sleep in our room in a bassinet. (Truth be told, she slept mainly in bed with me. When she woke to nurse, I latched her on and went back to sleep.)

Our plan was that when our younger daughter turned six months old, we'd move her into the crib in the nursery and move our older daughter into her big girl bed. I think my older daughter's first memory is being kicked out of her crib!

—*Patricia S. Brown, MD, a mom of two daughters, ages nine and seven, and a three-year-old son and a psychiatrist at Columbia-New York Child and Adolescent Telepsychiatry and in private practice in Cresskill, NJ*

Early into my pregnancy, I found out I was having triplets. We already had a daughter. My husband and I knew we needed to buy three more cribs, but we had no place to put them. We had just built a new house, and we never imagined we'd have four kids. Our master bedroom was downstairs, and we had three bedrooms upstairs. So we all moved upstairs. My husband and I took over the guest bedroom, we put our daughter in the second bedroom, and we put the triplets' new cribs into the third bedroom. We use our downstairs master bedroom closet and bathroom, but I won't feel comfortable sleeping downstairs while the babies are upstairs until I know that they are old enough to know how to escape from a fire or any other emergency.

—*Sadaf T. Bhutta, MBBS, a mom of a three-year-old daughter and 18-month-old triplets and an assistant professor and the fellowship director of pediatric radiology at the University of Arkansas for Medical Sciences and Arkansas Children's Hospital, both in Little Rock*

We chose a room in our home for our daughter's nursery and prepared it for her arrival, but she didn't actually get to see it until a few months after she was born.

I live in the town that Hurricane Katrina hit on August 29, 2005. We evacuated a few days before the hurricane, when I was seven months pregnant.

Our home was not destroyed, thank goodness. There were only two out of six homes in my family that made it. But we couldn't go back there for months. We evacuated to another town in Louisiana, and my family rented a house there for a few months.

I hoped we could return home in time for Christmas, and we made it! I was so happy that my baby could finally sleep in her nursery. I was grateful that the house wasn't damaged and her nursery was intact. I had chosen everything in her room with great care—the bedspread, the furniture, and the decorations.

The hurricane taught me two things. First, no *thing* matters as much as the bonds of family and the safety of the people we love. Second, many of the things we try so hard to control really are out of our control.

—*Christy Valentine, MD, a mom of one, a specialist in pediatrics and internal medicine, and the founder of the Valentine Medical Center in Gretna, LA*

Having an Alpha-Fetal Protein Test

The alpha-fetal protein (AFP) test isn't performed in all pregnant women. It used to be part of the triple screen test, which is often now replaced by the first trimester screening. (See "Getting the First Trimester Screening" on page 131.)

If you have an AFP test, it's usually done between 14 and 18 weeks. This test measures a protein called alpha-fetaprotein that is produced by your baby's liver and passes into your bloodstream. Some of your blood is drawn, and the amount of the protein is measured.

Higher levels of the protein in your blood can suggest twins, that you're farther along than you thought, or problems with the baby, such as a neural tube defect including spina bifida or a central nervous system deficit called anencephaly. Lower levels of the protein in your blood could mean you're at increased risk of having a baby with Down syndrome.

❧

I decided to have an alpha-fetal protein test because I'm one of those people who would sleep better knowing it was normal, as opposed to someone who might rather not know if there's bad news. Fortunately, the test came back just fine.

—*Ellen Kruger, MD, a mom of two teenagers and an ob-gyn in an academic and clinical practice in New Orleans, LA, with Ochsner Health System*

❧

During one of my pregnancies, we had an abnormal alpha-fetal protein test result that suggested there might be a problem, which really terrified me. My doctor recommended having an amniocentesis. My feelings at that point were that I was really attached to the baby, and the results of the amnio wouldn't cause me to change my direction, so I didn't want to have an amniocentesis. My husband, on the other hand, wanted to have the amnio so that we would know the situation and could prepare for it.

That's a stressful time: How do you navigate a situation as a couple when you each have unanticipated reactions to the test results? Thank goodness, we didn't have to deal with it because things worked out. I did have the amnio, and it turned out to be normal.

—*Nancy Rappaport, MD, a mother of two teenaged daughters and a teenaged son, an assistant professor of psychiatry at Harvard Medical School, an attending child and adolescent psychiatrist in the Cambridge, MA, public schools, and the author of* In Her Wake: A Child Psychiatrist Explores the Mystery of Her Mother's Suicide

Enlisting Help

This might be less about *enlisting* help, than about *accepting* help. Chances are good that people *want* to help you right now, but it can be hard to accept help, even when it's offered. Try to let down your guard, accept help, and even ask for it when you need it. Just say *yes*.

❧

It's hard as an independent woman to have someone help you. I didn't require too much of my husband, except during the last four to six weeks of my pregnancy. He really had to help me do basic things, like turning on water faucets, because I had such severe carpal tunnel syndrome that I couldn't use my hands.

But I was very grateful for my husband's emotional support. And throughout my pregnancy, he did kind things for me like bring me pillows or breakfast in bed. He's not really a cooker or a cleaner, but he tried.

—*Monica Lee-Griffith, MD, a mom of one, an ob-gyn, and senior staff, Henry Ford Health System in metropolitan Detroit*

During my pregnancy, my husband and I grew so much closer. We had just come back from our honeymoon, and we were still in the newlywed phase. My husband was so supportive, considerate, and thoughtful of my needs. I didn't have to ask for help; he just gave it. One thing that helped a lot was that we went out for dinner quite a bit because we didn't have the time to prepare and cook meals. He didn't even mind driving me across town to get my must-have craving: wonton noodle soup.

—*Diane Truong, MD, FAAP, a mom of one daughter and one son and a pediatrician in a multispecialty group practice in Southern California*

My first pregnancy wasn't an easy one. I was so tired. I was working 28-hour shifts twice a week, and 14-hour shifts the other days. Plus I had such severe morning sickness I had to take medication.

But my husband was very caring, and he stepped in and took care of everything else. Even though he worked long hours too, in commercial real estate, he took care of our home and made sure that I had dinner to eat each night.

—*Joanna Dolgoff, MD, a mom of a seven-year-old son and a four-year-old daughter, a board-certified pediatrician/child obesity expert with practices in Manhattan and Roslyn Heights, NY, creator of an online child weight loss program (www.DrDolgoff.com), and author of the book* Red Light, Green Light, Eat Right

My family and my husband's family both live in Pakistan. We're pretty much on our own here. But when we found out I was pregnant with triplets, my mom, who's also a physician, flew here and stayed with us for three months prior to the delivery. She took over the house work, cooking, and cleaning and caring for our older daughter.

This gave me the much-needed opportunity to rest, which was critical because I was on bed rest after week 25. My mom stayed with us until the babies were five weeks old.

—*Sadaf T. Bhutta, MBBS*

Preventing and Treating Urinary Tract Infections

During pregnancy, urinary tract infections (UTIs) are very common, especially between weeks 6 and 24. Some women who've never had a UTI develop their first one in pregnancy.

UTIs are more common in pregnancy because progesterone relaxes your urinary tract, slowing your urine's flow. This puts out a welcome mat for bacteria to enter your urethra and reach your bladder. There, they cause inflammation or infection. Because of the pressure on your bladder, it might be hard to empty it completely, which gives that bacteria plenty of time to set up camp.

To prevent UTIs, go to the bathroom when your body tells you to, and empty your bladder completely. It might help to lean forward on the toilet to push out all the urine.

It's critical to treat UTIs in pregnancy promptly because your bladder is relaxed, and the infection can easily spread to your kidneys. Symptoms of a kidney infection include a high temperature, shivering, and kidney pain. Kidney infections are serious; they can cause permanent kidney damage.

One simple home remedy to help prevent UTIs is drinking cranberry juice. Researchers think that tannins in cranberries might keep the bacteria from attaching to the urinary tract, and prevent an infection.

❦

During my first pregnancy, I had a lot of urinary tract infections. I think it was because during that pregnancy, I was very constipated. That caused urinary retention, which lead to urinary tract infections. I had terrible burning when I went to the bathroom. During my second pregnancy, I only had one UTI, and I think it was because I didn't have the constipation then.

I was given Keflex by my internist, and he said I could start taking it whenever I had symptoms, so I treated the UTIs myself with antibiotics and did not have to go in to see a physician. I worked in the emergency department at the time, and I tested my urine myself, and then later sent a sample to my obstetrician to confirm the results. My boss didn't mind; I think she preferred that to having me take a day off to go to the doctor!

—Sonia Ng, MD, a mom of seven-year-old and one-year-old sons and a pediatrician and expert in sedation at Children's Hospital of Philadelphia Pediatric Care at Princeton Health Care System in Princeton, NJ

> ## ? When to Call Your Doctor or Midwife
>
> If you have the frequent urge to urinate, experience burning when you go, pain in your back or lower abdomen, fever or chills, or cloudy, or dark or bloody urine, call your doctor or midwife right away. These could be signs of a urinary tract infection.

∽

During my last pregnancy, I tried to drink a lot of water because I kept feeling like I had a urinary tract infection. I felt like I had to go to the bathroom all of the time, and it burned when I did.

I took a urine test, and it turned out that I didn't have a urinary tract infection. My symptoms were all caused by a stent that my doctors had to put in to clear my kidney when I had a kidney stone. Fortunately, all of the symptoms went away after my baby was born and the doctors took the stent out.

—Dianna K. Kim, MD

Chapter 16
Week 16

Your Baby This Week

YOUR BABY'S SIZE
Your baby now measures around 4⅓ to 4⅔ inches long, about the size of a skittle ball. She's gearing up for a big growth spurt over the next few weeks.

YOUR BABY'S LATEST DEVELOPMENTS
Soft downy hair called lanugo covers your baby's body and head. It's thought that this hair helps to keep your baby warm until she has developed fat stores. Your baby's eyebrows and eyelashes are beginning to develop.

Around this time, your baby might turn away from bright lights. Even though her eyes are still shut, they are now forward enough on her face and able to see light through her lids. Plus, around now her retina is light-sensitive because nerve connections to the brain have been established.

Your baby's heart beats about twice as fast as your own. And her heart grows stronger with each passing day.

As your baby's skeleton hardens and her back muscles strengthen, her neck begins to straighten out. She can now move her head up and down and from side to side, as if she's saying *yes* and *no*.

Sometime around this week, your baby's legs grow longer than her arms. She can now bend and straighten her knees and fan and flex her feet and toes.

YOUR LATEST DEVELOPMENTS

In general, many women feel healthier and more energetic this week. You've probably gained around five pounds, but more or less is perfectly normal. Around now, you might feel the top of your uterus around four or five inches under your belly button.

Your breast pain might be going away around now. But your breasts might be continuing to grow. Their increased size might be a pain in the neck—literally. Doing stretching exercises, maintaining good posture, and wearing a supportive bra should help.

There's about 7½ ounces of amniotic fluid cushioning your baby. Between the weight of the fluid, the weight of your baby, and the size and weight of your uterus, your abdomen and back likely ache.

Heartburn might be making it hard to eat a lot at one sitting. Try eating several small meals a day instead of three larger ones.

During your second trimester, you'll experience the largest increase in your blood volume. Up until this point, the blood flow to your kidneys has continued to rise. But around now, it levels off. Your kidneys are working overtime to reabsorb the nutrients that pass through them. So your urine might contain small amounts of sugar and protein.

For a few weeks, you might not have to urinate as often. Your uterus is shifting, and it's no longer pressing as much on your bladder. This restroom respite is temporary. In the third trimester, you'll likely have to urinate frequently once again.

You could find it harder and harder to sleep. Both growing concerns and your growing belly might make it hard for you to settle down at night. Unfortunately, this news might make it even harder: This week marks a critical time to stop lying on your back because it can interfere with the baby's blood flow. It's okay to recline in a chair or prop up on pillows.

Don't worry if you haven't felt your baby move. Every woman is different, and every baby is different. Some babies are far more active than others. *Whenever* you feel your baby move, it will be well worth the wait.

JUSTIFICATION FOR A CELEBRATION

Your baby is aware of bright light beyond your abdominal wall.

Thinking about Names

There's a reason why an Amazon search on "baby names" gets 23,000 results: Our names are our identity. One recent study found that naming boys unpopular or uncommon first names might make them more likely to become criminals! The researchers think that the social factors of being tagged with an offbeat moniker "increase the tendency toward juvenile delinquency."

So it turns out parents-to-be have good reason to agonize about those baby names. Fortunately, talking about your baby's name is a lot of fun.

In addition to dozens of baby name books, you'll find many websites all about names. One helpful site is www.BabyNames.com. In addition to lists of the top 100 most popular names for the past 10 years, you'll find many unique lists, such as biblical names and reality TV show names. For a fee, they even offer baby name consulting.

While some parents-to-be readily share their name picks, others choose to keep their babies' names secret. If you tell people, you risk getting their opinion, which you might or might not want. Also, some people will call your baby by the name right away, which might feel awkward to you.

What's in a name? Everything!

My husband and I began thinking about names way before I was pregnant. We discussed names endlessly.

—*Elizabeth Berger, MD, a mom of two, a child psychiatrist, and the author of* Raising Kids with Character

My son's name is Max. It was my husband's grandfather's name. My husband used to crawl up in his lap as a kid, and he always thought he'd name his baby Max if he had a boy.

—*JJ Levenstein, MD, FAAP, a mom of one son in college and a pediatrician in private practice in Southern California*

When I told my older daughter that I was expecting twins, I asked her what she would name them. She said she would call them Nikki (which is also her name) and Adam (which was her best friend's name). When I asked her who would come when I called "Nikki" if we had two Nikkis, she said, "Nobody."

—*Susan Wilder, MD, a mom of an older daughter and twin girls, a primary care physician, and CEO and founder of Lifescape Medical Associates in Scottsdale, AZ*

⌒◦

My husband chose our oldest son's name, Aaron, the day I went into labor. My husband and our son have the same initials. The funny thing is that no one realized at the time that Aaron rhymes with my name, Karen!

We chose my second son's name, Nathanial, simply because we liked it. By the time I was pregnant with our third son, it got harder because we were running out of boy names we liked. Our third son is named Jesse after a grandparent. And we chose our youngest son's name, Matthew, so his initials were the same as my oldest sister's. We chose several of their middle names to honor relatives.

—*Karen Heald, MD, a mom of four boys and a board-certified family physician in private practice outside Atlanta, GA*

⌒◦

My husband picked all of our kids' names. I was fine with that. Our daughter is named Jillian, and our twin sons are Owen and Kyle. All of their middle names were after men in his family. I thought it was nice to name them after someone, but I didn't want it to be their first names. I wanted them to each have their own identities.

—*Kelly Campbell, MD, a mom of three and an ob-gyn in private practice at Women's Healthcare Physicians in West Bloomfield, MI*

⌒◦

We named our daughter Isabella. People think she was named after the hurricane. But she wasn't. We just liked the name.

My husband actually picked all three of our girls' names. In fact, he even picked the dog's name!

—*Rebecca Kazin, MD, a mom of three girls and the medical director of the Johns Hopkins Dermatology and Cosmetic Center at Green Spring Station in Lutherville, MD*

⌒◦

My husband and I decided not to find out our baby's gender ahead of time during all three pregnancies. So we had both boy and girl names ready for each.

Interestingly, we had family names each time for boys: William, Nathaniel, and Clarke. I didn't have any family names for girls. I liked the names Mary and Leigh. My two younger sons both have my maiden name for their middle name: Cote. My eldest is a junior.

—*Kathie Bowling, MD, a mom of three grown sons and an ob-gyn in private practice in Providence, RI, who's also on the clinical faculty at the Warren Alpert School of Medicine at Brown University*

I liked baby names that can be for both a boy and a girl. I had heard the name Kennedy a few years back, and while I've never heard it for a boy, it sounded like it could be for a boy or a girl. I just really loved it!

My husband is a junior, so if we had a boy, though, his name would have been Johnny III. Because we didn't know if we were having a boy or a girl, we had names picked for each.

—*Monica Lee-Griffith, MD, a mom of one, an ob-gyn, and senior staff, Henry Ford Health System in metropolitan Detroit*

My husband and I decided not to choose our babies' names until we actually met them. We weren't totally set on any names. But we did have some ideas. My maternal grandmother's name was Natalie, but everyone called her Nettie. We decided to name our older daughter Nettie Rose. We named our younger daughter Daisy Grace.

Customarily, people choose Hebrew names to honor family members who have passed away, but because Nettie's American name honored my grandmother, we chose her Hebrew name, Shira Vered, because we liked the way it sounded. But coincidentally it means "song of the rose."

Daisy is named after my grandfather Daniel. Her middle name, Grace, is after George, my husband's grandfather. Her Hebrew name is Efrat Lior, which means "golden light," and that was for Emil and Louis (my husband's and my grandfathers on the other side of the family).

Interestingly, my husband and I couldn't agree on boys' names. Good thing we had girls!

—*Janet Lefkowitz, DO, a mother of two girls and an ob-gyn in private practice in Rhode Island*

Deciding If You Want to Know the Sex of Your Baby

Because you'll soon likely be given the opportunity to discover the sex of your baby either through ultrasound or amniocentesis, you'll want to start thinking about whether that's information you want to know or not.

Some things in life hold no room for compromise. Finding out if you're having a boy or a girl is one of them! You either find out, or you don't. There's no middle ground.

In a 2007 Gallup poll, 51 percent of Americans said that they would wait until the baby was born to find out if they were having a boy or a girl, while 47 percent said they would like to know ahead of time. The rest of the folks said that they have no opinion. You might have guessed that the folks polled weren't actually pregnant at the time! Interestingly, older folks probably skewed those numbers higher. Among 18- to 34-year-olds, more than 60 percent said they would want to find out ahead of time if they're having a boy or a girl. Older folks said that they'd rather wait and be surprised. Perhaps age brings wisdom—or at least patience.

My husband and I found out ahead of time that we were having girls. I think a lot of men hope to have sons, to carry on the name. But my husband was excited to have girls. He's completely crazy about them. Even our dog, Zoe, is a girl.

—*Rebecca Kazin, MD*

We didn't find out the sex of our first baby before she was born. But with my second, I had an amniocentesis. I felt it would be more practical to know if the baby was a girl or a boy so I could either reuse my daughter's clothes or give them all away.

—*Susan Schreiber, MD, a mom of a son and daughter in their twenties and a pediatrician in Los Angeles, CA*

My husband and I didn't find out the sex of either of our babies. We felt that there are so few surprises in life. Because of our family tradition of not bringing things into the home before the baby is born, we couldn't do much to prepare anyway!

It was fun not knowing! I predicted our first baby was a boy and that our second would be a girl. My husband thought that they would both be girls. I was totally wrong, and he was only half right!

—*Michelle Paley, MD, PA, a mom of a six-year-old daughter and a two-year-old son and a psychiatrist and psychotherapist in private practice in Miami Beach, FL*

I had an amniocentesis during my pregnancy and many ultrasounds because I was taking part in a research study. But my husband and I had decided we didn't want to know the sex of our baby. The doctors who did my amnio and ultrasounds are very good friends of mine, and they could clearly tell, but I asked them not to let me know. They all remained stone-faced and didn't let on whether we were having a boy or a girl.

I really didn't want to know. I felt that the surprise when the baby is born is one of the biggest joys in life.

—*Monica Lee-Griffith, MD*

With our first two babies, my husband and I didn't find out the sex. We weren't going to find out with our third, either, but our two daughters were very excited about the baby, and they really wanted to know if they were going to have a baby brother or sister. They wanted to be able to plan and pick out a name.

It worked out well because we were building a new home at the time. We were picking out paint colors and assigning bedrooms, and it was handy to know we were having a boy.

—*Patricia S. Brown, MD, a mom of two daughters, ages nine and seven, and a three-year-old son and a psychiatrist at Columbia-New York Child and Adolescent Telepsychiatry and in private practice in Cresskill, NJ*

My husband and I decided not to find out the sex of our first baby. There are so few surprises in life that I wanted to enjoy that big surprise of finding out when the baby is born. For our second and third babies, we decided to find out at the ultrasounds. That was the practical thing to do.

—*Judy Dudum, MD, a mom of three, an ob-gyn, and a senior staff physician at Henry Ford Health System in Detroit, with interests in nutrition and adolescent gynecology*

My ex-husband definitely wanted to know the sex of our first baby, but I definitely didn't want to know. I thought I had it figured out, though. When I was having my ultrasound and it was time for the sonographer to look for the baby's sex, she asked me to turn my head. I had worked with this woman for years, and when she said, "Okay, you can look back now," 10 seconds later, I thought for sure that the baby must be a boy if she had determined the sex so quickly.

When my baby was born, and they announced she was a girl, I started to cry. I was so happy; I think that I secretly really wanted a girl first.

—*Melanie Bone, MD, a mom of four "tweens" ages 15 to 12, a gynecologist, the founder of the Cancer Sensibility Foundation, and the author of the syndicated column* Surviving Life *and the book* Cancer, What's Next?, *in West Palm Beach, FL*

We decided not to find out. This is somewhat unusual for an ob-gyn with ultrasound machines in her office. Sometimes I had to leave my office at the same time my staff did because I knew the temptation would be too great. If I had wanted to know at any time, I could have simply done an ultrasound.

But I had promised my husband I wouldn't find out, and I knew that it was easier not to know what the gender was than to lie to my husband about it for the rest of my life. That's what kept me strong.

Interestingly, my maternal instinct about my baby's gender was correct both times. Both my associate and my mom had predicted that each child was the other gender! My husband went along with my instincts. For my first baby, I had a dream she was a girl. My second baby I just knew in my heart was a boy. For both, we went to the hospital with two names, just in case.

For me, not knowing my baby's gender was like having a birthday present. You *could* open it before your birthday, but you don't want to. You *want* to be surprised. I think the anticipation is part of the excitement.

Plus, I would have been over the moon with either a boy or a girl both times, and there are so few events in life that end up being wonderful whichever way the outcome goes. What a wonderful surprise to have!

I have certainly had patients who do not find out the gender but their husbands do, or vice versa. It's possible for one partner to keep the secret but so difficult. It would make it an interesting nine months, that is certain! Perhaps you could agree to find out the gender this time but keep it a secret with the next pregnancy. Or maybe keep the secret until the baby shower.

—*Lauren Hyman, MD, a mom of two and an ob-gyn at West Hills Hospital and Medical Center in West Hills, CA*

Working with Your Health Insurance Company

Having a baby is expensive. Between your prenatal visits, hospital or birth center stay, and your baby's pediatrician checkups, it will total thousands of dollars. Check in with your insurance company about your coverage and any deductibles. It's also important to find out when and how you add your baby to your health insurance policy. Read the fine print because some policies only have a small window of time that a baby can be added to a policy after her birth. After that, no coverage will be provided.

Many insurance companies offer special programs for moms-to-be, such as free books, informative websites, or even nurses who call to check in periodically over the phone. Find out what services your company offers so you don't miss out on them.

⤸⤹

Many health insurance companies offer great prenatal programs, especially for high-risk women. It's well worth the time calling your insurance company to ask what they offer.

I remember that my health insurance company sent me a free book, *What to Expect When You're Expecting*. Insurance companies really do want you to be as healthy as you can be.

—*Mary Mason, MD, a mom of a nine-year-old girl and six-year-old boy, an internist, and the chief medical officer for a multi-state managed care company that coordinates care for about 70,000 pregnant Medicaid moms a year*

⤸⤹

Partway through my pregnancy, I left my job. Because my health insurance was tied to my former employer, I suddenly found myself without health insurance. The company didn't qualify for Cobra, which is a government program that provides certain former employees, retirees, spouses, former spouses, and dependent children the right to temporary continuation of health coverage at group rates.

I quickly realized that no one wants to insure a pregnant woman! It was scary. Thank goodness, I found out that I could get coverage from my state because I lost my insurance through no fault of my own. It was very expensive, but at least it was insurance.

—*Christy Valentine, MD, a mom of one, a specialist in pediatrics and internal medicine, and the founder of the Valentine Medical Center in Gretna, LA*

Trying Pregnancy Yoga and Pilates

Both yoga and Pilates are excellent during pregnancy. They foster relaxation, strength, and flexibility. Be sure to find a class, DVD, or online routine tailored specifically for pregnancy.

I think it's very important in pregnancy to do something to keep your muscles toned, such as yoga, Pilates, or even lifting free weights. For me, yoga was a great stress reliever and workout in one.

—*Gina Dado, MD, a mom of two daughters and an ob-gyn with Arizona OBGYN Affiliates, Paradise Valley Branch, in Scottsdale, AZ*

It's very important in pregnancy to do moderate exercise. I went to a few prenatal yoga classes. Both yoga and Pilates can be modified to be safe in pregnancy.

—*Jennifer Kim, MD, a mom of three girls, ages eight, five, and four; an ob-gyn in private practice in Evanston, IL, at the Midwest Center for Women's Healthcare; and a clinical assistant professor at the University of Chicago, Pritzker School of Medicine*

When I found out I was pregnant, I bought a pregnancy yoga video. It's still in the package. I chalked it up to a contribution to Denise Austin's Christmas fund. I think pregnancy yoga is a great idea, and I wish I would have tried it!

—*Diane Connelly, MD, a mom of a six-year-old daughter and an ob-gyn in HMO practice in Riverside, CA*

Yoga is a tool I've used over the years for relaxation. I find it to be super helpful.

I cannot do it at home; I'm not disciplined enough. I do three Downward Dogs, and I'm done. Plus my dog comes over and starts checking me out and licking my face, which is just too weird. Instead, I go to a yoga studio where I know the teacher well. When I'm *really* stressed out, I combine yoga with meditation.

—*Nancy Rappaport, MD, a mother of two teenaged daughters and a teenaged son, an assistant professor of psychiatry at Harvard Medical School, an attending child and adolescent psychiatrist in the Cambridge, MA, public schools, and the author of* In Her Wake: A Child Psychiatrist Explores the Mystery of Her Mother's Suicide

As a longtime student of yoga before babies, it was wonderful to be able to take prenatal yoga classes, which I did religiously through both my pregnancies. Going to the classes marked a special time during the week to honor being pregnant, and to also meet and socialize with other pregnant women—many of them are still my good friends years later! I felt the yoga poses helped me have fulfilling pregnancies and easy births.

I was fortunate to spend time with Gurmukh, a well-known prenatal teacher who introduced me to the natural parenting world, including such experiences as 40 days rest period following birth, family bed, and attachment parenting.

—*Lauren Feder, MD, a mom of two sons, a nationally recognized physician who specializes in homeopathic medicine, and the author of* Natural Baby and Childcare *and* The Parents' Concise Guide to Childhood Vaccinations, *in Los Angeles*

I'm a big fan of prenatal yoga and Pilates. However you can do yoga and Pilates is great.

Studios offer classes, and DVDs are helpful to do at home. Yoga helps you to stretch and strengthen your body and also to make you more aware of your posture. Pilates helps pregnant women to maintain core muscle strength and prevent a lot of the strain that comes with weakness of your abs and lower back.

—*Stephanie Ring, MD, a mom of two sons, ages six and two, and an ob-gyn at Red Rocks Ob-Gyn in Lakewood, CO*

During my third pregnancy, I did Pilates right up until the latter part of my second trimester. I loved it! I took a class at a nearby gym, and the teacher was very good. She helped me and the other participants who were pregnant to modify the exercises. It felt so good to stretch. I didn't feel so enormous!

—*Lezli Braswell, MD, a mom of one daughter and two sons and a family medicine physician currently working in an emergency room fast track in Columbus, GA*

RALLIE'S TIP

I didn't try yoga or Pilates when I was pregnant because I had a crazy work schedule, but I had a couple of friends who did. They always seemed so much more serene and radiant than me. It could have been because they weren't working as many hours, or it could have been the yoga and Pilates.

Pregnant women need exercise, for their own health and also for the health and well-being of their babies. There are only so many types of exercise you can enjoy when you're pregnant, and yoga and Pilates are probably two of the most beneficial, especially when they're tailored to pregnant women.

Chapter 17
Week 17

Your Baby This Week

YOUR BABY'S SIZE

This week, your baby's grown to 4½ to 4¾ inches crown to rump, about the size of a candlepin bowling ball. Your baby is growing rapidly. Around this week, he starts to accumulate fat deposits. Just think of those sweet little baby cheeks!

YOUR BABY'S LATEST DEVELOPMENTS

The fat that your baby is developing will help him to stay warm after he is born. If you breastfeed, the fat will also sustain him for a little while until your milk comes in.

Around this week, your baby's eyebrows are forming in a tiny little arch. Your baby's scalp continues to fill in with hair. What color will it be?

Around now, your baby starts to store up meconium in his intestines. This stool is sterile because it's made up of only lanugo and other things that your baby digests after he starts to swallow amniotic fluid.

Your baby is starting to develop his own internal clock. Depending on how often you feel him move, you might start to get a sense of when he's asleep and when he's awake.

If you could peek in on your baby, you might see him blinking, sucking, and swallowing. These are all reflexes that he's developing now that will help him after he's born. Blinking will help to keep his eyes moist and free from foreign material, and sucking and swallowing will help him to drink milk. At birth, most babies have a repertoire of around 70 reflexive behaviors.

Your baby's placenta and umbilical cord continue to grow. Right now, your baby and the placenta are around the same size. But soon your baby will grow larger than the placenta. Because blood is rushing through the umbilical cord with great force, it has about the same tension as a garden hose filled with water. This tension makes the umbilical cord resistant to knots, and it straightens itself out as your baby moves around.

YOUR LATEST DEVELOPMENTS

Because your baby is growing so rapidly, you probably are too. Your uterus is now around the size of a cantaloupe, and you might be able to feel it around 1½ to 2 inches below your belly button. Feel for your uterus while you're standing up because when you lie down, your uterus falls back toward your spine. If you're not already wearing maternity clothes, you soon will be.

Due to your growing body, and in particular your growing circulatory system, you might feel hotter and sweatier and experience more hot flashes. Dressing in layers might help.

You might feel hungrier than ever, partly because you can eat only small meals at a time. It's helpful to always pack a snack.

Dry eyes are a common complaint around this time. Talk with your doctor or midwife about trying an over-the-counter lubricant. Amazingly, your eyeballs might have changed shape. If your contact lenses are uncomfortable, you might want to switch to wearing glasses for a while.

Dizziness continues to be a concern. Be especially careful getting into and out of cars, chairs, and tubs.

Perhaps even before now, the skin around your vagina might have taken on a violet or blue color. This is called Chadwick's sign, and it's likely caused by the increased blood flow to the area.

JUSTIFICATION FOR A CELEBRATION

Hopefully, you're enjoying the "honeymoon" of pregnancy—the period after the first trimester complaints have passed and before the third trimester issues kick in.

Buying Maternity Clothes

It might be tempting to try to stave off buying clothes by using rubber bands to extend your waistbands. But you're going to need to buy maternity clothes at some point. Why not buy them now and get the most use out of them?

～〇～

I have the best work wardrobe: scrubs. I wore scrubs throughout my pregnancy, and they're so forgiving I don't even think I had to change sizes.

For home, I bought some maternity clothes at Japanese Weekend (www.JapaneseWeekend.com), which I love. Their clothing has a great waistband with good abdominal support.

—*Diane Connelly, MD, a mom of a six-year-old daughter and an ob-gyn in HMO practice in Riverside, CA*

～〇～

Because of the way my hips spread during pregnancy, I couldn't wear any of my usual clothes. I shopped at Motherhood Maternity because they sold many different styles and had great prices. It actually took me around three months after my babies were born for my hips to go back to normal and for me to be able to wear my regular clothes again.

—*Dianna K. Kim, MD, a mom of three and an ob-gyn in private practice in Vernon Hills, IL, at the Midwest Center for Women's Healthcare*

～〇～

When you're looking for affordable, comfortable work clothes, Old Navy tops my list. Several of the slacks are made to grow with you: from barely a belly to enormous. Most of Old Navy's maternity clothes mimic its women's line. If you check the sales rack, you can usually find slacks from $10 to $30 and buttoned shirts from $5 to $20. The website has more options than the store. Visit the store to try on your size, and then buy the rest online.

—*Tyeese Gaines Reid, DO, a mom of one, an emergency medicine resident physician at Yale New Haven Hospital in Connecticut, and the author of a time management book,* The Get a Life Campaign

～〇～

With my first daughter, I didn't start wearing maternity clothes until I was 7 months pregnant. But with my third daughter, I started to show practically immediately. I wore maternity clothes by 12 weeks. I carried her like a torpedo—straight out in front of me. By the end of my pregnancy, even XL maternity shirts didn't cover the underside of my belly. I just let my belly stick out for the final few weeks. I was too disgusted to go buy more and larger maternity shirts.

—*Marra Francis, MD, a mom of three daughters and an ob-gyn who's based in The Woodlands, TX*

Back when I was pregnant, they didn't sell the cute maternity clothes that they do now. I actually saved a lot of money by not buying a lot of maternity clothes. Because my friends and sister-in-law were also pregnant around the same time as me, we swapped clothes back and forth. Still, I quickly got sick of those maternity clothes. By the end of my pregnancy, I never wanted to see some of that clothing again.

—*Elissa Charbonneau, DO, a mom of an 18-year-old son and a 16-year-old daughter and the medical director of the New England Rehabilitation Hospital in Portland, ME*

During my second pregnancy, I was having triplets, and so I outgrew my clothing very quickly. I was full-term size by week 22. My pregnancy clothing from my first pregnancy lasted until around week 25. After that I wore my husband's big shirts. When I outgrew my husband's clothing, for the last 8

Mommy MD Guide–Recommended Product
Timex Indiglo Watch

You won't find these watches in the maternity department, but they should stock them there. A Timex Indiglo digital watch is a very handy item to add to your maternity wardrobe.

When you go into labor, your watch will be key to use to time your contractions. After your baby is born, the timer will be perfect to use to keep track of your baby's feedings. You'll be grateful for the light when your baby cries in the middle of the night. *Not again! What time is it?* And when your baby grows into a defiant toddler, the timer will be invaluable for timing his time-outs.

to 10 weeks of my pregnancy, I wore hospital scrubs—size XXL. I never want to see them again!

Fortunately, I was housebound by then, so it didn't matter much. I didn't have to wear cute pregnancy clothes because I didn't get out of the house much, except to go to my ob appointments!

—*Sadaf T. Bhutta, MBBS, a mom of a three-year-old daughter and 18-month-old triplets and an assistant professor and the fellowship director of pediatric radiology at the University of Arkansas for Medical Sciences and Arkansas Children's Hospital, both in Little Rock*

Preventing and Treating Back Pain

Back pain is the bane of many women's pregnancies. Between weight gain, hormonal surges, and a shifting center of gravity, back pain is pretty inevitable.

If the pain is in your tailbone, it might help to sit on a donut pillow. This gives some space between your tailbone and the seat. Exercise might help, in particular walking. Prenatal massage often can ease the pain. Rest whenever you can. If need be, talk with your doctor or midwife about taking Tylenol.

One particular type of back pain is especially troublesome. Sciatic nerve pain is an excruciating pain that you feel in your butt and radiating down the back of one or both legs. Sciatic pain might be caused by your uterus pressing on your sciatic nerve. The nerve can become inflamed, which causes pain, pins and needles, and even numbness. You might try hot or cold compresses to manage the pain. But the good news is, it should go away after your baby is born.

Trying to prevent back pain now can go a long way to keeping you comfortable later.

❧

During my pregnancy, I was seeing 35 patients a day. I was having some troubles with back pain, and I found that swimming helped a lot.

—*Mary Mason, MD, a mom of a nine-year-old girl and six-year-old boy, an internist, and the chief medical officer for a multi-state managed care company that coordinates care for about 70,000 pregnant Medicaid moms a year*

I'm 4 feet 11 inches tall, and I was not one of those ideal weight gainers. I put on 40 pounds with each pregnancy. (The ideal is 25, and most women gain between 35 and 40 pounds.)

That was a lot of weight to lug around on my frame. I had bad sciatic pain. One thing that helped was to rest lying on the side opposite of my pain.

—Kathie Bowling, MD, a
mom of three grown sons and
an ob-gyn in private practice in
Providence, RI, who's also on
the clinical faculty at the Warren
Alpert School of Medicine at
Brown University

Around 28 weeks, I started to have some mild back pain. I found that stretching helped, and I also went to see a physical therapist. The physical therapy exercises plus the stretching really kept the back pain at bay.

—Diane Connelly, MD

During the third trimester of one pregnancy, I had sciatica, which is pain in the lower back that runs down the leg. There's not much you can do for that when you're pregnant. I went to a massage therapist who specialized in treating pregnant women and had a massage.

The massage did help a bit—temporarily. But better yet was the hour of relaxing and being pampered.

—Lezli Braswell, MD, a mom of one daughter and two sons and a
family medicine physician currently working in an emergency room fast
track in Columbus, GA

? When to Call Your Doctor or Midwife

You should let your doctor or midwife know if you are experiencing back pain during pregnancy. If the back pain is severe or if you are feeling numbness, call your doctor or midwife right away. Back pain can be a signal of premature labor. Other symptoms of premature labor include vaginal discharge, contractions, abdominal pain, and menstrual-like cramps. You should call your doctor or midwife right away if you think you are having preterm labor.

During my pregnancy, I wore one of those belly support bands. You can buy them at maternity stores for around $25. You can wear them under or over your clothes. The bands definitely help with back pain. When I wore mine, I felt that I could move quicker and easier. That was a must for long nights at the hospital.

—*Nancy Thomas, MD, a mom of a 22-month-old son who practices general obstetrics and gynecology in Covington, LA, with Ochsner Health System*

Many women have back pain in pregnancy. You're gaining weight, you're walking in a new way, and your hormones are relaxing the muscles and ligaments throughout your body.

One thing that helped me to minimize my back pain was to wear good shoes. I wore the hospital-type shoes that doctors and nurses wear. I wore those clunky shoes everywhere—with everything. They have orthotic support and are wider than regular shoes. Now I guess many people have found a benefit in wearing these shoes because you can find them in many major department stores.

I see a lot of pregnant women wearing flip-flops or slip-on shoes to accommodate their wider feet. I don't think that this is a good idea because these shoes don't offer support. Wearing them might make your back hurt more. When I tried to wear shoes other than my hospital-type shoes, my back hurt.

—*Christy Valentine, MD, a mom of one, a specialist in pediatrics and internal medicine, and the founder of the Valentine Medical Center in Gretna, LA*

RALLIE'S TIP

The further along I got in my pregnancy, the more my back ached. Placing a pillow in the small of my back while I was seated helped my lower back, but it didn't touch the muscle tension and aching that had settled in my neck and between my shoulders. It finally occurred to me that my growing breasts were responsible for much of the strain on my upper back, and my slightly flimsy pre-pregnancy bra just wasn't providing enough support.

I wasn't quite ready to graduate to a nursing bra, but I did find that by wearing a sturdy sports bra most of the time, my heavier breasts didn't put such a big strain on my neck, shoulders, and upper back. I bought a few extra sports bras in my new size, and found that when I wore them at home and at work, I was a lot more comfortable, and my muscles weren't nearly as tired or as tense by the end of the day.

◦◯◦

Some degree of back pain is almost a certainly during pregnancy, just from the added weight and distortion of your anatomy. There might not be a lot to do about it, except for lying down and resting in a comfortable position (preferably on your left side). Many massage therapists can give an excellent massage during pregnancy, thanks to a special pillow with a cut-out for your belly.

During my pregnancies, I had back pain, and I even had some nerve entrapment in my upper back from my breasts being so big. It was a sharp, shooting pain that went down the length of the nerve, which in this case was in my arm. You can also get numbness or tingling in your

Mommy MD Guide-Recommended Product
Loving Comfort Maternity Support

"The first time you put this contraption on, you'll probably have a hard time deciding which way is up," said Tyeese Gaines Reid, DO, a mom of one, an emergency medicine resident physician at Yale New Haven Hospital in Connecticut, and the author of a time management book, *The Get a Life Campaign.* "However, this brace is the main reason I was able to work so far into the pregnancy and also how I could go shopping for more than 20 minutes. It decreases the fatigue caused from the heavy baby resting on your veins and cutting off circulation. The brace also kept my back from aching.

"Remember that your muscles, ligaments, and tendons are stretched out in anticipation of delivery. Your back doesn't have its normal strength, and you can injure it severely."

You can buy Loving Comfort Maternity Support back braces online for around $30.

fingers or in your toes, depending on which nerves are involved.

My ob-gyn gave me a referral to a physical therapist. This was enormously helpful. The best part was that the physical therapy office had a pool. I floated in that pool as often as I could. The only downside to swimming while pregnant is getting back out of the pool. You feel like you weigh 700 pounds.

—*Kristin C. Lyle, MD, FAAP, a mom of three girls and the disaster medical director at Arkansas Children's Hospital and an assistant professor of pediatrics at University of Arkansas for Medical Sciences, both in Little Rock*

∽

My job requires me to be on my feet a lot, and I had a difficult time with back strain during my pregnancies. The way that a pregnancy changes your body mechanics really predisposes women toward back strain.

During my pregnancies, I tried to stand up straight and to be more aware of my posture. A heavy belly causes your pelvis to tilt forward, which is a very stressful position for your lower back. Doing the yoga cat stretch really helps to counteract the lordosis (commonly known by the lovely name "swayback") that pregnancy causes.

Along the same lines, prenatal Pilates helps pregnant women to maintain core muscle strength and prevent a lot of the strain that comes

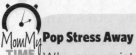
with weakness of your abs and lower back. Working with an instructor can be helpful, both to avoid injury as well as to ensure you're getting the most from your workout. Failing that, there are a number of high-quality DVDs on the market specifically for pregnancy.

—Stephanie Ring, MD, a mom of two sons, ages six and two, and an ob-gyn at Red Rocks Ob-Gyn in Lakewood, CO

Having an Amniocentesis

Currently, amniocentesis is the most commonly performed invasive test in pregnancy. It's usually done between 16 to 18 weeks, but it can be done up to week 26. Women who are older than 35, who have a family history of Down syndrome or other chromosomal abnormality, or who had an abnormal nuchal translucency scan are often advised to have amniocentesis.

The procedure takes around 20 minutes. Using ultrasound, the operator finds the best place to insert the amniocentesis needle, without touching the baby or placenta. You might first be given some local anesthetic into your skin, but the needle is so thin you won't likely feel it going in. The needle is inserted, and it draws out a sample of around four teaspoonfuls of amniotic fluid from around your baby. (If you're carrying fraternal twins, fluid might be taken from each gestational sac.) The operator will remove the needle and scan the baby carefully with the ultrasound to make sure that all is well. If you're Rh-negative, you should receive RhoGAM at your amniocentesis to prevent sensitization.

After an amnio, you might have a bit of spotting, and you might feel sore for a few hours. It takes around three weeks to get the results of the test. There is a slight risk of miscarriage with the procedure, around 1 percent.

An amniocentesis can identify around 10 percent of the 400

abnormalities that a baby can be born with, including fetal infections such as herpes, skeletal diseases such as osteogenesis imperfecta, and chromosomal disorders such as Down syndrome. More than 90 percent of women who have amnios learn that their babies *don't* have the disorder that the test was done for.

෴

I had amnios during my second, third, and fourth pregnancies. They all came back normal. I didn't think that the procedure was physically uncomfortable. I didn't even feel the needle going in! When they were taking the fluid out, it felt weird, like a little vacuum cleaner sucking out some fluid. But the procedure was over before I knew it.

—*Melanie Bone, MD, a mom of four "tweens" ages 15 to 12, a gynecologist, the founder of the Cancer Sensibility Foundation, and the author of the syndicated column* Surviving Life *and the book* Cancer, What's Next?, *in West Palm Beach, FL*

෴

I decided to have an amnio. I was 36 years old when I was pregnant, and my mom had me at age 40. I figured I started from old stock, which probably adds up, chromosomally.

Also, I'm the type of person who believes that more information is better than less. For one thing, if there is to be a problem, the more counseling you can have up front and understand how to cope, the better prepared you'll be. Plus, I think it's best to know what you're dealing with. You might need to start preparing for an entirely different journey than the one you set out on. It's very hard if you're packed up for one vacation and end up going somewhere else.

—*Susan Wilder, MD, a mom of an older daughter and twin girls, a primary care physician, and CEO and founder of Lifescape Medical Associates in Scottsdale, AZ*

෴

Because my screening test for Down syndrome was abnormal during my second pregnancy, I decided to have an amnio. I do amnios on people every single day, and I was a little nervous about having one done on myself. It is always hard to entrust the fate of your pregnancy to someone else. I was very nervous about the small risk of losing the pregnancy from the procedure.

But I was surprised at how painless it was. It didn't hurt. It felt weird more than anything else.

—Ashley Roman, MD, MPH, a mom of two daughters, ages three years and six months, and a clinical assistant professor in the department of obstetrics and gynecology at the New York University School of Medicine in New York City

⌒⌒

Because I was over age 35 during my second pregnancy, I had an amniocentesis. Also the doctors had seen some markers on my ultrasound that were concerning.

There are certainly risks involved in an amniocentesis. Plus, if you receive bad news, what will you do? But I believe that you have to trust that you're having the test for good reasons. I don't think my husband and I would have had the test done if I hadn't had those concerning markers on my ultrasound. But we chose to do the test because if something was indeed wrong, we wanted to have the information as early as possible, instead of waiting until the baby was born.

The amnio wasn't as painful for me as you might have heard. It felt like a bee sting when the needle went in. I also felt quite crampy during the procedure and for a little while afterward.

Thank goodness I had worked the night shift the night prior to my test, so I had that whole day off. (I don't think women necessarily need to take the day off after the procedure. I had just been up the night before and didn't want to have to go back to work.) After we got the results that the baby was healthy, it was a huge relief.

—Janet Lefkowitz, DO, a mother of two girls and an ob-gyn in private practice in Rhode Island

Joining a Support Group

A support group could simply be your circle of friends. It's not uncommon for several friends to be pregnant at the same time, making a ready-made support group! This can be a wonderful experience, enjoying and celebrating your pregnancy with a dear friend.

You could also simply Google "pregnancy support groups." A recent search netted 22 million hits! They don't call it the "worldwide web" for nothing!

You could join a formal group, either in your community or online. Websites such as www.babycenter.com offer birth clubs grouped into due date months. No matter which year and month your baby is due in, there's a group for that.

⌘

During my first pregnancy, I had a ready-made support group. I had a circle of friends who each already had two or three kids. I respected them and admired the way they were parenting their kids. I turned to them for advice and relied on them for support. Besides my friends being very supportive and helpful, it was also a great bonding experience with them.

—*Michelle Paley, MD, PA, a mom of a six-year-old daughter and a two-year-old son and a psychiatrist and psychotherapist in private practice in Miami Beach, FL*

⌘

I subscribed to the BabyCenter.com April 2005 babies board and read the posts every day. It was months before I got the guts to ask a question. But you know what? When you have very weird things happening that you don't want to tell your doctor for fear of being labeled another crazy preggo, there's someone on the board going through it too and you can vent (like my weird phenomenon of not being able to pee in a straight line late in pregnancy, which became important when aiming for that cup and trying not to pee on seats . . .).

—*Tyeese Gaines Reid, DO*

⌘

A friend of mine and I were pregnant at the same time. We also went shopping together, and we were

MommyTime — Join a Local MOMS Club

If you plan to be a stay-at-home mom, you might consider joining the International MOMS Club, which is an organization for at-home moms. In 1983, a stay-at-home mom in California named Mary James started the first MOMS Club. A few decades later, there are more than 2,100 chapters in the United States alone and more than 110,000 members.

The groups meet during the day, and they are focused on stay-at-home moms. Children are welcome to attend the meetings. Visit their website, **WWW.MOMSCLUB.ORG**, to learn more and to find a chapter near you.

"beauty buddies," hanging out together, supporting each other, and being there for each other during hard times. A UCLA study showed that women who hang out together have an increase in levels of the hormone oxytocin, which helps them to relax and feel calmer. The benefits of having close female friends aren't only psychological; they're also physiologic.

    —*Debra Luftman, MD, a mom of a teenaged daughter and a teenaged son, a board-certified dermatologist in private practice, a coauthor of* The Beauty Prescription, *the developer of the skincare line of products Therapeutix, and a clinical instructor of skin surgery and general dermatology at UCLA*

RALLIE'S TIP

I didn't join a formal support group while I was pregnant, but you can bet I had an informal one! I worked in a hospital as a resident during my last two pregnancies, and there was no shortage of support from other residents, nurses, doctors, and patients who were either mothers or mothers-to-be.

    Most women are wonderful like that. We try to love and nurture and encourage others who are facing a journey we've already made or who share similar challenges. If you're lucky, you'll find lots of these people right under your nose, but if you don't, joining a support group is an excellent way to bring them into your life.

Chapter 18
Week 18

Your Baby This Week

YOUR BABY'S SIZE

This week, your baby has grown to around 5 to 5½ inches long, about the size of a 12-ounce Klean Kanteen. Her growth is slowing a bit now. But she will continue to gain weight at a steady rate until she is born.

YOUR BABY'S LATEST DEVELOPMENTS

Your baby is constantly entertained by a symphony of your heart beating, your belly gurgling, and the blood rushing through your arteries. In a few months, when your baby cries, if you hold her on your left side, she'll hear the familiar, comforting sound of your heart beating, which might calm her down.

Your baby's skin is starting to secrete a protective covering called vernix. This waxy coating protects her from fingernail scratches and long-term exposure to the amniotic fluid. It also helps to lubricate her body to make it easier to pass through the birth canal.

Your baby's nervous system is developing quickly. Around this time, your baby's neurons are being covered by myelin, which is a white substance that allows for efficient transfer of electrical impulses. Your baby's myelin will continue to develop up to her first birthday. Your baby's skin is now responsive to touch.

If your baby is a girl, her fallopian tubes and uterus are now in their proper positions.

Around this time, your baby learns a new skill: yawning.

YOUR LATEST DEVELOPMENTS

You can probably feel your uterus just below your belly button. You might have gained 10 to 13 pounds so far.

With each passing day, you're more likely to feel your baby move as she grows larger and stronger.

Many women find that their allergies act up more during pregnancy. Nearly 10 percent of pregnant women have seasonal allergies. If yours start to worsen, talk with your doctor or midwife about it. If possible, avoid your allergy triggers by keeping windows closed and wearing a mask when you vacuum—or better yet, having someone else do the vacuuming for you. Drinking lots of water might help too.

If your back is aching, you have plenty of company. Half of all pregnant women have back pain. This can begin early in pregnancy, and it can unfortunately last for a few months after your baby is born.

Swelling is very common during pregnancy, and you might find that your feet and ankles are already beginning to swell.

Your linea nigra might be continuing to darken. This line marks the point where your right and left abdominal muscles meet. This line is usually more noticeable in women with olive or dark skin.

Around this time, you might have developed the "pregnancy walk." As your uterus grows and pushes your belly out, your center of gravity shifts, and you unconsciously walk with your feet farther apart.

Now's a great time to get those feet moving because it's perfectly okay—in fact, it's beneficial—to exercise. By this point, if you were a runner, you've probably switched to walking or swimming.

Because you might generally be feeling better, your sex drive might have revved up. But if not, don't dismay. That's perfectly normal too.

It's not too early to sign up for prenatal and/or breastfeeding classes. Some of them fill up far in advance. Ask your doctor or midwife for suggestions, and you might also want to ask friends who have kids. (See "Taking Prenatal and Breastfeeding Classes" on page 363.)

JUSTIFICATION FOR A CELEBRATION

Your baby's taste buds are formed enough that she can distinguish between sweet and bitter flavors.

Having an Ultrasound

Your mom probably calls this test a *sonogram*. But these days, they're more commonly called *ultrasounds*, although the technicians who perform them are still often called sonographers.

Although insurance companies, doctors, and midwives disagree on when, or even if, pregnant women should have ultrasounds, most women are offered an ultrasound between 18 and 20 weeks. This is sometimes called a fetal anatomy scan. Your baby's organs and major body systems are all developed enough by now that they can be carefully checked for most structural abnormalities. Once you have your ultrasound scheduled, it's probably written in big letters and circled on your calendar!

There are no known risks associated with ultrasounds. An ultrasound machine projects high-frequency sound waves via a transducer through your abdomen into your pelvis. The sound waves bounce off tissues, and they're reflected back toward the machine's transducer. This process works sort of like radar on an airplane.

Ultrasounds provide valuable information during a pregnancy. They help to show the size and growth of your baby and help to measure how far along you are. They can identify abnormalities such as hydrocephalus and microcephaly and concerns about internal organs such as the kidneys. They can identify some babies with Down syndrome. They can also help to check the location, size, and maturity of the placenta. If your ultrasound suggests there might be cause for concern, your doctor or midwife might recommend having an amniocentesis. (See "Having an Amniocentesis" on page 203.)

Most ultrasound tests are two-dimensional. However, three-dimensional ultrasounds offer advancements such as more accurate measurements and better images.

While all of this is important to you, perhaps the part of your ultrasound that you're anticipating the most is finding out whether you're going to have a son or a daughter.

⤜⤏

I was very nervous during both of my pregnancies. When I had my 20-week ultrasound, though, I was able to breathe a huge sigh of relief. I'm a radiologist, and I asked the technologist if I could see the images as well. I looked at every body part, very carefully, and I was so relieved to see that everything looked perfect with no structural abnormalities.

I think many parents-to-be are simply delighted to see their cute babies on the ultrasounds, and that is wonderful. But most people don't realize just how much you can see on an ultrasound. You can rule out structural abnormalities. You can even rule out certain genetic diseases that have patterns that can be seen on an ultrasound.

—*Sadaf T. Bhutta, MBBS, a mom of a three-year-old daughter and 18-month-old triplets and an assistant professor and the fellowship director of pediatric radiology at the University of Arkansas for Medical Sciences and Arkansas Children's Hospital, both in Little Rock*

RALLIE'S TIP

I didn't have an ultrasound with my first pregnancy, so I had no idea whether I was going to have a boy or a girl, and I couldn't wait to find out. When I finally delivered the baby's head, I blurted out, "Is it a boy or a girl?" He laughed and said, "We won't know until you push this baby all the way out!" I had ultrasounds with my next two babies, and I was glad I did. I took a lot of comfort in knowing that they were healthy before they were born.

⟳

I chose not to have any ultrasounds during either of my pregnancies, even though I was age 34 and 38 when my sons were born. My husband and I decided that no matter what the ultrasound found, we wouldn't terminate a pregnancy. And so we decided that we didn't want to have an ultrasound, which I believe is invasive and interrupts the natural pregnancy experience. I figure my mother didn't have an ultrasound, and neither did her mother, or her mother before that.

My midwife is very well versed in observation skills and palpation, and I knew that my babies were in good hands. She could touch my abdomen and measure and determine what position the baby was in. Rather than being focused on the machines, the midwife was focused on the life itself.

—*Lauren Feder, MD, a mom of two sons, a nationally recognized physician who specializes in homeopathic medicine, and the author of* Natural Baby and Childcare *and* The Parents' Concise Guide to Childhood Vaccinations, *in Los Angeles*

Discovering the Sex of Your Baby!

If you're curious whether you're having a boy or a girl, you could try this test devised by the ancient Greek physician Hippocrates. If your right eye is brighter and your right breast is firmer, you're having a boy. If your left eye is brighter and your left breast is firmer, you're having a girl.

Thankfully, medicine has come a long, long way since then. Now you can go a more modern route and get a sneak peek at your baby via ultrasound.

This seems almost too obvious to say, but if a penis is seen, you're having a boy. However, if a penis *isn't* seen, that doesn't necessarily mean you're having a girl because the penis could be hidden. Truth be told, depending on how your baby is positioned during the scan, the genitals could be hidden from view. For a much more accurate answer, an amniocentesis or chorionic villus sampling will give 99 percent accurate gender information.

               ✎

During my second pregnancy, I found out very early that I was having a boy. At my 12-week ultrasound, the ultrasound resolution was clear. It was a boy.

> —*Amy J. Derick, MD, a mom of one 15-month-old son who is 17 weeks pregnant with her second son. Dr. Derick is a dermatologist in private practice at Derick Dermatology in Barrington, IL*

               ✎

During my second pregnancy, I knew that I was having twins, and after my amniocentesis, I found out that they were both girls. We went to visit my family for my nephew's wedding, and my daughter and I got out of our car. My sister came out to meet us, and she gave my daughter a present. It was a big sister doll with two baby sister dolls! I told my sister, "You're psychic!"

> —*Susan Wilder, MD, a mom of an older daughter and twin girls, a primary care physician, and CEO and founder of Lifescape Medical Associates in Scottsdale, AZ*

               ✎

Because I had a complicated pregnancy, I had to have an amniocentesis. When the hospital called with the results, and the sex of our baby, I wasn't home. My husband answered the phone, but the nurse refused to tell him the results of the test.

My husband tried his best to reason with her, explaining, "I made this baby along with her!" but to no avail. Finally, my husband asked the nurse, "Should I go out and buy a baseball?" to which the nurse replied, "Yes."

That evening, when I came home from work, the house was dark. The only light was focused brightly on our dining room table, illuminating a tiny baseball mitt and ball. My husband had even managed to buy a brand of mitt called "Max," which is the name we had chosen for our son.

—*JJ Levenstein, MD, FAAP, a mom of one son in college and a pediatrician in private practice in Southern California*

We didn't find out the sex of our first baby before she was born. But with my second, I had an amniocentesis. I felt it would be more practical to know if the baby was a girl or a boy so I could either reuse my daughter's clothes or give them all away.

It's funny, though. I remember that getting that phone call and hearing "It's a boy!" was so very similar to the moment in the delivery room when I heard "It's a girl!" I had worried that it might take away a lot of the excitement finding out ahead of time, but it didn't diminish the excitement at all. It merely came earlier.

—*Susan Schreiber, MD, a mom of a son and daughter in their twenties and a pediatrician in Los Angeles, CA*

Coping with Leg Cramps

Leg cramps, which go by the unusual name *Charley horses*, are common in pregnancy. As your uterus grows, it puts increasing pressure on the veins that return the blood from your legs back to your heart. This can cause painful leg cramps—so painful that they can jolt you from a deep sleep.

To prevent Charley horses, it might help to avoid standing for long periods. Rest on your side as much as possible. Eating foods rich in potassium, such as bananas and raisins, might help. Because Charley horses can be exacerbated by dehydration, drinking lots of water might be helpful too. You could also try soaking in a warm bath before bed.

To relieve a Charley horse, try to push your toes up toward your knees. This stretch can ease the cramp, decrease the tension, and release the spasm.

∽

I've never had Charley horses in my life—until my pregnancies. I'd wake up in the middle of the night yelping in agony. My poor husband!

The Charley horses became more frequent as my pregnancy went along. The one thing I found that eased the pain was walking. I'd walk around my room to loosen the cramped muscle. Thankfully, I could fall back to sleep easily.

—*Rebecca Kazin, MD, a mom of three girls and the medical director of the Johns Hopkins Dermatology and Cosmetic Center at Green Spring Station in Lutherville, MD*

∽

I had Charley horses mostly in my last pregnancy. I'm not sure why, but during that pregnancy I had a kidney stone, and I was drinking less, and I think dehydration increases the leg cramps.

Charley horses are extremely painful. I'd wake from a deep sleep yelling, "My leg, my leg!" When I had one, my husband would help me stretch my leg in the other direction. Then the pain went away, and I could go back to sleep.

—*Dianna K. Kim, MD, a mom of three and an ob-gyn in private practice in Vernon Hills, IL, at the Midwest Center for Women's Healthcare*

Minimizing Swelling

Remember your ankles? Even if you *could* bend down to look at your ankles, they might be so swollen you don't want to. Swelling is very common in pregnancy, especially toward the end. To meet the needs of your developing baby, your body produces approximately 50 percent more blood and body fluids. All of this extra blood and fluid causes swelling. Normal swelling, which is also called edema, is seen in the hands, face, legs, ankles, and feet.

Swelling normally kicks in around the fifth month of pregnancy, and it often increases from there. Swelling can be worsened by heat, standing, getting too little potassium, and drinking too much caffeine.

Toward the end of my pregnancy, I had mild swelling, which is quite common.

I simply wore support hose, which are helpful, but take forever to put on!

—Diane Connelly, MD, a mom of a six-year-old daughter and an ob-gyn in HMO practice in Riverside, CA

RALLIE'S TIP

I had horrible swelling toward the end of my pregnancies. My cankles had cankles. I was so swollen that I couldn't fit into any dress shoes, so I simply wore tennis shoes or clogs with everything.

Also, socks with elastic at the top left deep, painful impressions in my calves. Instead, I wore soft fuzzy socks that didn't have any elastic on top. And just forget the panty hose. That's crazy!

These days, I see pregnant women wearing tighter clothing than they used to. I think it's great that women are proud of their baby bumps and not hiding their pregnancies under tents! But fashion isn't more important than comfort.

During my pregnancies, I lived in sweats and stretch pants when I was at home. And at work I wore scrubs, which are great because they have expanding drawstring waistbands.

During my pregnancy, I had a tremendous amount of swelling. In just two weeks, I gained 10 pounds. My hands were swollen, and my feet looked like puffer fish. The nurses took a picture of my feet when I was in labor because they were so swollen. Even my nose was swollen.

My feet were so swollen I couldn't wear any of my shoes. I used to joke that this is what they meant by "pregnant and barefoot in the kitchen." I lived in flip-flops, even with nice dresses. Thank goodness I live in sunny Arizona.

—Gina Dado, MD, a mom of two daughters and an ob-gyn with Arizona OBGYN Affiliates, Paradise Valley Branch, in Scottsdale, AZ

During my pregnancy, I had bad swelling of my feet and fingers. Whenever I had the chance, I'd put my feet up, especially at night when I was watching TV. I think it's helpful to keep a foot stool nearby.

Also, it sounds counterintuitive, but it helps to stay hydrated. Don't stop drinking if you're swelling. I drank a lot of water during my pregnancy, and an occasional caffeinated soda.

—Aline T. Tanios, MD, a mom of three and a general pediatrician and hospitalist who treats medically complex children at Arkansas Children's Hospital in Little Rock

I had very swollen ankles toward the end of my pregnancy. I was in residency, and I was on my feet many hours each day.

My ankles swelled so badly that I could only wear sneakers with no shoelaces. I tried to put my feet up as much as possible. Even during the day at the hospital, I'd sit in one chair and put my feet up on another one.

—Elissa Charbonneau, DO, a mom of an 18-year-old son and a 16-year-old daughter and the medical director of the New England Rehabilitation Hospital in Portland, ME

During my pregnancies, I got terrible swelling. With both of my babies, my ankles swelled to the size of my thighs, despite the fact that with my daughter I was working at a desk and with my son I was on my feet all the time.

I wore support hose. I live in Florida, and it was very hot, but the hose helped to make my legs feel more comfortable.

—Michelle Paley, MD, PA, a mom of a six-year-old daughter and a two-year-old son and a psychiatrist and psychotherapist in private practice in Miami Beach, FL

As my pregnancy progressed, my ankles started to swell. It was uncomfortable, and I often had to sit down to ease the discomfort.

Compression hose helped. I found that when I wore them, my legs didn't swell, and I didn't have to sit down so much. You can buy compression stockings online and at medical supply stores.

—Amy J. Derick, MD

I'm on my feet 12 hours a day at work, and I think that really contributed to swelling during my pregnancy. My feet were so swollen that I went up two shoe sizes.

One thing I found that helped was wearing compression stockings called Jobst. Hospitals carry them to prevent embolism in patients. They come in different pressures and lengths. You can buy them from surgical supply stores or from Internet companies. I bought mine at www.allheart. com. I wore them under my clothes. Thank goodness I was pregnant in winter because it would have been far too hot in summer.

—*Sonia Ng, MD, a mom of seven-year-old and one-year-old sons and a pediatrician and expert in sedation at Children's Hospital of Philadelphia Pediatric Care at Princeton Health Care System in Princeton, NJ*

Mommy MD Guide-Recommended Product
Compression Stockings

"Because I was on my feet so much during my pregnancy, I had a little bit of swelling in my legs," said Debra Luftman, MD, a mom of a teenaged daughter and a teenaged son, a board-certified dermatologist in private practice, a coauthor of *The Beauty Prescription*, the developer of the skincare line of products Therapeutix, and a clinical instructor of skin surgery and general dermatology at UCLA. "I wore those stockings that people with blood clots in their legs wear, called T.E.D. stockings. Plus I elevated my legs every opportunity I had."

You can buy T.E.D. stockings for around $20 a pair online.

Chapter 19
Week 19

Your Baby This Week

YOUR BABY'S SIZE

Your baby measures around 5¼ to 6 inches long at this point, about the size of a mini beach ball.

YOUR BABY'S LATEST DEVELOPMENTS

Your baby's brain is developing at an amazing rate. His motor skills are beginning to develop as his brain is forming neurons that tell his muscles what to do. He's beginning to be able to make conscious movements, in addition to unconscious movements and reflexes.

Your baby's senses are developing because around now the part of his brain that is responsible for the senses is specializing.

Around now your baby has buds for his permanent teeth. These buds are located behind his baby teeth buds.

Your baby's hair follicles continue to form on his scalp, and his hair continues to grow.

YOUR LATEST DEVELOPMENTS

When you turn to the side, people can really notice a change in your body. At each visit, your doctor or midwife will measure your belly to check your fundus height. Generally the number of centimeters you measure will correlate to the number of weeks you are along. But if you measure large or small, don't panic. Your due date might have been miscalculated. This can be checked against your ultrasound results.

During your second trimester, colostrum, a thin yellow fluid, begins to form in the glands of your growing breasts. Also, each week your milk ducts expand, preparing to feed your baby if you choose to breastfeed.

The second trimester is prime time for round ligament pains. These feel like sharp pains in your abdomen or hip, and they can extend to your groin. You might feel round ligament pains on your left side, your right side, or both. They hurt, but they're normal. The round ligaments are attached to each side of your upper uterus and to your pelvic side wall. As your uterus grows, the ligaments are pulled and stretched. Just chalk it all up to growing pains. When you feel round ligament pain, it might help to lie down and rest for a bit.

It's a good bet your feet and ankles are swelling. Perhaps you need to buy new shoes already.

You might continue to spot skin changes, such as red splotches on the palms of your hands. Perfectly normal, this should go away after your baby is born.

JUSTIFICATION FOR A CELEBRATION
Your baby can now make purposeful, conscious movements.

Buying Baby Clothes

Impossibly small, impossibly cute, baby clothes are one of the great joys of pregnancy. Enjoy!

～

For both of my pregnancies, my husband and I chose not to find out the sex of our babies. I went with my mom to the store ahead of time and picked out the basics, such as the layette.

We picked out onesies and cloth diapers that are used for things other than diapers—and gender neutral things. If there was an outfit I particularly liked and it was gender specific, it was marked as a "maybe" until the call was made to the store to say that the baby was a boy or a girl.

—*Janet Lefkowitz, DO, a mother of two girls and an ob-gyn in private practice in Rhode Island*

～

I wanted to shop for baby clothes, but my mom urged me to wait until after the shower. It turns out she was right because I received so many clothes as gifts and passed down from my friends' babies that I didn't buy a stitch of clothing—except for a special Christmas outfit—for my daughter until she was nine months old.

—*Kerri A. Daniels, MD, a mom of one toddler daughter and an instructor in the department of pediatrics at the University of Arkansas for Medical Science in Little Rock*

～

For my pregnancy with my daughter, my friends and family held a baby shower for me. They knew what I needed, and so we got a lot of baby clothes for my daughter.

I was able to use quite a lot of the baby clothing for my son as well. That was a good thing because I was on bed rest the last seven weeks or so of my pregnancy, and I couldn't really shop. Truth be told, I didn't think my son would have minded wearing pink for his first few weeks if need be.

—*Diane Truong, MD, FAAP, a mom of one daughter and one son and a pediatrician in a multispecialty group practice in Southern California*

～

My friends and family hosted a baby shower for me and gave me lots of things for my first baby. To be honest, after I had my first baby, I refused to spend more money on onesies and tiny baby clothes that would only be worn a short time. My son wore pink for a long time.

—*Melanie Bone, MD, a mom of four "tweens" ages 15 to 12, a gynecologist, the founder of the Cancer Sensibility Foundation, and the author of the syndicated column* Surviving Life *and the book* Cancer, What's Next?, *in West Palm Beach, FL*

Don't buy too many zero- to three-month clothes! Especially with my first baby, I received so much clothing as gifts, and the baby only wears them for a few months, especially if you have a big baby. We hardly got through all of the clothes before my baby outgrew them.

Mommy MD Guide-Recommended Product
Dreft Laundry Detergent

As you buy baby clothes and receive them as gifts and hand-me-downs, you're probably diligently washing them, along with your baby's bedding and towels. You'll find several brands of laundry soap specifically made for babies, such as Dreft, which are especially helpful if your baby has sensitive skin.

You might find that it's convenient to wash your baby's clothing separately. Tiny little socks worm their way into adult's sleeves and pant legs, and grippy baby washcloths cling to any cotton clothing. Mesh lingerie bags are handy to zip these small articles into to wash and dry. Plus once your baby is born, you'll probably find that you do his laundry much more frequently than the rest of the family's.

One important laundry precaution: Don't use fabric softener on any infant or children's clothing or sleepwear that's labeled *flame retardant*. Fabric softener might reduce the clothing's flame retardance.

One brand of baby detergent that's readily available nationwide is Dreft. It costs around $9.50 in grocery stores for a 50-fluid-ounce bottle.

I remember receiving six- to nine-month clothes before my baby was born and thinking, *When is he going to wear those?* But moms with kids know: The time goes by so fast.

—*Dianna K. Kim, MD, a mom of three and an ob-gyn in private practice in Vernon Hills, IL, at the Midwest Center for Women's Healthcare*

⁓

Because we didn't know if we were having a boy or a girl for my first pregnancy, I bought clothes in neutral colors. I did buy some blue clothing, though, because I figured girls can wear blue clothes, but a boy can't wear pink.

This worked out well because our first child is a boy, but our second and third are girls. So our daughters could wear some of our son's clothes.

—*Judy Dudum, MD, a mom of three, an ob-gyn, and a senior staff physician at Henry Ford Health System in Detroit, with interests in nutrition and adolescent gynecology*

⁓

During my pregnancy, my husband and I were living in France. My friends had a lot of parties for me, not really baby showers, but they did gift me with many things for the baby, especially clothes. The styles were quite unusual in France. I remember one outfit looked like something an astronaut would wear! I thought that was so interesting that when we moved back to Colombia, I brought it home with me and passed it along to my sister's daughter.

—*Lilian Morales, MD, a mom of an 11-year-old daughter and a physician in Bogotá, Colombia*

Choosing a Hospital, Birth Center, or Home Birth

Today about 98 percent of babies are born in hospitals or birth centers, leaving just a few to be born at home.

The most common situation today is the mother-to-be delivers in a hospital delivery room, and then she moves into a private room after the baby is born. Some hospitals have birthing suites where the woman labors and delivers, all in one room.

Depending upon your insurance and your health care provider, you might have many options to consider, such as more than one hospital from which to choose. It's a great idea to take a tour of each one, ask questions, and gauge how you feel about them.

❦

I knew that I wanted to have my babies in a hospital. In particular, I wanted the hospital to have a neonatal intensive care unit (NICU). There were two hospitals in our neighborhood, one with a NICU and the other without. I chose the one with the NICU. The hospital had a birthing center as well, and that was the perfect atmosphere for me.

—*Debra Luftman, MD, a mom of a teenaged daughter and a teenaged son, a board-certified dermatologist in private practice, a coauthor of* The Beauty Prescription, *the developer of the skincare line of products* Therapeutix, *and a clinical instructor of skin surgery and general dermatology at UCLA*

❦

I chose to deliver at the hospital. There was a birthing center associated with the hospital, but the hospital was more comfortable for me. It's very important to feel comfortable where you are going to deliver your baby.

I was going to deliver at the hospital I worked at, and I spent so much time there it felt like home. I spent more hours in the labor room than in my own house at that point.

For my first delivery, I had a semi-private room. For my second delivery, I had my own room, and that was really nice. Sharing a room was a drag.

—*Ellen Kruger, MD, a mom of two teenagers and an ob-gyn in an academic and clinical practice in New Orleans, LA, with Ochsner Health System*

❦

All four of my deliveries were in hospitals. Had there been a birth center near my home, I might have considered that, but there are no birth centers near my home.

I would never have considered a home birth. I have delivered babies at women's homes, and it went fine. However, one thing I learned as an ob is that pregnancy is all nice and fun until it's bad, and 50 percent of things that go bad in labor happen in low-risk patients. There's no predicting it. That wasn't a risk I was willing to take.

—*Melanie Bone, MD*

I decided to have a home birth for both of my babies. I knew that I would be most comfortable at home—and I was.

—Lauren Feder, MD, *a mom of two sons, a nationally recognized physician who specializes in homeopathic medicine, and the author of* Natural Baby and Childcare *and* The Parents' Concise Guide to Childhood Vaccinations, *in Los Angeles*

My choice of where to deliver is not in a hospital. I do not think that hospitals, where normal childbirth is treated as an intensive-care experience, are the best places to have low-risk babies. My choice is at a birth center or at home within 10 minutes of a hospital, with supported skilled attendants—midwives who have backup and training. Midwives need support so that they are ready and able to call for help if they need it, without repercussions or judgment.

My older daughter was born in the Ozarks of Missouri at a birth center, and my younger daughter was born on the Farm in Tennessee in a cottage in the woods.

When I was pregnant with my first baby, I was living in a town outside Columbia, Missouri. I went to the local hospital to check it out. I asked if I could keep my baby in my room with me. This was 1972, and they said, "Absolutely not! The only way you could keep your baby in your room would be if that baby was born outside of the hospital, such as on the way here. Then we'd consider it to be contaminated, and so it would have to stay with you."

Their attitude that it would be better for my baby to be elsewhere away from me, not to mention that they believed my baby would be contaminated, totally freaked me out. I didn't want my baby to be taken away from me. So I checked into other options.

I found a doctor around 60 miles south who was associated with a birthing clinic. If he needed to, he could do a C-section. I knew that I would feel safe there. So even though it meant driving 60 miles, this doctor felt like the best option. I made that 60-mile trek each way every month for my prenatal visits.

The decision of where you have your baby should be based on where you feel safe. If someone tells you that home is the best place, but you don't feel safe having your baby at home, you shouldn't do it. But on the other hand, if you're terrified of hospitals, then you shouldn't have your baby in one. No one can have a healthy delivery if they're scared or feel unsafe.

—*Stacey Marie Kerr, MD, a mother of two grown daughters, a family physician with strong roots in midwifery, and the author of* Homebirth in the Hospital, *in Santa Rosa, CA*

My two older children were born at home, but my two younger children were born in the hospital for several reasons—one was because I was age 38 and 40, a bit higher risk. But I was careful to identify a doctor for their deliveries who understood that I was pregnant, not diseased. I needed to trust that my medical provider would honor my wishes to allow me to have my baby as I chose but be present just in case I needed him but not interfere with the process.

Before I went to medical school, I lived on a spiritual commune called the Farm. They have been doing home births there for more than 30 years, and their C-section rate is less than 2 percent. (According to the Centers for Disease Control in Atlanta, in 2006, the latest statistics available, 31.1 percent of babies in the United States were delivered by Cesarean section.)

On the Farm, everyone was having babies at home with midwives. I didn't want to have medical intervention because the birth process is a natural and sexual and intimate process. Just imagine, it's impossible to have an orgasm in front of unfamiliar people; likewise, it's difficult to progress through labor when unfamiliar people are in the "audience."

When I was in labor with my first baby, someone came into the room that I didn't know, and my labor stopped. I asked my husband to ask them to leave, and then my labor restarted when I was comfortable in my environment.

The important thing is to find the place to give birth where you will feel comfortable, surrounded by people you trust.

—*Hana R. Solomon, MD, a mom of four, ages 35 to 19, a board-certified pediatrician, the president of BeWell Health, LLC, and the author of* Clearing the Air One Nose at a Time: Caring for Your Personal Filter

Resting Despite Restless Legs Syndrome

Around 15 percent of pregnant women develop a mysterious condition called restless legs syndrome (RLS). This neurological condition causes you to have a strong urge to move your legs, especially in bed at night or when you're resting. Some people say that RLS feels like creeping, itching, pulling, crawling, or tugging. *All* of them would agree that RLS feels uncomfortable. The best news is, it usually goes away after your baby is born.

Some people with RLS find that it helps to eliminate caffeine and to take a warm bath and massage their legs before going to bed. If you're having a hard time falling asleep, it might help to get up and walk around for a few minutes, and then try to sleep again. You might want to talk with your doctor or midwife about your iron levels because some research suggests a link between iron deficiency and RLS.

You can learn more about RLS at the Restless Legs Syndrome Foundation's website, www.rls.org.

During my pregnancy, I couldn't stop moving my legs, especially at night. It was hard to sleep. My husband couldn't sleep in the same bed because I kept kicking him.

I found that sleeping with a pillow between my legs helped. And thank goodness, the restless legs syndrome went away after my baby was born.

—*Sonia Ng, MD, a mom of seven-year-old and one-year-old sons and a pediatrician and expert in sedation at Children's Hospital of Philadelphia Pediatric Care at Princeton Health Care System in Princeton, NJ*

? When to Call Your Doctor or Midwife

If you are having problems falling or staying asleep because of restless legs, talk with your doctor or midwife about it at your next appointment.

During my pregnancies, I had a bit of restless legs syndrome (RLS). I just put up with it. RLS is a big problem in pregnancy, and it's a major contributor to poor sleep.

Sometimes RLS can be caused by low iron stores, so it can be a symptom of anemia. It might be helpful to ask your doctor or midwife to check your iron levels.

Yoga and exercise in general might be helpful to treat RLS. Try to release as much tension during the day as possible. The best news is, the RLS will likely go away after the baby is born.

—*Stephanie Ring, MD, a mom of two sons, ages six and two, and an ob-gyn at Red Rocks Ob-Gyn in Lakewood, CO*

Easing Braxton Hicks Contractions

Braxton Hicks contractions were named for an English doctor, John Braxton Hicks, who first described the contractions in 1872. They're also sometimes called practice contractions or false contractions. But what they are *not* is in your imagination: These *are* contractions of your uterus.

You might have had Braxton Hicks contractions in your first trimester, but you probably couldn't feel them until now. Some women feel Braxton Hicks contractions in the second trimester, and they're most common in the third.

Braxton Hicks contractions feel like a slight tightening and releasing in your abdomen. Your uterus will tighten for around 30 to 60 seconds, or for as long as 2 minutes.

How can you tell a Braxton Hicks contraction from the real thing? Braxton Hicks contractions probably began in your lower abdomen. This is in contrast to the contractions that signal real labor, which usually start at the top of the fundus and roll downward. Or contractions that indicate you're in labor might begin in your lower back and spread to your lower abdomen. During a contraction, your uterus feels hard to the touch.

Some women describe labor as feeling like bad intestinal cramps or menstrual cramps. Other women experience backache. Once labor starts, you might get diarrhea. You also might feel that you have to urinate a lot. If your water breaks, you'll feel warm fluid running down your leg.

Braxton Hicks contractions are irregular, infrequent, unpredictable, nonrhythmic, and nonpainful. They don't increase in intensity or frequency, and they taper off and then disappear. *Real* contractions, on the other hand, are regular, frequent, predictable, rhythmic, and painful. They *do* increase in intensity and frequency, and they don't taper off or disappear until you have your baby—or your epidural when at least you won't *feel* them anymore!

❧

I had Braxton Hicks contractions toward the end of my pregnancy. They didn't bother me because I knew what they were.

But if you're feeling contractions that are regular, frequent, predictable, and rhythmic, especially if they're painful and increasing in intensity or frequency, pay attention and call your doctor or midwife.

—*Mary Mason, MD, a mom of a nine-year-old girl and six-year-old boy, an internist, and the CMO for a multi-state managed care company that coordinates care for about 70,000 pregnant Medicaid moms a year*

❧

? When to Call Your Doctor or Midwife

Let your doctor or midwife know right away if you experience intense Braxton Hicks contractions before 37 weeks.

Braxton Hicks contractions feel like a tightening of your uterus. They aren't painful, just tight. They're very normal after 20 weeks. Some women are more sensitive to them than others. What's important is to monitor their frequency. If you're having more than four or five of them in an hour, let your doctor or midwife know. Otherwise, just go on with your life.

I found that increasing my hydration eased them. Being dehydrated makes them worse

—*Ann LaBarge, MD, a mom of four children, ages 16 to six, and an ob-gyn in private practice at the Midwest Center for Women's Healthcare in Park Ridge, IL*

I did have quite a bit of Braxton Hicks contractions in my pregnancies, but it's difficult to know whether contractions are Braxton Hicks or real contractions. It's important to call your doctor right away if you're not sure.

—*Kristie McNealy, MD, a mom of seven- and four-year-old daughters and a two-year-old son, who's pregnant with another son, and a blogger at www.KristieMcNealy.com, in Denver, CO*

Chapter 20
Week 20

Your Baby This Week

YOUR BABY'S SIZE

By the end of this week, your baby's head is in much better proportion to the rest of her body. Her head now makes up less than one-third of her total length. Her crown-to-rump length is 5⅔ to 6½ inches, about the size of a small playground ball.

YOUR BABY'S LATEST DEVELOPMENTS

Around this time, all of your baby's hair follicles have formed, both on her head and on her body—all told around 5 *million* follicles. The hair on your baby's head is forming. Right now, all of your baby's hair is unpigmented—totally white.

You might be able to hear your baby's heartbeat with a stethoscope around this week. But you might not want to run out and buy one. Some of them cost more than $100. Your baby's heartbeat sounds like a swishing sound, and it's fast, usually 120 to 160 beats per minute. *Your* heartbeat sounds more like a beating sound, and it's slower, around 60 to 80 beats per minute.

If your baby is a girl, her uterus is fully formed, and her vaginal canal is starting to hollow out. If you're having a boy, his testes haven't descended yet, but you can see a scrotal swelling alongside a developing penis. Once your baby's scrotum is developed, his testicles will drop.

Prior to now, you probably felt your baby's gentle fluttering movements. Sometime around now, your baby starts to stretch her legs—and kick.

You now have around 11 fluid ounces of amniotic fluid. The fluid remains a constant 99.5°F, slightly higher than your body temperature, to keep your baby warm.

YOUR LATEST DEVELOPMENTS

You're probably looking quite pregnant! Your uterus is just about level with your belly button. Up to now, your growth has come in fits and starts, but around this time, it will start to even out.

By as early as this week, your breasts might be producing milk.

As your baby grows, your abdominal muscles are stretched and pushed apart. The muscles might separate in the middle. When this happens, it's called a diastasis recti. This happens to around one-quarter of pregnant women. If you lie down, raise your head, and tighten your abs, you might be able to see this separation. It will look like there's a bulge in the middle of your abdomen, and you might be able to feel the edge of either muscle on either side of the bulge. If this happens, don't be alarmed. It isn't harmful to you or your baby, and it isn't even painful. A few months after your baby is born, the muscles will tighten and return to their usual positions. Here's a spot of good news: If you do have a diastasis recti, you might feel your baby's movements more easily there.

For quite a while now, you've probably had vaginal discharge, and if anything, you might be noticing it more than ever.

You've probably never been more in tune with your body than you are now, noticing every twinge and ache. This is actually very beneficial because you will be alert for any changes that could be a cause for concern. One thing that's important to watch out for as your pregnancy progresses is a condition called preeclampsia. (See "Preventing and Treating Preeclampsia" on page 235.)

JUSTIFICATION FOR A CELEBRATION

You're halfway through your pregnancy! In another 20 weeks or so, you'll be able to hold your baby in your arms.

Celebrating the Halfway Mark and Enjoying Your Pregnancy

You're halfway there! The second trimester is often a time of increased energy, so now is a great time for a celebration. It's easy to get caught up in the concerns and worries of pregnancy. Give yourself a break and really enjoy this wonderful time. Forty weeks sounds like a long time, but when you look back, it will feel like it went by in the blink of an eye.

❧

I loved being pregnant. I was fascinated by the whole process—medically as well as spiritually. I was in awe of the fact that I was two people. I thought that was really neat. I enjoyed people asking me about the pregnancy, people touching my belly, and everyone being excited around me because I was pregnant. People love pregnant people.

—*Rebecca Kazin, MD, a mom of three girls and the medical director of the Johns Hopkins Dermatology and Cosmetic Center at Green Spring Station in Lutherville, MD*

❧

I had three very easy pregnancies. Despite feeling a little queasy for a week or so, I never threw up. After that passed, I felt really good. I loved being pregnant. Especially during my third pregnancy, which I knew would be my last, I really took the time to enjoy being pregnant and to cherish that time.

—*Lezli Braswell, MD, a mom of one daughter and two sons and a family medicine physician currently working in an emergency room fast track in Columbus, GA*

❧

I enjoyed being pregnant, and I loved having babies. I'd have 15 of them if I could. Being pregnant was fun for me.

I remember once during my second pregnancy, we went out to a fancy hotel. I'm not a fancy hotel kind of girl, but it was lovely. A woman came to our room to turn down the bed, and she smiled at me and looked at my belly, and said, "This is a blessed event that's about to happen."

—*Nancy Rappaport, MD, a mother of two teenaged daughters and a teenaged son, an assistant professor of psychiatry at Harvard Medical School, an attending child and adolescent psychiatrist in the Cambridge, MA, public schools, and the author of* In Her Wake: A Child Psychiatrist Explores the Mystery of Her Mother's Suicide

During my pregnancy, my husband and I were living in France. I enjoyed my pregnancy immensely! I went to many different parties and celebrations for my pregnancy, hosted by my dear friends.

Pregnancy is such a wonderful time. It's a time to celebrate and enjoy.

—*Lilian Morales, MD, a mom of an 11-year-old daughter and a physician in Bogotá, Colombia*

My second baby was born nine weeks early. And so when my third pregnancy reached—and passed—31 weeks, my husband and I quietly celebrated that and were glad to move forward.

—*Kristie McNealy, MD, a mom of seven- and four-year-old daughters and a two-year-old son, who's pregnant with another son, and a blogger at www.KristieMcNealy.com, in Denver, CO*

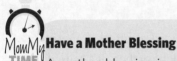

Have a Mother Blessing

A mother blessing is a celebration of new life. They're sometimes called Blessingways. Some people believe that this tradition was begun by Native Americans.

Unlike baby showers, a mother blessing can be hosted by the mom-to-be herself. The focus at a mother blessing is on spending time with family and friends, making memories, honoring the mom-to-be, and celebrating her becoming a parent.

Generally, a mother blessing includes very close female friends and family members, such as sisters, cousins, and sisters-in-law. Some women, however, also invite their doulas and midwives—even their doctors.

Mother blessings can include many different activities. For example, friends and family members might read poems or say prayers, the women might light candles and say blessings, everyone could bring a bead for the mom-to-be to string on a necklace to wear during labor, and moms-to-be can make casts of their bellies.

During my pregnancy, I didn't have any special celebrations; the whole pregnancy was a celebration. I was living on a spiritual commune called the Farm, and we were a bunch of young childbearing people making a community together, and so many of us were making babies. Pregnancy was fully supported and celebrated as a total process, but not with any particular ritual. We didn't light a candle or anything. Pregnancy was a big part of our life. There was such joy when women got pregnant, and we cared for the pregnant women as if they were queens.

When a woman went into labor, the word went out on the Farm, and the whole community would hold that space. It wouldn't be with any fear; it was more like, "Theresa is going to have her baby today! Awesome!"

—*Stacey Marie Kerr, MD, a mother of two grown daughters, a family physician with strong roots in midwifery, and the author of* Homebirth in the Hospital, *in Santa Rosa, CA*

Dealing with Vaginal Discharge

Throughout pregnancy, you might have noticed a white, sometimes creamy, thick, mild-smelling discharge called leukorrhea. It's caused by high estrogen levels and increased blood flow to the vaginal area.

Vaginal discharge serves several important purposes. It cleanses the birth canal, keeps infection-causing bacteria out, and maintains the proper pH balance in the vagina.

? When to Call Your Doctor or Midwife

Although large amounts of leukorrhea are quite normal, green, yellow, or foul-smelling discharge is not. If you experience that, talk with your doctor or midwife right away. It could signal an infection or a sexually transmitted disease.

During pregnancy, this discharge can be so copious that it's not uncommon to go through as many panty liners as you would when you have your period. It's just fine to wear pads or liners, but never douche or use tampons while you're pregnant. Using a douche might cause you to bleed or even cause air to get into your bloodstream. This is very rare, but it can cause some quite serious problems.

Even though I didn't have any vaginal infections during pregnancy, I had extra discharge, which is normal during pregnancy. I wore panty liners during my entire pregnancy because of it.

—*Dianna K. Kim, MD, a mom of three and an ob-gyn in private practice in Vernon Hills, IL, at the Midwest Center for Women's Healthcare*

RALLIE'S TIP

I had minor vaginal discharge with pregnancy, which my obstetrician assured me was perfectly normal. I found it to be mostly annoying, but it was good preparation for the major discharge that followed childbirth. After I had my baby, I also had the milk letdown to contend with. I felt as if my body was springing leaks all over the place, and I changed my own clothes almost as often as I changed my baby's diapers!

Preventing and Treating Preeclampsia

Preeclampsia is a condition that happens only during pregnancy and the postpartum period. It occurs in 5 to 8 percent of pregnancies. It's characterized by high blood pressure and proteins in the urine. Typically, it begins after 20 weeks, but it can happen earlier.

Preeclampsia is very serious, and it can progress very rapidly. Some women are more prone to it than others, including women who are overweight, who are pregnant with multiples, who already have high blood pressure or diabetes, who have never been pregnant before, and paradoxically women who are pregnant in their early teens *or* past age 40.

Your doctor or midwife will check your blood pressure at each visit because high blood pressure often has no symptoms. If you experience headache, blurred vision, upper abdominal pain, and/or unexplained anxiety, call your doctor or midwife right away. Part of the reason why preeclampsia is so insidious is that women who have it often feel fine.

Blood pressure is well named: It's the amount of force that your blood exerts against your artery walls. According to the American Heart Association, normal blood pressure is less than 120/80. (Both the first number, which is called the systolic pressure, and the second number, which is called the diastolic pressure, need to be under 120/80.)

Prehypertension is 120 to 139/80 to 89. High blood pressure is a reading of 140/90 or greater.

If your blood pressure was high before pregnancy, you have a greater chance of complications during pregnancy. You might want to buy a blood pressure monitor to check your blood pressure at home.

Usually, mild preeclampsia can be managed with bed rest and more frequent doctor visits. But the only effective *treatment* for it is delivery. (For more information about preeclampsia, visit the website of the Preeclampsia Foundation, www.preeclampsia.org.)

❮—❯

I had high blood pressure in both of my pregnancies. When I was pregnant with my daughter, it was diagnosed about halfway through the pregnancy. With my twins, it was diagnosed at 12 weeks.

I was put on medications both times. I wasn't really concerned about the medications harming my babies because they have been studied extensively. What I was concerned about was that the medication would make me so exhausted it would affect my work because I was still working full-time. But it all worked out fine.

—*Kelly Campbell, MD, a mom of three and an ob-gyn in private practice at Women's Healthcare Physicians in West Bloomfield, MI*

? When to Call Your Doctor or Midwife

As we mentioned before, high blood pressure often has no symptoms, but if you experience headache, blurred vision, upper abdominal pain, and/or unexplained anxiety, call your doctor or midwife right away. These are signs of preeclampsia.

Around 10 percent of pregnant women who develop preeclampsia go on to develop a related condition called HELLP syndrome. It's a cluster of conditions, including hemolytic anemia, elevated liver enzymes, and low platelet count. It can cause severe complications to both you and your baby. Symptoms include constant, all-over itching, lethargy, nausea, vomiting, and pain and/or tenderness in your upper right side. Call your doctor or midwife right away if you experience these symptoms.

In my first pregnancy, around 36 weeks, I developed preeclampsia. I was having swelling, and then my blood pressure went up. I didn't have headaches or visual changes, which are other symptoms.

I have to admit, I wasn't a very good patient. Even though my doctor wanted to put me on bed rest, I continued to work. "I'm fine, just swollen. You're overreacting," I told him.

In hindsight, this was not the right thing to do. Preeclampsia is serious. Lots of times women don't think bad things will happen to them. But you need to take care of yourself. I tell my patients that if they're coming apart at the seams, working full-time and pregnant, they need to cut back. We try to be superwomen and do everything, pushing until our bodies or brains give out. But instead, it's important to relax. Go to a movie, take a bubble bath, and put your feet up. The stress on your body has an impact on your baby.

—*Gina Dado, MD, a mom of two daughters and an ob-gyn with*
Arizona OBGYN Affiliates, Paradise Valley Branch, in Scottsdale, AZ

The day I went into labor, I had gone to the doctor for a regular appointment. I wasn't feeling well that day. I felt tired and achy—very nonspecific signs. I didn't recognize those as symptoms of preeclampsia, which is high blood pressure in pregnancy, because my symptoms were so mild. That's one of the tricky things about preeclampsia. Many signs and symptoms of it mirror other regular symptoms of pregnancy.

My doctor discovered that my blood pressure was elevated, and she sent me to the hospital. I was induced with Cytotec and Pitocin. It was a long labor. I went in Thursday afternoon, and my daughter wasn't born until Saturday at 4 am.

—*Diane Connelly, MD, a mom of a six-year-old daughter and an ob-*
gyn in HMO practice in Riverside, CA

Receiving a Concerning Diagnosis

Pregnancy can affect all parts of your body, often in unpredictable ways. No one knows your body better than you: You are the world's foremost expert on yourself—and on your baby. Pay attention to what your body is telling you, and report any unusual symptoms to your doctor or midwife.

A part of pregnancy is the fear that you don't know that your children are normal. We feared that one of our twins might have cerebral palsy. He's fine—beautiful, lovely, and smart. But at the time, we didn't know that.

During my pregnancy, I decided that whatever these babies were, it was okay with me. What I learned is that whatever situation you're given, you'll love that child fully. The journey isn't about having perfect children. Let's face it: None of them are ever perfect anyway! We all struggle, and we all have challenges to face. And we love our children through all of that.

—*Ruth D. Williams, MD, a mom of twins—a boy and a girl—and another boy, and an ophthalmologist in private practice at the Wheaton Eye Clinic in Wheaton, IL, who specializes in the diagnosis and treatment of glaucoma*

I had a very scary thing happen during my second pregnancy. My older daughter was diagnosed at five months with cerebral palsy, so everyone was nervous during my second pregnancy.

One Friday when I was around five months pregnant, I went to the doctor, and he said that my baby was too small and that even for a *small* baby, her head and brain were too small. I was hosting a surprise 40th birthday party for my husband that weekend, and it was the worst weekend of my life. I spent most of the weekend in bed. I was devastated.

I had to wait until the following Tuesday, when I had an appointment with the best sonographer in Florida. It took around an hour for him to measure every single part of my baby. After that, he said, "Everything is fine. Your doctor is crazy. There's nothing wrong with this baby. Get back up on your feet."

I was so relieved, but my doctor was still not convinced, so he put me on modified bed rest. It made for a very stressful end to my pregnancy. My daughter was born tiny, but thank God she was born well.

—*Eva Ritvo, MD, a mom of two teenaged daughters, an associate professor and vice chairman at the Miller School of Medicine of the University of Miami, and a coauthor of* The Beauty Prescription

With my first two pregnancies, at 36 weeks I was diagnosed with low amniotic fluid. So in my third pregnancy, I went for an ultrasound to check my fluid around that time. During the ultrasound, I knew something was wrong. The ultrasound technician kept peering at the screen. Then she called in one of the doctors, then another, and then the head of the ultrasound department. It was very scary.

It turned out my son had a mass on his adrenal gland. Until he was born, there was no way to know what the mass was. On the one hand, it could have been a blood clot that would simply go away on its own after birth. But on the other hand, it could have been a neuroblastoma, which is a type of tumor that would have required him to have surgery very soon after he was born.

I really wanted my labor to be induced early because the waiting and not knowing was the hardest part for me. But my midwife wanted me to wait and go into labor naturally. In the end, she did induce me early so that we could find out what was wrong.

Thank God, the mass was a blood clot, and my baby was fine.

—*Siobhan Dolan, MD, MPH, a mom of three, a consultant to the March of Dimes, and an associate professor of obstetrics and gynecology and women's health at Albert Einstein College of Medicine/Montefiore Medical Center in the Bronx, NY*

Chapter 21
Week 21

Your Baby This Week

YOUR BABY'S SIZE

This week, your baby measures around 7¼ inches crown to rump, about the length of a horseshoe. Around this time, some professionals begin to measure head to feet instead because the baby can be easily measured that way now too. Your baby probably measures around 10½ inches long from head to heels.

YOUR BABY'S LATEST DEVELOPMENTS

Your baby looks like a miniature newborn now, albeit a skinny one. Right now, he has only about 1 percent body fat. He continues to build fat stores under his skin.

Your baby's eyelids have finished forming, as have his impossibly tiny lashes.

Around this week, babies begin to swallow amniotic fluid. The water in the fluid is absorbed by your baby's body, and the unabsorbed matter goes through his digestive system all the way to his large bowel. This material is called meconium. Because it contains only undigested debris, and no bacteria, it's sterile. It's sticky and greenish-black or light brown to black in color. Your baby will either pass it before delivery, during labor, or after birth.

Your baby gets a little nutrition from the amniotic fluid, but his swallowing is mainly practice for nursing and bottlefeeding. He still gets most of his nutrition through the placenta—from you.

If your baby is a girl, her vagina is completely formed by now, but it will continue to develop until she is born.

By this week, your baby's legs are catching up in size with the rest of his body. Soon you'll feel every inch of those legs kicking you.

Your baby's white blood cells, critical to his immunity, are forming.

Your baby's skin is becoming thicker and less transparent as it develops into three layers, the deepest fatty subcutaneous layer, the middle dermis layer, and the surface epidermis layer. As your baby develops more fat, he is looking less wrinkly. The fat that your baby is developing is a particular type of fat called brown fat, which provides insulation and heat. By the time your child is an adult, he'll have only a trace of this brown fat left.

Your latest developments

Welcome to the second half of your pregnancy! You no longer have a waistline, and it would be difficult to hide your pregnancy now. You're probably gaining about a pound each week, and you've probably gained 10 to 15 pounds so far.

If you notice that your teeth look a little gray, take that as a huge hint that you need to get more calcium in your diet. Milk and other dairy products are the best food sources.

You might notice that your nails break more easily now. It could help to wear gloves when doing the dishes and other chores. Better yet, have someone else do them!

Some women find that their hair grows thick and shiny during pregnancy. Most women shed less hair during pregnancy, and because of your increased metabolic rate, your hair is growing faster than usual. But other pregnant women's hair is dry and splits. If this describes your hair, try using a mild shampoo and don't brush it too often.

Before now, your body was producing more progesterone than estrogen. Around now, levels of the two hormones even out. You might notice that your moods are running less amok.

Your blood volume continues to increase. By now, it's around 11 pints.

Justification for a celebration

Your uterus has now passed your belly button!

Signing Up for Your Baby Registry

This is a great time to register for baby things. Stores such as buybuy Baby make it easy and fun to register.

Even though registries aren't new, they still make some moms-to-be uncomfortable, as if they're asking for gifts. The key is, you don't *have* to tell anyone that you've registered, but if you register, then you'll be prepared if someone asks. And many people *will* ask because it's so easy to buy a gift from a registry with the reassurance that you're buying something a person wants, and something that there's a good chance no one else has yet purchased.

One day, I took my husband to a baby store. We walked in the door, saw the incredible amount of stuff, fell into a complete panic, and walked out.

For the first few months of their lives, my girls slept in their car seats and lived in diapers and gowns that I could pull up and easily change. I'm not one to spend a lot of time and money on gear and clothes.

Babies really don't need all that much. My mom had seven kids in 20 years, and she ran her own business all the while. When she came to visit after my twins were born, she saw the baby monitor. She asked, "What on earth is this?" When I explained it was a monitor so that I could hear them cry, she asked, "Why would you want to?"

—Susan Wilder, MD, a mom of an older daughter and twin girls, a primary care physician, and CEO and founder of Lifescape Medical Associates in Scottsdale, AZ

During my first pregnancy, I had no idea what to buy for the baby. It really helps to take a trusted friend who has kids along to register. When you go into one of those big baby stores, it feels like a foreign country at first. You look at 20 different strollers and have no clue which one is the best. I asked my friend to help, and she took me aisle by aisle around the store. She had been through this already with her kids, and she knew exactly what I needed and what were the best buys.

—Dianna K. Kim, MD, a mom of three and an ob-gyn in private practice in Vernon Hills, IL, at the Midwest Center for Women's Healthcare

Mommy MD Guide-Recommended Product
Baby Buddy Closet Organizer

Teeny tiny onesies, itty bitty pants—all of those baby clothes sure look cute, but if they're not organized well, they can turn into a fabric jumble quicker than you can say "Hold onto your hat!"

Here's a simple solution to the closet conundrum: Baby Buddy closet organizers. You simply slip these circular, plastic size dividers onto your baby's closet rod to keep clothing in different sizes separate and organized.

One Baby Buddy set includes five plastic size dividers, removable labels for 15 sizes ("newborn" through "size 8"), and six blank, write-on labels. The dividers come in four colors: pink, light blue, royal blue, and yellow.

You can buy Baby Buddy closet organizers at buybuy Baby stores or at OneStepAhead.com, for around $8 a set.

My family has a superstition about buying things before the baby arrives. My husband and I went to the baby stores and registered for what we wanted. But we didn't bring anything home until after the baby was born.

While I was in the hospital, my brother and his wife went to the store and picked everything up. The stores had already gathered it all up and packaged it for them.

After I got home with the baby, my parents told me, my husband, and our baby to go to sleep. By the time I woke up, my parents had unpacked, washed, and arranged everything. It was so nice!

—*Joanna Dolgoff, MD, a mom of a seven-year-old son and a four-year-old daughter, a board-certified pediatrician/child obesity expert with practices in Manhattan and Roslyn Heights, NY, creator of the online child weight loss program (www.DrDolgoff.com), and author of the book* Red Light, Green Light, Eat Right

Preventing and Treating Spider Veins and Varicose Veins

During pregnancy, many women develop spider veins and varicose veins.

When to Call Your Doctor or Midwife

If you notice any varicose veins, talk with your doctor or midwife about it at your next visit. Occasionally, varicose veins can make you more susceptible to blood clots, so your doctor or midwife will want to monitor them carefully.

If your mother had them, you're more likely to get them too.

The extra volume of blood in your body as well as the extra weight you're carrying put pressure on the blood vessels in your legs. Spider veins and varicose veins develop when blood pools in a vein, causing the vein to bulge. They are more common in later pregnancy. In addition to looking unsightly, they can ache and cause discomfort.

Spider veins look like bright red lines radiating from a central point. Spider veins and varicose veins can appear on your breasts, stomach, and legs. They can also appear on your vagina. When they appear on your rectum, they're called hemorrhoids. (See "Preventing and Treating Hemorrhoids" on page 354.)

Elevating your legs, wearing support hose and low-heeled shoes, changing positions frequently, and exercising might help to prevent spider veins and varicose veins. Some experts caution against crossing your legs—though sitting cross-legged will be less and less comfortable anyway.

If you get spider veins or varicose veins, there's not much you can do about them except perhaps try to consider them a badge of honor—and hope that they go away after your baby is born!

❧

I had mild spider veins before I got pregnant, but by my fourth pregnancy, they were very uncomfortable. They were mainly pelvic and vulvar varicose veins. They were especially painful after a day of standing.

As soon as I finished working, I'd sit on the couch and put an ice pack on my bottom. Thank goodness, they went away after my baby was born.

—*Melanie Bone, MD, a mom of four "tweens" ages 15 to 12, a gynecologist, the founder of the Cancer Sensibility Foundation, and the author of the syndicated column* Surviving Life *and the book* Cancer, What's Next?, *in West Palm Beach, FL*

I didn't get any varicose veins in my pregnancy, and I think perhaps that was because I was very physically active. We had no running water, and no electricity. I hiked three miles to do laundry. We were farm people, and I think that helped.

—*Stacey Marie Kerr, MD, a mother of two grown daughters, a family physician with strong roots in midwifery, and the author of* Homebirth in the Hospital, *in Santa Rosa, CA*

Coping with Unusual Complications

These types of things are called unusual for a reason. They're not common. But it's always important in pregnancy to keep an eye out for the unexpected and to let your doctor or midwife know right away about any unusual symptoms.

During my second pregnancy, I was bitten by a red ant. I've had ant bites before—and after—my pregnancy, and they're no big deal.

But when I was bitten while I was pregnant, my ankle swelled to the size of a watermelon! I couldn't walk on it at all for days. Likely it was because during pregnancy, your immune system is altered.

During pregnancy, weird things like that happen. You have to be patient with yourself and know that odd symptoms will most likely go away. But if something unexpected like this happens to you, call your doctor or midwife. My husband is a dermatologist, so I asked him to check it out for me.

—*Eva Ritvo, MD, a mom of two teenaged daughters, an associate professor and vice chairman at the Miller School of Medicine of the University of Miami, and a coauthor of* The Beauty Prescription

My second pregnancy was blissfully uneventful—up until the end anyway. When I was seven months pregnant, I developed a kidney stone. Then I went into premature labor. That was not so much fun.

One morning I was driving into work. A new physician was starting that day, and we had planned a welcome reception for him. All of a sudden, I felt this terrible pain in my flank area. I thought, *Oh my God, what is this? Back labor?* By the time I got to work, the pain was so intense that I could barely stand. I hobbled into the room, and the new doctor looked at me.

"Are you okay?" he asked.

A few of the doctors I work with quickly ushered me into another room, checked me out, and then drove me straightaway to the hospital. The doctors there gave me pain medication and a lot of fluids. Once the kidney stone passed, the pain was gone. And then my labor stopped.

—*Elissa Charbonneau, DO, a mom of an 18-year-old son and a 16-year-old daughter and the medical director of the New England Rehabilitation Hospital in Portland, ME*

? When to Call Your Doctor or Midwife

If you were born before 1971, it's possible that your mom could have taken a medication called diethylstilbestrol (DES) when she was pregnant. (The medication was prescribed between 1938 and 1971.) Unfortunately, that drug could have affected the children who were born to those women, including causing an incompetent cervix. When this happens, the cervix prematurely opens because of pressure from the uterus.

An incompetent cervix can also be caused by previous damage to the cervix. If your mom might have taken DES or if your cervix has been damaged, talk with your doctor or midwife about it. He or she might stitch your cervix shut.

During my last pregnancy, when I was around 26 weeks pregnant, I had a lot of back pain. It was unilateral, which means it was only on one side of my back. I thought it was just a muscle ache, and I tried to put up with it. I got a massage and put a heating pad on it. But it kept getting worse.

I thought, *This is not normal for me.* I went to our office and had a kidney ultrasound. The doctor discovered that my kidney was double its normal size, and he diagnosed an obstruction. I had kidney stones. The next day, I started having severe nausea and vomiting. They put in a ureteral stent, which provided an opening for the urine to go from the kidney to the bladder. Once my kidney drained, my intense back pain went away.

Unfortunately, the stent had to stay in for the rest of my pregnancy, and I had a lot of burning and had to go to the bathroom all of the time. It felt like I had a urinary tract infection, and it was very uncomfortable.

I took a bit of Tylenol for the pain, but other than that I just coped with it. I really couldn't wait to have that baby! After I had the baby, they were able to take out the stent, and I felt like a new person.

—*Dianna K. Kim, MD*

⁙

Around 11 weeks into my pregnancy, I started bleeding. It wasn't a whole lot of blood, but it was plenty to get me worried. My doctor did an emergency ultrasound and determined that the baby was fine.

I had a cyst on my ovary. My doctor monitored it weekly, but it grew and grew until it was the size of a grapefruit. By that point, it would have threatened my pregnancy, so I had to have it surgically removed at 16 weeks under spinal anesthesia. Thankfully, the surgery went well, and the remainder of my pregnancy went without a hitch.

—*JJ Levenstein, MD, FAAP, a mom of one son in college and a pediatrician in private practice in Southern California*

Preventing and Treating Vaginal Infections and Yeast Infections

Both bacterial vaginitis and yeast infections are more common in pregnant women. To make matters worse, they can be more difficult to control in pregnancy.

Vaginitis is an umbrella term that covers conditions that cause burning, irritation, itching, and abnormal discharge of the vagina. Two common causes of vaginitis are bacterial vaginosis (BV) and trichomoniasis.

About 15 percent of pregnant women get BV during pregnancy. It's caused by an overgrowth of bacteria. Your doctor or midwife can diagnose BV by testing the discharge for bacteria, and it's treated with antibiotics. Untreated, BV can make you more vulnerable to pelvic inflammatory disease, urinary tract infections, and sexually transmitted diseases.

Trichomoniasis is caused by an organism called *Trichomonas vaginalis*. Your doctor or midwife will check for it with a vaginal swab or cervical smear. It too needs to be treated with antibiotics. Some experts believe that trichomoniasis can cause preterm labor.

Yeast infections are never fun. If it's possible, they're even more of a pain during pregnancy. They are more common during pregnancy than at any other time in a woman's life. Interestingly, they're most common in the second trimester. One reason why is that pregnancy hormones alter the pH balance in the vagina, which the yeast take full advantage of.

The symptoms of a yeast infection are a white, curdy vaginal discharge that often causes itching, burning, or irritation. In most cases, yeast infections don't negatively affect pregnancy.

If you have a yeast infection when your baby is born, he can develop thrush, which is caused by the growth of a fungus, called *Candida albicans*, on the tongue and elsewhere in the mouth. It's rather common in nursing babies.

One food that might help to prevent yeast infections is yogurt. It contains healthy bacteria called probiotics that help to maintain the delicate pH balance in your vagina and prevent yeast infections. It might also help to cut down on the amount of sugar you eat. It might help to wear cotton underwear rather than nylon to allow for more air circulation. Washing with baking soda can help too. Simply sprinkle some on your washrag.

❧

When I was 19 weeks pregnant, my husband and I took a trip to Costa Rica. I know that pregnant women, especially pregnant women lounging around in wet bathing suits, are prone to yeast infections. Because I had no idea if they sold

? When to Call Your Doctor or Midwife

If you think you might have a yeast infection during pregnancy, talk it over with your doctor or midwife at your next appointment—or perhaps sooner if the itching is making you crazy. Your doctor or midwife might recommend an over-the-counter treatment.

If you have a discharge with more of a fishy odor, that may be another type of vaginitis, called bacterial vaginosis. A heavier discharge with no odor and no symptoms is quite common in pregnancy and does not need to be treated unless infection is found.

Monistat in Costa Rica, I took some along. It's a good thing because I did develop a yeast infection. (Talk with your doctor or midwife before taking this or any medication.)

—*Jennifer Kim, MD, a mom of three girls, ages eight, five, and four; an ob-gyn in private practice in Evanston, IL, at the Midwest Center for Women's Healthcare; and a clinical assistant professor at the University of Chicago, Pritzker School of Medicine*

Before I got pregnant, I had never had a yeast infection. During pregnancy, I had one, and I didn't know it. It turned up on my Pap test. The yeast infection wasn't symptomatic enough for me to feel it, but I treated it anyway with a three-day treatment.

My yeast infection wasn't uncomfortable. I mainly found it to be proof of what the textbooks say: Yeast infections are common in pregnancy. That's because pregnancy decreases your immune response. Your baby has DNA that is foreign to yours, and so your immune response has to decrease a bit to allow the pregnancy.

—*Diane Connelly, MD, a mom of a six-year-old daughter and an ob-gyn in HMO practice in Riverside, CA*

Chapter 22
Week 22

Your Baby This Week

YOUR BABY'S SIZE

Crown to rump, your baby is around 7⅔ inches, about the size of a neoprene hand weight.

YOUR BABY'S LATEST DEVELOPMENTS

Around this week, your baby's cartilage is starting to form in her nose. Her lips are becoming more defined, but they'll still be thin until she puts on more weight. Your baby's taste buds are becoming more sensitive, and she might react to different foods you eat.

Even inside the womb, your baby is learning. She can hear, taste, and now touch, and she's discovering how to use her new senses. Her hands and fingers are in near constant motion, touching everything within her reach.

Your baby's fingernails have grown, and they now cover her fingertips.

When babies sleep, they tend to favor certain positions, just like we do, and they settle into their comfiest position before sleep. Some babies sleep with their chins resting on their chests. Other babies sleep with their heads tilted back. You might get a clue to what your baby's favorite positions were after she's born.

YOUR LATEST DEVELOPMENTS

Around this week, your uterus is about ¾ inch above your belly button. Fascinating transformations are going on in your body. As your uterus moves upward in your abdomen, your rib cage will move up too, by a few inches, and your lowest ribs begin to spread outward.

Your growing belly might be making you uncomfortable when you're sitting or lying down. It might help to support the small of your back with a pillow strategically placed behind you.

You might feel more and more nasal congestion, and around now it might be accompanied by postnasal drip. Running a humidifier when you sleep might help. You could even prop the head of your bed up on blocks to raise your head and make it easier to breathe. (This is also a handy trick to know when your baby is born and has her first cold.)

Abdominal pain is common in pregnancy. Aches in the lower abdomen are quite normal because of the strain your ligaments are under. However, if you're experiencing severe, persistent abdominal pain, call your doctor or midwife right away because that can be a sign of a bigger problem such as a uterine fibroid, appendicitis, or a urinary tract infection.

It's common around this time to start leaking urine, especially when you cough, laugh, or sneeze.

Some pregnant women develop an itchy rash called a heat rash. This is very common, and it often appears on the chest and stomach. It might help to wear cotton clothing, which breathes better than synthetic fabrics. Also taking an oatmeal bath could help. You can buy oatmeal bath products at drugstores for a few dollars. Or try sprinkling baby powder on the rash to absorb perspiration.

If you're having a hard time sleeping, it's not unusual. Insomnia often kicks in around now, which is so ironic because just a few short months ago you probably couldn't get *enough* sleep.

If you're feeling excessively tired, however, it might be a warning sign of anemia. Talk with your doctor or midwife about having your iron levels checked because anemia can be dangerous for you and your baby. (See "Preventing and Treating Anemia" on page 257.)

JUSTIFICATION FOR A CELEBRATION
Your baby now weighs about a pound.

Coping with Bed Rest

Some estimates hold that as many as one in five pregnant women is put on bed rest at some point during pregnancy. Bed rest can be prescribed for any number of reasons, most commonly preeclampsia, cervical changes, premature labor, and vaginal bleeding. Unfortunately, bed rest is one thing you *do* have to take lying down.

⌒

After I went into early labor, my doctor sent me home for two days of bed rest. I spent those days cleaning and organizing my house and doing everything I shouldn't have been doing. In hindsight, I should have tried to rest and had someone else come help clean and organize.

—*Patricia S. Brown, MD, a mom of two daughters, ages nine and seven, and a three-year-old son and a psychiatrist at Columbia-New York Child and Adolescent Telepsychiatry and in private practice in Cresskill, NJ*

⌒

During my second pregnancy, I was having twins. I was put on bed rest for the last 9 or 10 weeks. Even though I was stuck in bed, I was still working seven-hour days answering e-mails and participating in phone meetings. But at one point it struck me that I normally did those things *in addition* to a full-time patient care schedule. I thought if I could be on bed rest eight weeks each year, with no new babies at the end of it, that would be great!

One funny thing, my older daughter used to come into my room and ask me to get her things, such as a drink. Then she'd tattle on me to her father that I'd gotten up.

—*Susan Wilder, MD, a mom of an older daughter and twin girls, a primary care physician, and CEO and founder of Lifescape Medical Associates in Scottsdale, AZ*

⌒

When I was pregnant with my first daughter, I was living in Manhattan and working around the clock as a second-year resident. I went in for an ultrasound at around 36 weeks because I was measuring slightly small and my doctor was concerned about my fluid. I was wearing scrubs and had three beepers on my belt! The doctors looked at the amniotic fluid level. It was too low, so they promptly took my beepers away from me and sent me home on bed rest.

It was so abrupt that I didn't know what to do with myself. All I had known was working! When I went home that day sans beeper, it took me a while to make myself relax. It turns out I had a few weeks of bed rest, and then I had my eldest daughter right around her due date.

—Siobhan Dolan, MD, MPH, a mom of three, a consultant to the March of Dimes, and an associate professor of obstetrics and gynecology and women's health at Albert Einstein College of Medicine/Montefiore Medical Center in the Bronx, NY

During my first pregnancy, I started to feel contractions at around 22 weeks. When they put me on the monitor, they saw that indeed I was booming out contractions.

My doctors gave me medicine to stop my contractions, and then they sent me home on bed rest. My mom came and kept me from going crazy. She cooked and cleaned, and my husband was able to go to work. It was a scary time. I was in medical school, and I knew just enough to scare myself half to death.

Ironically enough, after that lengthy bed rest, my baby was born five days *after* her due date!

—Ann LaBarge, MD, a mom of four children, ages 16 to six, and an ob-gyn in private practice at the Midwest Center for Women's Healthcare in Park Ridge, IL

I had a wonderful pregnancy. I didn't have a single day of nausea. But the one pesky part of my pregnancy was my doctor put me on bed rest at 31 weeks. At that time, I had no cervix left, which means my cervix was shortening and dilating before it should have.

I wasn't very good at bed rest. I kept getting up to do things, like laundry. That's what we women do; we keep going. At the time I was on bed rest, I was studying for my boards, so I tried to make myself stay off my feet as much as possible, and at least I had something very productive to do.

It's so important if you're put on bed rest to take that time and stay off of your feet because you want your baby to be as far along as possible when he or she is born.

—Jennifer Gilbert, DO, a mom of three-month-old twins and an ob-gyn at Paoli Hospital in Pennsylvania

I went into preterm labor with my son at 30 weeks. My doctor put me on strict bed rest. I had bathroom privileges, and I could take a shower once a week—that was it.

My ob wasn't messing around; she had me hooked up to a machine that was monitored by a nurse. She could see my contraction patterns. If I moved around and started to have contractions, she'd call me and ask, "What are you doing?" I had to behave.

I was on bed rest for seven weeks, incubating my son, and there wasn't much I could do to occupy the time. I watched a lot of TV. I'll never forget, Princess Diana died during that time, and it was on TV all of the time. I remember thinking to myself, *Couldn't there be something happier than this to watch?*

My husband is so supportive, and never more so than during that time. I was on an American Diabetes Association diet because of gestational diabetes, and he prepared special meals and brought them up to me. He helped me with everything that I needed because I couldn't get out of bed.

—*Diane Truong, MD, FAAP, a mom of one daughter and one son and a pediatrician in a multispecialty group practice in Southern California*

I had two very difficult pregnancies, and I had to be bedridden at the end of both of them. The funny thing is, at first I thought I'd fill my days doing interesting things like learning how to play the piano and building an Internet community. I ended up watching soap operas and reading stupid novels. One productive thing I did was sew baby clothes. It must have been some sort of a hormonal surge, though, because today I can hardly sew on a button.

During my second pregnancy, I needed some help caring for my son. I was born in France, so I called some friends there and asked for the names of teenaged girls to come help me in New York. I had a lot of candidates, and the 16-year-old girl who finally arrived really saved me during that period! An au pair might not be an option for everyone, but the point is, don't be afraid to ask for help.

—*Nathalie Stern, MD, a mom of two and a French-born pediatrician practicing in New York City and in Southampton, NY*

My preparations for my triplets were made challenging because my ob-gyn said I was full-term size at 22 weeks and needed to go on bed rest. I pushed it another three weeks and kept on working, but at week 25, he put his foot down and insisted I stop working. He asked me, "What are you trying to prove? You're a rat in a rat race! If you have these babies prematurely and they get complications from prematurity, you'll feel guilty about it for the rest of your life." In hindsight, he was right: I was putting my babies at risk just to work another few weeks! And so I went on modified bed rest at home.

It's a good thing my specialty is radiology because I was able to set up a reading room in my laundry room at home. My boss and the rest of my colleagues were extremely supportive, and they were all rooting for me to go all the way to full-term gestation. If I had been a clinician, this wouldn't have worked. I couldn't have patients coming over to my house! I was able to work at least four hours a day. I continued to work until a week before the babies were born.

—*Sadaf T. Bhutta, MBBS, a mom of a three-year-old daughter and 18-month-old triplets and an assistant professor and the fellowship director of pediatric radiology at the University of Arkansas for Medical Sciences and Arkansas Children's Hospital, both in Little Rock*

Caving In to Cravings

Pregnancy and cravings go together like pickles and ice cream.

Common cravings are ice cream and also very salty foods such as pretzels. No one knows for sure why pregnant women have cravings. Perhaps they're linked to the hormonal and emotional changes you're going through. Cravings are very normal in pregnancy. Just the word *craving* has sent many a husband scurrying to the store.

⌒⌒

During my pregnancy, I craved eggs. They're good for you, so I ate a lot of them!

—*Patricia S. Brown, MD*

⌒⌒

During my pregnancy, my husband and I went out for wonton noodles a lot. I don't eat them at all anymore, but during my pregnancy, that was the thing I needed to have. I think it must have been a comfort food for me when I was a child.

—*Diane Truong, MD, FAAP*

Initially in my pregnancy, I craved spicy foods. But as my pregnancy went along, I craved carbs. I'd ask my husband to make waffles for dinner—and not those frozen ones. I'd call from work and request *homemade* waffles.

—*Diane Connelly, MD, a mom of a six-year-old daughter and an ob-gyn in HMO practice in Riverside, CA*

I tend to be lean, especially prior to pregnancy, and while I was pregnant with my sons, I was very hungry. Sometimes my body told me to eat things that weren't good for me. I craved French fries and cheeseburgers. I'm an expert in nutrition, so I tried to focus on more wholesome choices, but occasionally I did give in to the high-calorie food cravings.

I also craved watery, sweet fruits such as watermelon, cantaloupe, and pineapple. Those cravings were easy to give in to.

—*Ann Kulze, MD, a mother of four children, ages 20, 19, 18, and 14, a nationally recognized nutrition expert, motivational speaker, physician, and the author of the critically acclaimed book* Dr. Ann's 10-Step Diet: A Simple Plan for Permanent Weight Loss and Lifelong Vitality

I think it's important to listen to your body. Cravings are a normal part of pregnancy. They're not a sign that anything is wrong. If you're craving something unhealthy, try to eat something healthier, such as yogurt instead of ice cream. But if you really *must* have that ice cream, eat it.

—*Erika Schwartz, MD, a mom of two and the director of www. DrErika.com, who's been in private practice for more than 30 years in New York City, specializing over the past 15 years in women's health, disease prevention, and bioidentical hormones*

? When to Call Your Doctor or Midwife

Sometimes pregnant women crave nonfood items. This condition is called pica. If you're craving nonfood items, such as dirt, copper, or detergent, don't indulge those. And call your doctor or midwife about it right away.

I gained 70 pounds during my pregnancy, so don't take the following advice to the extreme. But if you have morning sickness, and your body craves something that is not completely harmful, eat it. If you go along with what your body wants, you're a lot less likely to throw up. Yes, I know, it might be junk food or your 1,000th taco, but sometimes you have to follow the cravings—or else. If your tummy wants ice cream and you're eating salad and cottage cheese in the midst of nausea, what's gonna happen? Please indulge from time to time.

—*Tyeese Gaines Reid, DO, a mom of one, an emergency medicine resident physician at Yale New Haven Hospital in Connecticut, and the author of a time management book,* The Get a Life Campaign

RALLIE'S TIP

With each of my pregnancies, I developed a huge appetite, and I had cravings for foods that I usually wouldn't allow myself to eat when I wasn't expecting— salty foods like hot dogs, French fries, and potato chips, and sweet treats like cinnamon rolls, doughnuts, and chocolate bars. With my first pregnancy, I didn't hold back: I ate whenever I was hungry and whatever I craved. I ended up feeling miserable, both physically and emotionally. Not only did I have a lot of indigestion, I hated feeling fat! By the time my first son was born, I had gained around 60 pounds, which wasn't good for me or my baby.

When I found out I was pregnant with my second son, I vowed to eat less and gain less weight, but that didn't stop me from craving crazy foods, and it certainly didn't blunt my appetite. Because I was working in the hospital full- time, I had easy access to an unlimited supply of junk food in vending machines, hospital coffee shops, and the doctors' lounge.

Finally, I made a healthy compromise. I started bringing a small cooler to work with me every day, packed with nutritious foods such as yogurt, nuts, granola bars, boiled eggs, and fresh fruits and veggies. At work, I would allow myself to eat whenever I was hungry, but I limited my selection to the foods that were in my cooler. As a result, I never felt hungry or deprived. Although I snacked regularly throughout the day, I ended up eating a more nutritious diet and gaining a lot less weight than I had with my previous pregnancy.

Preventing and Treating Anemia

Iron is essential for producing hemoglobin, which is the protein in red blood cells that transports oxygen throughout your body. When you don't have enough iron in your blood, it's called iron-deficiency anemia.

Pregnant women need more iron than nonpregnant women do, partly because you have more blood volume now, which means you also have more red blood cells, which means you need more iron. At the same time as you have more red blood cells, you also have more plasma, which is the fluid in blood. This increase in plasma can cause anemia.

Anemia makes you feel tired or just generally unwell. Around 20 percent of pregnant women are treated for anemia during their pregnancies.

Pregnant women need a total of 18 milligrams of iron each day from supplements and food. Your prenatal vitamin contains iron, and a quick check of the label will tell you how much it offers. It's also important to eat plenty of foods rich in iron, such as beans, fortified breakfast cereals, and red meat.

If your doctor or midwife thinks you might be anemic, he or she will give you a hemoglobin test and check your hematocrit reading, which measures the percentage of your blood that is red blood cells. Anemia is defined as hemoglobin less than 12 and a hematocrit lower than 33 in pregnancy.

If you're anemic, your doctor or midwife might advise you to take additional iron supplements. They can come with side effects, such as stomach upset, nausea, constipation, and vomiting. If this happens to you, talk with your doctor or midwife about adjusting your dosage.

❧

Pregnant women are usually tested for anemia early in pregnancy, and then again in the early part of the third trimester. I'm always anemic in pregnancy, so I took a special iron supplement in addition to my prenatal vitamins.

—*Ashley Roman, MD, MPH, a mom of two daughters, ages three years and six months, and a clinical assistant professor in the department of obstetrics and gynecology at the New York University School of Medicine in New York City*

❧

During my pregnancy, I craved crushed ice from the machine at work. This was probably a sign of a mild form of pica, which is when you crave nonfood items like dirt. I think it was due to mild anemia. I had my routine blood tests, which were reassuring, so I just kept up with the usual prenatal vitamins, which contain iron.

—*Diane Connelly, MD*

❦

During my third pregnancy, I had to stop taking my prenatal vitamins because their extra niacin was giving me migraine headaches. But then I got weak and felt tired all of the time. My doctor checked my blood hemoglobin level for anemia with a finger stick in the office. It was low, and so he followed up with more tests. No doubt, I had iron-deficiency anemia. I started to take extra iron and felt much better.

—*Patricia S. Brown, MD*

❦

? When to Call Your Doctor or Midwife

If you're feeling especially tired or a little dizzy on occasion, talk with your doctor or midwife about it at your next visit. He or she might check your iron levels. If you're very dizzy or dizzy a lot, call right away.

When I had a hemoglobin test during my pregnancy, it indicated borderline low iron levels. This might have contributed to the light-headedness I often felt. It's a good idea to have a hemoglobin test in pregnancy because around 10 percent of women are anemic even *before* they get pregnant, and anemia often worsens during pregnancy.

I took iron supplements during my pregnancy. Because they can cause constipation, I was careful to ease into taking them. For a few days, I only took half a dose every other day, then for a few days I took half a dose every day, then for a few days I took a full dose every other day, and then finally I worked up to taking a full dose every day.

I also ate more lean red meats and leafy greens. They're some of the best food sources of iron.

—*Katja Rowell, MD, a mom of a four-year-old daughter, a family practice physician, and a childhood feeding specialist with www. familyfeedingdynamics.com, in St. Paul, MN*

❦

When I got pregnant, I was very nauseated and sick. I got extremely anemic. My hematocrit levels were in the 20s, and anything less than 33 in pregnancy is defined as anemia.

I didn't feel good; I was wiped out. I went to my doctor, and he told me it wasn't worth it to get iron shots, which was fine with me because I didn't want them anyway!

I wasn't a doctor back then, which I think was good because we have a saying, "MD equals Major Disaster." I'm grateful I knew so little at the time I was pregnant. If I had been more cerebral about my pregnancy, I probably would have had more trouble. I know now that my anemia put me at risk for complications. Had I been my own doctor, I would have recommended nutrition counseling and a high-iron diet. But I didn't do any of those things. I just went into labor terribly anemic! And I actually did just fine.

—*Stacey Marie Kerr, MD, a mother of two grown daughters, a family physician with strong roots in midwifery, and the author of* Homebirth in the Hospital, *in Santa Rosa, CA*

Leaking Urine

This is a well-kept secret: It's very common in pregnancy for women to leak when they laugh, cough, or sneeze. No one told you that before you got pregnant? No one told us either!

Here's how to fight back: Start doing Kegels. These exercises strengthen the muscles at the bottom of your pelvis, which might help prevent urinary incontinence. As a bonus, Kegels could even make labor easier.

You could ask your doctor or midwife how to do Kegels, or you could simply learn on your own. Sometime when you're going to the bathroom, stop urination midstream. Notice which muscles you use to do that? Now contract those same muscles when you're not urinating.

Why not kill two birds with one stone and do Kegels while you're urinating? It might seem easier and logical—not to mention really efficient!—to just do Kegels while you're urinating. But frequently stopping and starting urinating midstream like this might cause other bladder problems. Always empty your bladder completely.

RALLIE'S TIP

When I was expecting my third son, I was well prepared for the leaky bladder that accompanies the later stages of pregnancy, especially with coughing, sneezing, and climbing stairs. I kept a few maxi-pads and a spare pair of undies stashed in my car, my purse, and at my desk at work. On more than one occasion, they saved the day!

୧⌒⌒

I wore Serenity Pads the last month of my pregnancy. I was so fat you couldn't see them, and I didn't want to laugh and pee myself.

A friend of mine did have an "accident" at a party, and she was rushed to the hospital because she didn't want to tell anyone that she peed. I told her to tell everyone that the amniotic sac resealed and the fluid reaccumulated, and the baby is fine.

—Sonia Ng, MD, a mom of seven-year-old and one-year-old sons and a pediatrician and expert in sedation at Children's Hospital of Philadelphia Pediatric Care at Princeton Health Care System in Princeton, NJ

? When to Call Your Doctor or Midwife

If you're noticing that you're leaking, it might be just urine. But it can be distressing to fear that you're leaking amniotic fluid.

It's pretty easy to tell the difference on your own. Urine will look yellowish and smell like ammonia. Amniotic fluid can be clear, brown, green, or pink, and it will have little to no scent. If you're not sure, call your doctor or midwife right away. He or she can do a simple test in the office to confirm that it's not amniotic fluid.

If you have a gush of fluid or a steady leak from your vagina, your bag of waters might have broken. Call your doctor or midwife immediately.

Chapter 23
Week 23

Your Baby This Week

YOUR BABY'S SIZE

Already, your baby has grown to around 8 inches crown to rump, around 11¼ inches head to heel, about the size of a Frisbee. In the next month, your baby will almost double in weight.

YOUR BABY'S LATEST DEVELOPMENTS

The downy lanugo that covers your baby might begin to darken. Your baby's eyebrows and the hair on his head continue to grow. Don't get too attached to that hair after your baby is born, though. Lots of babies lose their hair a few weeks after they're born, and it's replaced by coarser, thicker hair.

Your baby's middle ear and, along with it, his sense of balance are forming. He might conduct little science experiments with this, flipping around inside of you. The three bones in the middle ear are the smallest bones in the human body, so they're *really* tiny in your baby. They're called the hammer, anvil, and stirrup.

Around this week, your baby's pancreas is developing. It has the very important job of producing insulin and other hormones. The pancreas will continue developing even after your baby is born. It won't be completely developed until he's two years old.

YOUR LATEST DEVELOPMENTS

You probably have a beautiful, round belly. Your uterus is now around

1½ inches above your belly button. By now, you've probably gained around 12 to 15 pounds, but more or less is likely just fine too.

As your belly grows, sex might become challenging or uncomfortable. With a little creativity, you can continue to have sex during your pregnancy, which, unless your doctor or midwife told you not to, has benefits to you and your partner. Let your comfort be your guide.

If you notice small growths on your gums, don't panic. These harmless growths are called pregnancy tumors, or pyogenic granulomas. They generally go away after the baby is born.

Every now and again, you might feel pins and needles in your fingers and toes, or even in your hands and feet. This is very normal, though uncomfortable. As the fluid builds up in your body, it can put pressure on nerves, causing that pins-and-needles feeling. It might help to move around more frequently and to elevate or shake your hands and feet.

As your skin stretches, your belly might itch. Try keeping your skin moisturized with lotion.

Because your uterus is sitting right on top of your bladder, you probably feel that you have to urinate a lot more frequently again.

You're probably getting a good feel for your baby, such as how and when he moves. You might even be noticing patterns of times he's usually active or quiet. *You* know your baby better than anyone else.

JUSTIFICATION FOR A CELEBRATION
If not now, soon your partner will be able to feel your baby move.

Enjoying Your Baby Shower!

Baby showers started after World War I, when many families were too poor to afford everything that they needed for a new baby. Women brought the growing family homemade food, clothing, and even furniture.

Baby showers are common in the United States, but they're held in other countries as well, such as in Europe—and even Africa and Asia. Traditionally, baby showers were held only for first babies, but people do hold showers for subsequent babies. They're sometimes called diaper showers. Some people even hold Grandma's showers to help outfit the Grandma-to-be's home to welcome the new grandbaby.

~

My friends had a baby shower for me. It wasn't a surprise because they asked me up front if it was okay to have one. I was so excited about it. It was held at a friend's house right after a hurricane. She didn't have any electricity that day because of the storm, but it didn't matter one bit.

—*Rebecca Kazin, MD, a mom of three girls and the medical director of the Johns Hopkins Dermatology and Cosmetic Center at Green Spring Station in Lutherville, MD*

~

My friends had a baby shower for me during my first pregnancy. The venue was a private room in a restaurant. We had so much fun. I was grateful because as a first-time mom, I didn't know what I needed. I hadn't registered for any baby things. I routinely use many of the practical gifts from that shower.

—*Amy J. Derick, MD, a mom of one 15-month-old son who is 17 weeks pregnant with her second son. Dr. Derick is a dermatologist in private practice at Derick Dermatology in Barrington, IL*

~

I worked until just a few days before my son was born. My last work day was a Friday, and he was born on a Monday.

At the time, I was on an endocrinology rotation at Good Samaritan Hospital. The two attending physicians I worked with were like Papa bears, very protective of me. On my last day of work, they threw a surprise baby shower for me. The entire staff gave me gifts. It was so dear.

—*JJ Levenstein, MD, FAAP, a mom of one son in college and a pediatrician in private practice in Southern California*

I'm Jewish, and in Jewish tradition, we don't do a lot of preparations until the baby is born safe and healthy. Generally, we try not to bring any baby things into the house until the baby arrives.

I didn't have a baby shower. Instead, we had a baby naming after the baby was born. Our friends and family came, and that's where our baby received her Hebrew name.

—*Janet Lefkowitz, DO, a mother of two girls and an ob-gyn in private practice in Rhode Island*

Instead of having a baby shower while I was pregnant, my family had a celebration after our baby was born. They all came to our home to meet the baby and brought him presents.

Mommy MD Guide-Recommended Product
Rechargeable Batteries for All Those Toys

AA, AAA, C, D—that's the way *parents* say their ABCs. Now would be a really good time to buy stock in Duracell.

Just about every baby toy that comes through your door requires batteries—lots of them. You can save yourself a lot of money, a lot of time in trips to the store, and a lot of crying that will result if you don't have the right kind of batteries on hand when your baby's favorite toy isn't working, by buying rechargeable batteries and a charger *today*.

Now that even mainstream battery companies—such as Duracell—have their own lines of rechargeable batteries, they're easier to buy than ever, in stores and online. Sure, rechargeable batteries cost around twice as much as regular ones, but you can use them over and over again—often hundreds of times. Rechargeable batteries are also better for the environment. They're the *real* energizer bunny.

You'll have to buy a charger as well. They vary greatly in price, from a few dollars on up to close to $100. Before purchasing a charger, consider how many batteries you can charge at a time, and how many different types of batteries the charger can charge. Some chargers can charge A, AA, C, and D batteries.

Even though they all came to our house, it wasn't a lot of work for me. I only served coffee and sweets.

—Judy Dudum, MD, a mom of three, an ob-gyn, and a senior staff physician at Henry Ford Health System in Detroit, with interests in nutrition and adolescent gynecology

❧

It's important to keep in mind that people don't expect you to write those thank-you cards the second you open their gifts. They just want to know that you got it in a reasonable amount of time. I was so fried from thank-you note writing!

—Michelle Paley, MD, PA, a mom of a six-year-old daughter and a two-year-old son and a psychiatrist and psychotherapist in private practice in Miami Beach, FL

Adjusting to Your Changing Center of Gravity and Preventing Falls

As your baby grows, your center of gravity changes, and it's easy to lose your balance. Falls are the most common cause of minor injury during pregnancy. Rest assured, your baby is well protected by the amniotic fluid, your uterus, and your abdominal wall.

Be especially careful if you're walking outside in bad weather when sidewalks and parking lots might be wet or icy. Take your time and hold the railing when you're walking up and down stairs. Try not to carry bags or other things that might throw you further off balance. Consider downsizing your purse if you tend to carry a big, heavy bag, which could throw you off balance. Eliminate tripping hazards in your home, such as throw rugs, electrical cords, and things left on staircases.

❧

During my pregnancies, I wore only sturdy, low-heeled shoes. When you're pregnant, your balance and center of gravity are off. This is not the time to wear high heels! It really is time to do everything to keep you safe. Falls can be largely prevented.

—Aline T. Tanios, MD, a mom of three and a general pediatrician and hospitalist who treats medically complex children at Arkansas Children's Hospital in Little Rock

I wear practical and sensible shoes all of the time. I'm fortunate that I get to wear scrubs to work, so there's no need for fancy shoes. I didn't have to buy anything new for my pregnancy. It's important to wear safe shoes while you're pregnant to prevent falls.

—Diane Connelly, MD, a mom of a six-year-old daughter and an ob-gyn in HMO practice in Riverside, CA

? When to Call Your Doctor or Midwife

If you fall, you might want to let your doctor or midwife know so that he or she could examine you. Be on the lookout for any bleeding, gush of fluid from the vagina, or severe abdominal pain. Any of those warrants an *immediate* call to your doctor or midwife.

RALLIE'S TIP

As my belly expanded during pregnancy, I found that I had more trouble keeping my balance, especially when I carried my purse or my briefcase slung over one shoulder. I once fell in the middle of the hospital parking lot for no apparent reason, and it was so embarrassing because two elderly ladies insisted on helping me up. I think I weighed more than both of them put together.

Packing the contents of my purse and my briefcase in a backpack helped distribute the weight more evenly, and it allowed me to keep both hands and arms free for better balance. In the final trimester, when the backpack was too heavy to carry comfortably, I transferred everything to a roll-behind briefcase. I could easily pull it wherever I went without struggling to keep my balance or straining to bear the extra weight.

Pacing Yourself

Pregnancy is a marathon, not a sprint. At times you might feel overwhelmed by how much you have to do to get ready for the baby. But just about every time, working steadily toward a goal will complete it faster than racing through it.

∾

Lots of women go a little nutty nesting during their pregnancies. Don't feel that you have to get everything done in your life at this time! Your to-do list isn't going anywhere. For example, why bother cleaning out your cupboards?

I was pretty easy on myself as far as that was concerned, especially during my pregnancies. I figured some things could wait for another day.

—*Kelly Campbell, MD, a mom of three and an ob-gyn in private practice at Women's Healthcare Physicians in West Bloomfield, MI*

With my twins, I was put on bed rest for a few months, and I delivered them at 29 weeks. On bed rest, I was forced to slow down and rest. But it's important for women who continue to work to rest as well. Slow down your body, and slow down your brain. Growing your baby is the most important thing you will do in your entire life.

—*Ruth D. Williams, MD, a mom of twins—a boy and a girl—and another boy, and an ophthalmologist in private practice at the Wheaton Eye Clinic in Wheaton, IL, who specializes in the diagnosis and treatment of glaucoma*

If I could do it over again, I would have taken more time out of my schedule during my pregnancies and not worked so hard. I would have done more stress-relieving activities and cut down on my work load.

I really pushed myself during my first pregnancy, but with my second pregnancy, I took better care of myself. I stopped working at 36 weeks, and I did all the right things. I felt so much better.

—*Gina Dado, MD, a mom of two daughters and an ob-gyn with Arizona OBGYN Affiliates, Paradise Valley Branch, in Scottsdale, AZ*

During my first pregnancy especially, I was at work and on my feet a lot. I worried that I was putting myself and my baby at risk, but in the middle of a busy night on call, you can't just sit down and take it easy. I pushed myself very hard because I didn't see any other option.

I was lucky, and my baby was born healthy, but in hindsight I should have realized I could ask for help. Now when my colleagues are pregnant, I work hard to compensate for them. When I see that they're fatigued, I try to go out of my way to make it okay for them to take it easy.

—*Alicia Brennan, MD, a mom of three daughters and the medical director of inpatient pediatrics of Children's Hospital of Philadelphia Pediatric Care at Princeton Health Care System in Princeton, NJ*

Thinking about Pain Control Options in Labor

At some point during your pregnancy, it will hit you, *Uh-oh, this baby has got to come out of me somehow.* Your next thought will probably be, *How can I do that in the least painful way possible?*

Fortunately, medicine has come a long way since Prissy proclaimed in *Gone with the Wind*, "Cookie say effen de pain get too bad, jes' you put a knife unner Miss Melly's bed an' it cut de pain in two."

One important thing to remember is everyone has a different pain tolerance, and every labor is different. Pain in labor is caused mainly by uterine contractions. Women feel pain in different places. You might feel the pain in your abdomen, groin, and back. Some women feel it in their sides or thighs, and others just feel achy all over. Women also feel the pain itself differently. Some women feel pain like menstrual cramps, while others feel it as severe pressure or strong waves that feel like diarrhea.

Depending upon your situation, you might be given several different pain control options. When most women think of pain control, they think of epidurals. An anesthesiologist inserts a thin, tube-like catheter into your spinal canal in your lower back. Through this catheter, medication can be given and carefully regulated. Some medicine does reach the baby, but not as much as with intravenous medicine or general anesthesia. Almost three-quarters of women in labor have epidurals.

Another way to relieve pain in labor is with pain medications such as morphine. They are given intravenously or by an injection. These medications affect your whole body, and they also affect your baby. Tranquilizing medications such as Valium or Versed can be given to calm and relax you if you're anxious. They can also affect both you and your baby, so they're used very cautiously.

Because there's no way to predict what your labor will be like, it's a great idea to educate yourself about your options and perhaps to put your wishes in writing in a birth plan. (See "Making a Birth Plan" on page 387.) But it's best not to get your heart set on a particular scenario. The best-laid birth plans do *often* go awry.

⟡

I actually didn't want to ease the pain much during my labor because I wanted to feel what it was like. My mother gave birth to me naturally, and it was important to me to do the same. Plus, my midwife reminded me that you don't want to take away all of the painful contractions. It's the pain that allows you to give birth.

I did use some homeopathic remedies in labor that took the edge off: Caulophyllum and Cimicifuga.

—*Lauren Feder, MD, a mom of two sons, a nationally recognized physician who specializes in homeopathic medicine, and the author of* Natural Baby and Childcare *and* The Parents' Concise Guide to Childhood Vaccinations, *in Los Angeles*

౨ೲ

A lot of women are scared of having an epidural, afraid of feeling a shot in the back. But I think that when you're in enough pain to want an epidural, the fear of getting a shot is eclipsed by the pain of labor. The issue becomes null and void. If you're in that much pain, you most likely won't be concerned in the least about a tiny needle going into your back. You will probably barely notice it. But you will notice the pain fading away about five minutes later.

—*Lauren Hyman, MD, a mom of two and an ob-gyn at West Hills Hospital and Medical Center in West Hills, CA*

౨ೲ

I knew that when I went into labor, I wanted to learn what contractions feel like. I figured that as an obstetrician, it would be a good thing for me to know. When labor started, my plan was to give it some time before asking for the epidural, but I definitely got an epidural both times.

—*Ashley Roman, MD, MPH, a mom of two daughters, ages three years and six months, and a clinical assistant professor in the department of obstetrics and gynecology at the New York University School of Medicine in New York City*

౨ೲ

I thought that I would probably like to have an epidural. I knew I was going to deliver at the hospital where I had done my residency, so I was very familiar with it, and I knew many of the staff there. Before I went into labor, I talked with some folks there to get an idea of who the best anesthesia residents were. I wanted to know who was particularly good at epidurals. I didn't mind having a resident because I know those guys were putting in 8 or 10 epidurals a day, and so they were probably the most practiced. But I didn't want a first-year resident!

—Diane Connolly, MD

RALLIE'S TIP

Toward the end of my third pregnancy, I thought I might try to deliver without an epidural. Because I had delivered two babies before, I was under the impression that this last baby would just slip right out with minimal effort. Wrong! After laboring painfully for a few hours without any anesthetic, I found myself getting extremely testy with my husband.

To make the birth experience more pleasant for everyone, including my poor husband, I finally asked for an epidural, and it was wonderful! In retrospect, I realize that if I had wanted to deliver my baby without an epidural, I should have spent a lot more time and energy preparing myself, mentally and physically. As it was, I was working at the hospital and taking care of my other two children right up to the day of my son's delivery, and I think my mind and my body were worn down by the stress of it all. I'm sure that lowered my pain threshold considerably.

The pain of labor and delivery can be very intense, and if you're not well rested and really ready to take on this challenge, it can be overwhelming. There's really no shame in asking your doctor for a little help with the pain. I've never met any woman who wished she had experienced more pain during labor and delivery!

I think these days, people try so hard to plan ahead that they get locked into decisions. For example, a lot of people think it's bad to have an epidural. I tried very hard not to make any decisions about my labor ahead of time. I had some guidelines about what I thought I might want, but nothing was set in stone. Make a plan, but be prepared for it to fall apart!

For example, you might vow not to have an epidural, and sure you could have a three-hour-long labor and not need one. But on the other hand, you could have been awake for 20 hours, labored for 23 hours, and then pushed for 4 hours, and be totally exhausted. Somewhere back there, you probably should have had an epidural!

—Susan Schreiber, MD, a mom of a son and daughter in their twenties and a pediatrician in Los Angeles, CA

When my two daughters were born, I had epidurals. But when I was pregnant with my son, I talked to some women who told me about their experiences with natural childbirth: how amazing and empowering it was. They said it was the most unbelievable experience of their lives.

I wondered, was I missing something? So I started seeing a midwife and thinking about trying natural childbirth myself. I attended natural childbirth classes and prepared myself for my natural delivery. But as they say, the best-laid plans so often go awry.

During an ultrasound late in my pregnancy, my doctor discovered that my son had a mass on his adrenal gland. We couldn't tell if it was a cancerous tumor or a benign blood clot until my son was born. The waiting was very difficult, so I persuaded my midwife to induce me, and I was able to deliver my son naturally, without pain medicine or an epidural. I'm glad that I experienced natural childbirth so that I know what it's like. I don't think it was the most empowering experience of my entire life, as I've faced lots of great challenges, but I'm definitely glad that I did it.

—Siobhan Dolan, MD, MPH, a mom of three, a consultant to the March of Dimes, and an associate professor of obstetrics and gynecology and women's health at Albert Einstein College of Medicine/Montefiore Medical Center in the Bronx, NY

I had to have three C-sections because my babies were all so big. But my biggest problem wasn't with the delivery at all; it was with the anesthesia *before* the delivery. The problem was they put the epidural in the wrong section of my back. It went in too high, and I wasn't able to swallow.

My epidural was put in by the attending physician at the hospital. In theory, that should have been a good thing because at a teaching hospital, the attending is the highest-level person there. But the problem is, the attending physicians are not necessarily the most up-to-date on their skills. That's because, in a teaching institution, the residents do most of the procedures. So the person who would be the most up-to-date on his or her skills would be the senior-level resident. He or she has been doing those procedures all day every day for the past few months.

Truth be told, you might not have a choice who gives you your epidural. But it might be a good idea to ask your ob-gyn or midwife about the structure of the hospital you'll be delivering at. For example, you could ask if there are medical students or nurse practitioners working with your anesthesiologist. At least you'd know ahead of time! And you could ask whom your ob-gyn recommends. Every situation—and every hospital—is different, but you can at least ask about your options ahead of time and adjust your mind-set accordingly.

— *Kristin C. Lyle, MD, FAAP, a mom of three girls and the disaster medical director at Arkansas Children's Hospital and an assistant professor of pediatrics at University of Arkansas for Medical Sciences, both in Little Rock*

Chapter 24
Week 24

Your Baby This Week

YOUR BABY'S SIZE

Your baby's crown-to-rump length is about 8½ inches, about the size of a soccer ball, and she's around a foot long from head to heels. She'll undergo a growth spurt this week, putting on around six ounces of fat plus bone and muscle mass.

YOUR BABY'S LATEST DEVELOPMENTS

By this week, your baby's brainwave patterns are similar to those of a newborn. Her brain is developing, and it can be monitored electronically on an electroencephalogram (EEG).

Your baby can now open and close her eyes. You might notice that she notices bright lights more now because she moves around in response to bright lights shining on your belly.

This week, your baby's lungs are developing. Cells are forming that will eventually produce surfactant, which prevents the tiny air sacs in her lungs from collapsing when she inhales. Babies who are born prematurely often have difficulty breathing because their lungs aren't developed.

Under your baby's skin, she's started to develop sweat glands.

Your baby already is curled into the fetal position inside your uterus. It's starting to get crowded in there.

YOUR LATEST DEVELOPMENTS

Your uterus is now a bit bigger than a soccer ball, and it's 1½ to 2 inches above your belly button. Your fundal height should be around 24 centimeters. You're probably gaining about a pound a week.

It's oddly appropriate that your uterus is the size of a soccer ball because it might feel like you have a small soccer *star* in there. Your baby is getting bigger and stronger now, so you probably feel her kicking and punching you. Most babies kick around 250 times a day, but anything from 50 to 1,000 times is normal.

Heartburn might be making you quite uncomfortable. It often gets worse around this time because your uterus is pushing up on your diaphragm and esophagus. This, plus the hormone relaxin, causes your stomach acids to defy gravity and squeeze upward. Try eating smaller, more frequent meals and staying upright after eating them.

Around this time, a different type of back pain sometimes develops. It's called posterior pelvic pain, and it originates at the back of your pelvis and radiates out to your left buttock, your right buttock, or both. You might find sitting for long stretches of time makes it worse. Lying down, having a massage, and applying a heating pad might ease the ache.

This week there's a good chance that you're itching more than ever. Your skin is stretching over your breasts and abdomen, and stretched skin can become very dry and itchy.

Sometime around this week, your doctor or midwife will likely ask you if you wish to bank your baby's cord blood. He or she will also probably send you for a glucose tolerance test to check for gestational diabetes. This test is done around now because your placenta floods your body with hormones that might inhibit the production of insulin.

After this week, if you have any signs of preterm labor, your doctor or midwife might suggest you have a fetal fibronectin (fFN) test, which helps to predict risk of premature delivery. (See "Preventing and Treating Preterm Labor" on page 305.)

JUSTIFICATION FOR A CELEBRATION

Around this time, your baby's palms are developing creases and lines. She becomes better able to use her hands each day as she becomes more coordinated.

Checking into Child Care

Especially if your energy is high and you're feeling good, this is a great time to start thinking about child care. There are many options to consider, depending on your needs, such as a day care center or a nanny.

Even if you won't be going back to work after your baby is born, it's beneficial to find some people to help you with your baby after she is born. Perhaps a family member, a friend, or a local teenager could watch your baby for a bit while you nap, shower, or run errands. Lining this up now will save you time, energy, and stress later.

∽

I checked into several day cares for my older son, and I chose one that was high-end and recommended. But my son hated it. It was so high pressure; they had SAT prep—for *preschoolers*!

I didn't want my kid to be under that much pressure. I transferred him to KinderCare so that he could be a kid.

—*Sonia Ng, MD, a mom of seven-year-old and one-year-old sons and a pediatrician and expert in sedation at Children's Hospital of Philadelphia Pediatric Care at Princeton Health Care System in Princeton, NJ*

∽

I was very particular about choosing my daughters' day care. I knew very clearly what I was looking for. As a doctor, you often work on instincts, and I've learned to trust mine. I had to walk into the day care and right away feel comfortable. For one thing, it had to have lots of sunlight. And of course it had to be very clean, and the providers needed to be very interactive. I also wanted to make sure the other children seemed happy and well cared for.

In one day care, the area where the children slept looked like they were in little cages in a dark closet. I couldn't get out of that day care fast enough.

The day care I chose was more expensive than the others I had visited, but it had a great reputation for enhancing education, and they had very strict hiring requirements. I had talked with other parents who sent their children there and gotten good reports. My instincts about that place were very good.

—*Alicia Brennan, MD, a mom of three daughters and the medical director of inpatient pediatrics of Children's Hospital of Philadelphia Pediatric Care at Princeton Health Care System in Princeton, NJ*

We have a nanny. In fact, I've only had two nannies in 16 years. I went through an agency, and I feel that referrals are very important. But during interviews, you have to know how to read between the lines and read people well.

—*Ann LaBarge, MD, a mom of four children, ages 16 to six, and an ob-gyn in private practice at the Midwest Center for Women's Healthcare in Park Ridge, IL*

One of the biggest challenges I've had since having kids has been child care. It was very helpful to have my nanny start working before my baby was born. It was a lifesaver because I had so much anxiety surrounding the birth and adjusting to the nanny. It enabled me to get to know the nanny ahead of time, and it helped her to feel more invested in the baby when she was born. This might not be applicable for a day care, but it would certainly be great for a nanny or babysitter.

Even before my baby was born, there was plenty of stuff for our nanny to do. She helped me to set up the nursery and prepared some meals in advance for us to freeze and then eat after the baby was born.

Also, don't wait too long to start looking for childcare. You want to do it before you get too big, cranky, and tired. I started to interview for a nanny about three months before my baby was born.

—*Michelle Paley, MD, PA, a mom of a six-year-old daughter and a two-year-old son and a psychiatrist and psychotherapist in private practice in Miami Beach, FL*

Having Vivid Dreams

Do you dream in Technicolor? During pregnancy, your mind is working overtime, and some of that can spill over into sleep. It's very common for pregnant women to have detailed, vivid dreams and to remember them more often than usual. Some women dream about water, fish, or even the sex of their babies. Other women dream about labor and delivery and holding their babies in their arms.

Experts think that dreaming is your subconscious mind's way of working out feelings and replaying ideas and thoughts about what has happened to you. Dreaming might help you to sort out your feelings and concerns and prepare you for being a mom. Some experts think that—you guessed it—pregnancy hormones cause this increased dreaming. Another reason why you might be dreaming more is because you're sleeping more. Plus, you're waking up to go to the bathroom more, so the dreams might be easier to recall than if you slept the whole night through.

❧

During my pregnancies, I had very vivid dreams. I never dreamed about the baby. I just dreamed all sorts of other crazy things.

—*Gina Dado, MD, a mom of two daughters and an ob-gyn with Arizona OBGYN Affiliates, Paradise Valley Branch, in Scottsdale, AZ*

❧

One natural thing that happens during pregnancy is dreaming. I found that keeping my journal next to my bed and jotting down my dreams was very instructive.

—*Nancy Rappaport, MD, a mother of two teenaged daughters and a teenaged son, an assistant professor of psychiatry at Harvard Medical School, an attending child and adolescent psychiatrist in the Cambridge, MA, public schools, and the author of* In Her Wake: A Child Psychiatrist Explores the Mystery of Her Mother's Suicide

Considering Cord Blood Banking

Deciding whether or not to bank your baby's umbilical cord blood is a very personal decision. Because you have only one opportunity to bank your baby's cord blood, on the day she's born, it can also be a very difficult decision to make. The blood in the umbilical cord contains stem cells, which have the potential to treat leukemia and some inherited disorders now and have the possibility of treating more diseases in the future.

When the baby is born, the cord blood is collected by the doctor or midwife. The blood is placed into bags or syringes and carried by courier to a cord-blood bank. There the sample is given an identifying number and frozen in liquid nitrogen. Theoretically, the stem cells can last forever if stored properly. But because the research only began in the 1970s, no one knows for sure how long they'll last.

Cord blood banking comes with a cost, around $2,000 for the

initial collection and processing and an annual storage fee of around $125. You can donate your baby's cord blood to a public bank for free, but it is not reserved for your family's use.

~

My husband and I decided to bank each of our children's cord blood. We thought we would do that just in case something happened. Researchers are finding more and more applications for stem cells, so I think that in the future cord blood might be even more useful. It's like life insurance.

—*Dianna K. Kim, MD, a mom of three and an ob-gyn in private practice in Vernon Hills, IL, at the Midwest Center for Women's Healthcare*

~

I did not bank my babies' cord blood, but now I wish that I had. It's like insurance; you pay for it, hope you don't use it, but it's there if you need to.

Even if you don't bank your baby's cord blood, you can donate the cord blood and that could still help someone. Don't throw it away.

—*Jennifer Kim, MD, a mom of three girls, ages eight, five, and four; an ob-gyn in private practice in Evanston, IL., at the Midwest Center for Women's Healthcare; and a clinical assistant professor at the University of Chicago, Pritzker School of Medicine*

~

I banked all three of my children's cord blood. When I was pregnant with my oldest daughter, we had a very limited income. My husband originally said we couldn't afford to bank her cord blood. I said, "Wait a minute. How much do those Starbucks you buy each day add up to in a year?" When he came up with the figure, I replied, "You can drink Folgers at home for a year, and we can do cord blood banking." That's how important it was to me.

For my second and third daughters, I used Cord Blood Registry, and that's the company I recommend to my patients when they ask. I highly recommend cord blood banking. It costs a one-time banking fee and then a storage fee each year, which is locked in at a set rate when your child is born. You only have one opportunity to save your child's cord blood. I knew that someday if my child needed it, I'd never forgive myself if I hadn't saved it because it's the simplest thing I could have done.

The current statistics are that a child born today who lives to be 70 has a 1 in 400 chance she will use her cord blood. She has a 1 in 200 chance that she or her sibling will use it. If you consider the research that's being done on regenerative medicine, the chance that a child born today who lives to age 70 would have the *opportunity* to use her cord blood is 1 in 10.

You can donate your baby's cord blood to some public banks for free. If a public bank has your sample, then it's free to you. However, there's no guarantee that your child's cord blood will be there if you need it. If you didn't save it or if you have a match that isn't yours in a public bank, it costs between $25,000 and $40,000 to get a sample for use.

I believe that when our kids today are adults, if they go to an emergency room for a heart attack or stroke, the nurse will ask, "Do you have your cord blood banked?" The answer to that question will determine their first step in treatment.

—*Marra Francis, MD, a mom of three daughters and an ob-gyn who's based in The Woodlands, TX*

When I was pregnant 11 years ago, I checked into cord blood banking, and it sounded like very good technology. I didn't know much about it at the time, but I got a discount as a physician, and it sounded like banking my baby's cord blood could only help, not hurt. It turned out to be one of the smartest things I ever did.

The day before my older daughter turned seven, we were out of town, and she developed bruises on her legs. It looked like someone had been kicking her. The next day, I noticed she had spots on her chest that looked like petechiae, which look like tiny blood blisters. I knew that could be a sign of abnormal blood clotting, so I started to get very concerned. I called her doctor, and he said that it was either leukemia or a condition called Idiopathic Thrombocytopenic Purpura (ITP), which is a blood disorder where the platelets become dangerously low.

The next morning, I gave my daughter a bath, and she bumped her head on the faucet. The bump on her forehead started out the size of a nickel, and it quickly swelled to the size of a tennis ball. We raced home to Scottsdale.

Our pediatrician ran several tests, and he determined that it wasn't leukemia, but rather ITP. A normal platelet count is 150,000. My daughter's was 7,000. Thank goodness, the condition resolved on its own, and in a few months my daughter was back to normal. But I shudder to think how close we came to leukemia, and how desperately we would have wanted to have that cord blood.

I highly recommend cord blood banking. On the Cord Blood Registry's website, you'll find an eight-minute tutorial about it. Visit www.CordBlood.com and click the "Video Tour" tab on the bottom.

Certainly there's a cost to bank and store your baby's blood, but I can tell you it is well worth it. That cost pales in comparison to the cost of treating conditions with other means, such as physical therapy and occupational therapy. The peace of mind is truly priceless, knowing that if something should happen to your child, especially as science advances, you might have the ability to cure a disease by having those stem cells. Plus, there are payment plans available, such as $50 per month. If you're creative, it's not hard to come up with that.

—*Gina Dado, MD*

Having a Glucose Tolerance Test and Managing Gestational Diabetes

Often this week, doctors and midwives send moms-to-be for a glucose tolerance test. This test checks for gestational diabetes, which is the particular type of diabetes that women get in pregnancy.

During the test, you'll be given several ounces of a beverage containing glucose to drink. After an hour, your blood will be drawn to check the level of glucose, or blood sugar.

Gestational diabetes affects around 4 percent of pregnant women. You're at greater risk for it if you're older than age 25, overweight, have prediabetes, or have a parent or sibling with diabetes.

No one knows for sure what causes gestational diabetes, but experts think that the hormones from the placenta block the action of the insulin in your body. This is called insulin resistance, and it makes it hard for your body to use insulin. Without enough insulin, glucose can't leave your blood and be used for energy by tissues in the body. The glucose builds up in your bloodstream, where it can wreak havoc, causing complications such as kidney disease and blindness.

Gestational diabetes can affect your baby as well. That extra

? When to Call Your Doctor or Midwife

Gestational diabetes often has no symptoms at all. But if you have excessive thirst or increased urination, talk with your doctor or midwife about it at your next appointment.

glucose in your blood crosses through the placenta, giving your baby high glucose levels. This gives her more energy than she needs, and the extra energy is stored as fat. That's why babies of moms-to-be with gestational diabetes are closely managed for weight. These babies are also at risk for breathing problems, obesity, and type 2 diabetes themselves.

If your glucose tolerance test comes back with elevated levels, your doctor or midwife will recommend more testing to determine if you have gestational diabetes.

During each of my pregnancies, I had the glucose tolerance test. I remember it being horrible, and I was so grateful that I only had to do the one-hour test, and not come back for the three-hour test.

—*Lezli Braswell, MD, a mom of one daughter and two sons and a family medicine physician currently working in an emergency room fast track in Columbus, GA*

About halfway through my pregnancy, I had to take the glucose tolerance test, which checks for gestational diabetes, the type of diabetes women get in pregnancy. I had to fast and then drink that wretched orange stuff. I thought it was gross, but you just suck it up.

There are many things you tolerate during pregnancy simply because you have to for your baby and because you want everything to be okay for your baby.

—*Rebecca Kazin, MD, a mom of three girls and the medical director of the Johns Hopkins Dermatology and Cosmetic Center at Green Spring Station in Lutherville, MD*

I had the glucose tolerance test, and I thought it was gross. It's yet another thing we pregnant women have to endure. I really didn't like the taste of the stuff, but I drank it anyway. Fortunately, I didn't have diabetes, so I didn't have anything to worry about.

—*Ashley Roman, MD, MPH, a mom of two daughters, ages three years and six months, and a clinical assistant professor in the department of obstetrics and gynecology at the New York University School of Medicine in New York City*

⌒⌒

I wanted so badly to pass the glucose tolerance test that I took it after fasting. It's not always necessary to fast, but I didn't want to have a false positive, so I didn't eat anything eight hours before the test to make *sure* I'd pass it.

—*Dianna K. Kim, MD*

⌒⌒

I took the glucose tolerance test in my second trimester as is commonly done. I don't like sweets and having to drink all of that sweet liquid almost made me throw up. But I was a good girl and kept it down!

It turned out I did have mild gestational diabetes. My doctor put me on an American Dietetic Association diet to manage it.

—*Diane Truong, MD, FAAP, a mom of one daughter and one son and a pediatrician in a multispecialty group practice in Southern California*

⌒⌒

I managed to fail my one-hour glucose screening during my second pregnancy. They scheduled me to have the three-hour test, but the day I was supposed to have it, I was hospitalized because I had gone into preterm labor. The doctors gave me steroids to help mature my baby's lungs, and they said that the steroids would likely make the three-hour test show up with a false positive, because steroids can increase blood sugar levels. So while I was in the hospital, they put me on special IV fluids and tested my blood sugar each morning and after meals.

I think it was just a fluke that I tested positive for gestational diabetes during that pregnancy because I've passed the test in my other pregnancies with no problem.

—*Kristie McNealy, MD, a mom of seven- and four-year-old daughters and a two-year-old son, who's pregnant with another son, and a blogger at www.KristieMcNealy.com, in Denver, CO*

Chapter 25
Week 25

Your Baby This Week

YOUR BABY'S SIZE

This week, your baby is around 8¾ inches from crown to rump, around 13.6 inches from head to heels. He continues to put on weight rapidly, gaining around six more ounces this week.

YOUR BABY'S LATEST DEVELOPMENTS

Your baby's face is developing definition, making him look more like himself every day. His nostrils were plugged before, but they begin to open around now, and he can practice "breathing" through his nose.

Around this week, if your baby has hair, you might be able to tell the color and texture at this point if you could see him. What color will it be?

Your baby's lungs are continuing to develop blood vessels. Capillaries, which are the smallest blood vessels in your baby's body, are developing beneath his skin and filling with blood. This gives him a beautiful, rosy pink complexion.

This week, your baby is still swallowing amniotic fluid, although most of his nutrition comes from you. Studies show that what you eat *now* will influence what your baby will eat *later*. That's big incentive to choose a banana over bonbons.

Your baby continues to learn how to use his hands. He will develop a strong grip during this month.

Around this time, your baby's spine is developing. This will help him to become more flexible and also more coordinated.

Your baby's bones are continuing to harden, and you probably feel him kicking more than ever.

If you are having twins, they are beginning to interact with each other, reaching out to touch their brother or sister.

YOUR LATEST DEVELOPMENTS

The top of your uterus is now about two inches above your belly button, about halfway between your belly button and your sternum. By now, it's about the size of a volleyball. All of that extra weight is probably giving you plenty of aches and pains.

Your eyes might be more sensitive and dry now. Artificial tears can help keep your eyes moist.

You might still be experiencing nausea, along with heartburn, gas, and bloating. Eating smaller, more frequent meals might help.

If your itchy belly is driving you to distraction, try moisturizing it with lotion.

Around this time, carpal tunnel syndrome (CTS) can become a problem. Some women even experience it before now. Your fingers might feel numb and tingly, and you might find it hard to grasp and hold on to things.

You might be tempted to have a keepsake ultrasound performed, to have one more peek at your growing baby. Talk it over with your doctor or midwife first. Ultrasound uses high-frequency sound waves to produce those images, and it's wise to limit your baby's exposure to them as much as possible.

JUSTIFICATION FOR A CELEBRATION

There's a good chance that your baby can distinguish between your voice and your partner's voice at this stage.

Choosing a Theme for Your Nursery

Not everyone chooses a nursery theme, but it can be fun to do. Stores such as buybuy Baby make it very easy to create a nursery theme with their coordinating baby-room collections, including bedding, lamps, light switch covers, photo frames, and more.

∽

I chose a theme for my daughter's nursery, and I actually used that same theme for my sons' room as well. The bedding pattern had little lambs on it, and on the wall I stenciled "The Lord is my shepherd." It was very sweet.

—*Lezli Braswell, MD, a mom of one daughter and two sons and a family medicine physician currently working in an emergency room fast track in Columbus, GA*

∽

With my daughter, my plan was to have a very gender-neutral nursery theme. We didn't know if we were having a boy or a girl. So I decided to be practical and choose decorations that would suit a boy or a girl.

But once my daughter was born, I wanted everything to be pink! I went back online and bought a fun, girly, pink nursery set. Practicality went out the window.

—*Michelle Paley, MD, PA, a mom of a six-year-old daughter and a two-year-old son and a psychiatrist and psychotherapist in private practice in Miami Beach, FL*

∽

I'm very pragmatic, and I worked so much during my pregnancies that I didn't have any nursery themes. Plus in Judaism, you're not supposed to do much of anything to prepare for the baby until after the baby is born.

I'm not particularly religious and only mildly superstitious, so I did bring home the gifts I received from my baby shower. But my mother was very firm about not setting up the nursery ahead of time. At the last minute in my pregnancy, I just threw a crib into the room and painted the walls.

—*Melanie Bone, MD, a mom of four "tweens" ages 15 to 12, a gynecologist, the founder of the Cancer Sensibility Foundation, and the author of the syndicated column* Surviving Life *and the book* Cancer, What's Next?, *in West Palm Beach, FL*

Writing a Will

If you don't have a will, this is a great time to write one. If you have a will, now's the time to name a guardian for your child. Without a will, the courts will decide who will care for your child if something happens to you and your partner.

Once you have your will, you might consider giving a copy to the executor. Also find a secure place to store your will and your other important documents, such as in a fireproof safe at home or in a safe deposit box at a bank.

⁓

After our first baby was born, my husband and I wrote our wills. It's so important in case, God forbid, something happens to us.

—*Ann LaBarge, MD, a mom of four children, ages 16 to six, and an ob-gyn in private practice at the Midwest Center for Women's Healthcare in Park Ridge, IL*

⁓

Shortly after I found out I was pregnant, I put together a will. I needed to know that if something happened to me, there was someone to step in and care for my daughter. I needed to make sure that this person and I were of

(✓) Mommy MD Guide–Recommended Product
Quicken WillMaker Software

You could pay an attorney hundreds of dollars to write a will for you, or you could do it yourself. A program called Quicken WillMaker Plus makes it easy. The program promises that it "assembles your forms from among 40,000 document possibilities—but so easy to use, you'll have them finished in minutes."

You can buy Quicken WillMaker Plus online for around $30.

Even with a do-it-yourself system, you might want to hire an attorney to look the will over. However, before you go this route, talk with the attorney first. He or she might actually charge more to do this than to just draw up the documents in the first place.

the same mind and that she would be able to help my daughter develop and to reach her goals.

—Christy Valentine, MD, a mom of one, a specialist in pediatrics and internal medicine, and the founder of the Valentine Medical Center in Gretna, LA

∽

During my pregnancy, I wrote a living will to explain my wishes in case something bad happened to me. In my living will, I assigned the decision-making to my mom, not my husband. My brother passed away when he was 19 years old, and my mom made all of his end-of-life decisions. Because she's been there before, I knew she would be able to handle it if need be. I was afraid my husband would panic.

I didn't show my husband my living will, so he didn't know that my mom was the decision-maker. But when I was in labor, the medications they gave me knocked me out. A nurse had borrowed my living will to photocopy it, and she returned it by mistake to my husband. Fortunately, he didn't get upset after I explained why I had written it the way I did.

—Sonia Ng, MD, a mom of seven-year-old and one-year-old sons and a pediatrician and expert in sedation at Children's Hospital of Philadelphia Pediatric Care at Princeton Health Care System in Princeton, NJ

Treating a Stuffy Nose

As if you needed more challenges to breathing when you're expecting, pregnancy can cause a very stuffy nose. The extra progesterone and estrogen in your body cause the mucous membranes to swell. You might feel especially congested in the wintertime, when dry air circulates to heat the house, or if you have a cold or the flu. Your ears also might feel full or stuffy.

Nasal saline sprays are safe to use. (See "Mommy MD Guide–Recommended Product: Ocean

> **? When to Call Your Doctor or Midwife**
>
> If you're desperate for relief from a stuffy nose, talk with your doctor or midwife, who might recommend some OTC products. If a stuffy nose is joined by fever, flu-like symptoms, or pain, call your doctor or midwife right away.

Spray" on page 147.) They lubricate nasal passages. Running a humidifier in your room might help by preventing the air from becoming too dry. It also might help to dab some petroleum jelly in your nose. And it can never hurt to drink more water.

❧

During my pregnancy, I was congested a lot. I think it's very common. I tried to stay well hydrated by drinking a lot so that my mucus could come out. But nothing helped much!

—*Patricia S. Brown, MD, a mom of two daughters, ages nine and seven, and a three-year-old son and a psychiatrist at Columbia-New York Child and Adolescent Telepsychiatry and in private practice in Cresskill, NJ*

RALLIE'S TIP

I had a stuffy nose with each of my pregnancies, but I didn't want to use medicated nasal sprays. Breathing in the steam from a cup of hot tea worked wonders for me. When I didn't have time for tea, I got a lot of relief from a few squirts of a saline nasal spray.

I have a deviated septum, so I'm used to nasal issues. During one pregnancy, I had a wicked sinus infection. It was so bad I went on antibiotics and decongestants, and finally I got better. (Talk with your doctor or midwife before taking this or any medication.)

—*Melanie Bone, MD, a mom of four "tweens" ages 15 to 12, a gynecologist, the founder of the Cancer Sensibility Foundation, and the author of the syndicated column* Surviving Life *and the book* Cancer, What's Next?, *in West Palm Beach, FL*

Coping with Carpal Tunnel Syndrome

During pregnancy, your wrists might swell, and this extra fluid puts pressure on the nerve that runs inside the carpal tunnel from your arm to your hand, causing carpal tunnel syndrome (CTS). This can be quite painful. It might be so bad that it wakes you up at night.

Carpal tunnel syndrome affects around 25 percent of pregnant women. The symptoms are numbness, tingling, and pain or a burning sensation. Eight out of 10 pregnant women who get CTS develop it in both of their hands.

You could try over-the-counter splints to support your wrists. But the best remedy for this is time. It usually goes away the first week after the baby is born.

᠅

In my third trimester, I developed carpal tunnel syndrome. I felt fine during the day, but at night my hands felt numb. It would actually wake me up at night. The one thing that helped was that I bought a large body pillow and propped my hands up on it at night.

Thank goodness, the carpal tunnel syndrome went away completely on its own by the time my baby was around six weeks old.

—*Kerri A. Daniels, MD, a mom of one toddler daughter and an instructor in the department of pediatrics at the University of Arkansas for Medical Science in Little Rock*

᠅

I had tremendous swelling during my pregnancy, and that led to carpal tunnel syndrome. It was difficult because my hands got so numb it was hard to work. It's helpful to soak your hands in warm water or wear splints that keep your wrists in a resting position. Of course, I didn't do any of that.

I did see a friend who's a hand surgeon. He said if it got too bad, he could give me a steroid injection. That didn't sound too pleasant, so I loughed it out. Fortunately, about eight weeks after delivery, the carpal tunnel syndrome went away.

—*Gina Dado, MD, a mom*
of two daughters and an ob-
gyn with Arizona OBGYN
Affiliates, Paradise Valley
Branch, in Scottsdale, AZ

∽

During most of my pregnancy, I felt great! You can eat what you want, and people are nicer to you. For example, they give you their seats.

But toward the end of my pregnancy, I developed very bad carpal tunnel syndrome. It began toward the end of my second trimester with tingling and pain. It felt like my fingers were falling asleep. It got worse and worse, and then it progressed to the point that I couldn't move my fingers or use my hands. It was very difficult. My husband had to turn on the water faucet for me so I could brush my teeth. I had to stop performing surgeries and go on maternity leave a week early. This was a very unusual, severe case, and most women who get carpal tunnel syndrome in pregnancy don't get it this bad.

Generally, carpal tunnel syndrome in pregnancy goes away after the baby is born. But not mine! It actually got worse. It was easy not to worry or focus on it because the first few months with a newborn are so hectic. By about three months, it went away, and my fingers and hands have been fine ever since.

—*Monica Lee-Griffith, MD, a mom of one, an ob-gyn, and senior staff,*
Henry Ford Health System in metropolitan Detroit

Chapter 26
Week 26

Your Baby This Week

Your baby's size

Your baby measures around 9¼ inches from crown to rump. She is starting to fill out now, and she weighs almost two pounds already.

Your baby's latest developments

Your baby's lungs are still relatively immature. She's practicing breathing movements in preparation for birth.

Around this time, your baby probably has gotten into a rhythm of sleeping and waking. Can you discern the pattern?

All five of your baby's senses are developed: sight, smell, hearing, taste, and touch. She is busy exploring her tiny world with them.

Your baby is now surrounded by around 16 fluid ounces of amniotic fluid. The pool of fluid is recirculated every three hours.

Your latest developments

By now you've probably gained around 16 to 22 pounds. The top of your uterus is about 2½ inches above your belly button. Your uterus grows both outward and upward. It's compressing your stomach and intestines. Even if you have a healthy appetite, you might not feel able to eat large meals.

You're probably feeling a lot of movement from your baby, and you'll continue to do so until around week 30. Your baby is getting cramped, but she can still maneuver enough for somersaults and big position changes. If your baby is still upright, with her head up, you might feel a sharp pain if her head hits your rib cage. Ouch.

Another cause of rib pain is that your rib cage is pushed outward to make room for your uterus. You might feel especially uncomfortable when you're sitting because this position compresses things even more. Change positions frequently and try to use good posture.

In preparation for breastfeeding if you choose to do it, the veins on the surface of your breasts darken and become more prominent. Those veins are a good sign of increased activity in the breasts—tissue growth and development in preparation for milk production. Your breasts might start to feel fuller now. High levels of estrogen and progesterone block the hormones that trigger milk secretion, but you might leak a bit of fluid. Not every woman does, however, so don't panic if you don't.

If your to-do list is a mile long, you might feel a lot of pressure to get things done. Try to let yourself rest now, before your baby is born. Around this time, fatigue often sets in. Whenever you have the chance, lie down on your left side. This position is best because it provides the best circulation for your baby.

JUSTIFICATION FOR A CELEBRATION
You're two-thirds of the way through your pregnancy.

Spending Special Time with Your Family

What a wonderful time this would be to enjoy a celebration, such as a dinner with your parents, tea with your aunts, or a weekend getaway with your sister.

~

I'm very close with my mom and aunts, and pregnancy presented lots of opportunities for bonding, such as teas and lunches. I especially enjoyed quiet times with my mom. While I was rubbing my belly, she'd tell me about when I was a baby in her belly and her experiences when I was first born.

—*Joanna Dolgoff, MD, a mom of a seven-year-old son and a four-year-old daughter, a board-certified pediatrician/child obesity expert with practices in Manhattan and Roslyn Heights, NY, creator of an online child weight loss program (www.DrDolgoff.com), and author of the book* Red Light, Green Light, Eat Right

RALLIE'S TIP

My oldest son was 12 when I got pregnant again. Having been an only child for so long, his life was about to change dramatically. Throughout my pregnancy, I tried to prepare him for the emotions that he might experience once the baby was born—joy, jealousy, and everything in between.

To celebrate his upcoming status as big brother, my husband and I took him and his best friend to Walt Disney World and Universal Studios before the baby was born. Looking back, I realize that preparing my oldest son to be a big brother ahead of time was important, but it was even more important to spend time alone with him after the baby was born.

Planning for Your Maternity Leave

If you haven't already done so, you'll want to begin planning your maternity leave. Perhaps your company has a policy of paid leave. The federal Family and Medical Leave Act usually allows for up to 12 weeks of unpaid leave either during your pregnancy or after your baby is born. Each state has different rules for the FMLA. A lot of people don't realize that you can take those 12 weeks of unpaid leave any time during the first year after your baby is born. However, if you work for a small company of fewer than 15 people, you're not covered by the FMLA.

It's best to talk with your human resources department about your options.

✧

I was a late bloomer. I started medical school at age 30, and I was pregnant with my son in my junior year. I certainly didn't get a paid maternity leave, so I saved up all of my vacation time. I was able to stay home with my son for almost three months, and then I took a seminar for another month that was only three hours a day.

—*JJ Levenstein, MD, FAAP, a mom of one son in college and a pediatrician in private practice in Southern California*

RALLIE'S TIP

I am the poster child for what not to do when planning your maternity leave. Because I had already had one baby in my second year of residency, my residency director was a little put out that I had "decided" to have another baby in my third year of residency. Actually, this wasn't a planned pregnancy, but my residency director said that as a doctor, I should be fully aware what causes it.

He said that I could have two weeks off and still graduate on time, but I would have to schedule my maternity leave three months in advance. I crossed my fingers and scheduled it to begin on my due date. Of course this baby didn't cooperate, and after burning up two days of my maternity leave with no sign of the baby, I called my ob in a panic. He was so kind and understanding; he told me to come right in so that he could induce me. I made a mad dash to the hospital, and my baby was born the next morning. After all that drama, I ended up taking eight weeks off and graduating late. I couldn't stand the thought of leaving my precious new baby to go back to work when he was just two weeks old!

✧

When I found out I was pregnant, I was working in an emergency room. In that job, you treat people, and then they go away. They don't come back to tell you how they're doing. I always wondered how my patients were doing. Were they okay?

So during my pregnancy, I was changing jobs to work in a primary care position, where I would have more continuity with patients. Because I was starting a new job, I was in a unique position when planning my maternity leave. I was able to negotiate all of that into my job position. I made sure that I would have some paid maternity leave time and be covered by health insurance.

Even though I had my maternity leave all planned for, I still saved up money throughout my pregnancy as if I didn't have a paid maternity leave to look forward to. That turned out to be a good idea because when I was seven months pregnant, Hurricane Katrina made landfall in the town where I worked, so I didn't get that much-planned-for paid maternity leave after all! The money I had saved turned out to be critical for my family and me to have the things we needed.

My family had all come to my house on August 27th to celebrate my birthday with cake and ice cream. We all left together the next morning to evacuate. With a town full of people all trying to get out at the same time, this was not a quick process. I had to keep stopping to go to the bathroom. But finally we made it out of town safely. We rented a house in Baton Rouge for a few months.

Looking back, I treasure that experience. That's what motivated me to open my own medical center. Looking at our city under water, I was determined to do what I could to help bring our city back even better than it was before.

—*Christy Valentine, MD, a mom of one, a specialist in pediatrics and internal medicine, and the founder of the Valentine Medical Center in Gretna, LA*

I was so, so old by the time I got around to having children that I had already fulfilled many of my professional goals—teaching residents and fellows in several different medical schools and all of that. I had written papers, run various programs, and been in many different practice arrangements. I knew that I wanted to stay home with my children and raise them myself.

This was an easy decision for me to make because I was no longer full of those burning, youthful, frustrated professional ambitions. I was in this sense really prepared for motherhood.

I was also in a privileged financial position as a doctor married to a doctor. I was able to make pretty good money working a limited number of hours, so I felt I was using my mind professionally, serving the public, and contributing something to our household income.

I stayed home with each infant about a month. I thought I'd go crazy staring at the laundry and the dishes in the sink for 24 hours a day. I should have gone back to work the next week! But I only worked three hours each day until my children went to school. Sometimes I hired an outside helper to stay at home with my offspring for a couple of hours while I ran to the office. Sometimes my husband and I would just take shifts, and I would work a few evenings and Saturday mornings.

I never worked full-time until my children went away to college. I always wanted to be the one to put them on the yellow bus for school in the morning and chat with them when they got home right after school. From my children's perspective, they always had an "at-home Mom" because I was always there whenever they were at home. In between, I ran to the clinic and taught and fought for funding and played hospital politics—so I had the best of all worlds. This was the wisest decision I ever made as a parent.

Naturally, having two full incomes is not the same as having one income. Every family has to evaluate this math problem, and many families cannot even consider a solution that does not involve mother working full-time. Hardship forces many women into full-time jobs. But I know that many women wish that they could be the one to kiss the boo boo, to see that loose tooth finally wriggle out, to hear all about it when the child bursts in the front door, to mind the brood during those long afternoons in the backyard. In my mind, these are the most precious experiences that life has to offer.

I want to support women who feel this way, but who feel isolated in our job- and money-oriented culture, as if they were being disloyal to their professional ambitions or as if they were contemplating doom by reducing their potential family income by even a little. I can tell these women that I wouldn't trade being home for my children for all the private schools, big new cars, and luxury vacations in the world.

—*Elizabeth Berger, MD, a mom of two, a child psychiatrist, and the author of* Raising Kids with Character

Touring the Hospital or Birth Center

Chances are good that you're looking forward to touring the hospital or birth center where you'll be delivering your baby. Your doctor or midwife has probably encouraged you to do this. Some hospitals offer tours in conjunction with prenatal classes. This is a great time to look around and ask questions.

I chose to deliver at a hospital in my neighborhood with both a birth center and a neonatal intensive care unit. My husband and I took a tour of the hospital and birth center when I was pregnant to familiarize ourselves with it.

—*Debra Luftman, MD, a mom of a teenaged daughter and a teenaged son, a board-certified dermatologist in private practice, a coauthor of* The Beauty Prescription, *the developer of the skincare line of products* Therapeutix, *and a clinical instructor of skin surgery and general dermatology at UCLA*

I didn't take a tour of the hospital I was going to deliver at because I had done my residency there. I was very familiar with it, and I knew a lot of the nurses there. I do think a tour is a great idea so you know what to expect of the hospital.

—*Diane Connelly, MD, a mom of a six-year-old daughter and an ob-gyn in HMO practice in Riverside, CA*

I didn't need to take a tour of the hospital I was going to deliver at. I worked there!

—*Melanie Bone, MD, a mom of four "tweens" ages 15 to 12, a gynecologist, the founder of the Cancer Sensibility Foundation, and the author of the syndicated column* Surviving Life *and the book* Cancer, What's Next?, *in West Palm Beach, FL*

Checking on Your Life Insurance

Now's the time to check into your life insurance policy or to get one if you're uninsured. You need coverage for both you and your partner. The amount of insurance you need is a highly personal choice, but the U.S. government estimates it costs between $250,000 and $300,000 to raise a child to age 18. Some experts recommend purchasing 6 to 10 times your yearly salary in coverage.

You might also want to check on and update the beneficiaries for your IRAs and/or 401(k).

My husband and I made sure when I was pregnant that we had enough life insurance on each of us that if something happens to one of us, the other one could pay off the house. I wouldn't want my family to be out on the street! The economy is hard nowadays. You can't always make it in a single-income family.

—*Sonia Ng, MD, a mom of seven-year-old and one-year-old sons and a pediatrician and expert in sedation at Children's Hospital of Philadelphia Pediatric Care at Princeton Health Care System in Princeton, NJ*

⤳⤺

My husband and I have always had life insurance, but just this past year, we increased it. It's so important to have insurance.

—*Ann LaBarge, MD, a mom of four children, ages 16 to six, and an ob-gyn in private practice at the Midwest Center for Women's Healthcare in Park Ridge, IL*

⤳⤺

When I found out I was pregnant, it motivated me to get all of the pieces of my life in order. For the first time, I got life insurance. It was really important to me to know that if something happened to me, my daughter would be cared for.

—*Christy Valentine, MD*

Chapter 27
Week 27

Your Baby This Week

YOUR BABY'S SIZE

Crown to rump, your baby measures around 9⅔ inches. Head to heels, he's around 15¼ inches long. He weighs almost two pounds.

YOUR BABY'S LATEST DEVELOPMENTS

Your baby's senses are becoming even more refined. This is a great time to start reading him stories, singing him songs, or playing him music. No doubt about it, he's listening!

Around this week, your baby's retinas develop their layers, which receive light and transmit it to the brain for interpretation. Your baby can see his hands, the placenta, and the umbilical cord. He might even turn his head now to look at things. Your baby's eyes stay open more now than they did before.

Pigmentation has begun in your baby's irises.

By the end of your baby's second trimester, his heart rate slows from 180 beats per minute to around 140 to 150 beats per minute.

Your baby by now has produced enough air sacs and surfactant that he is capable of breathing air. This dramatically improves his chances of survival even if born prematurely.

Around this time, your doctor or midwife might ask you to do kick counts. There are a few ways to do them. In one method, you might note how long it takes for your baby to move 10 times. Another method is to count how many times your baby moves in an hour. Kick counts can be very reassuring, and a great reason to sit down, relax, and tune in to your baby.

Even though your baby still has room to stretch out, he's probably quite happy in the fetal position. He feels safe, comfortable, and warm.

Your latest developments

This week, your uterus measures around 2¾ inches above your belly button. Your uterus is about the size of a basketball. If it hasn't happened yet, your belly button might pop out this week! You might be able to see it through thin shirts.

As your uterus grows, it's really crowding your lungs. If you've had a respite from feeling out of breath, your breathlessness is probably coming back. Your uterus is so large that the top of it rests *in* your rib cage. Some women feel out of breath from this point until the end of their pregnancies.

If your fingers are swollen, you might need to take your rings off and store them in a safe place until after your baby is born. It's a good idea not to take them to the hospital when your baby is born.

Your uterus is pushing your bones out of its way to make room. This is causing you aches and pains from your shoulders to your feet. Change positions slowly and rest however—and whenever—you can.

If you feel the odd sensation that your heart has skipped a beat, rest assured that this is common. It's usually not a worry, but it's a good idea to mention it to your doctor or midwife just in case.

Progesterone is slowing the movement of food through your digestive system. Because of this, food sits longer in your stomach than it usually does. If it feels like you ate a brick for breakfast, that's why. Your digestion slows during pregnancy so that your baby can pull every molecule of nutrition out of each bite of food that you eat.

Justification for a celebration

You've reached the end of your second trimester!

Buying Some Special Outfits for Your Baby

Perhaps you received a lot of clothing as gifts or passed down from friends or family members. Even if you have a lot of clothing for your baby, it's fun to go shopping for one special outfit, such as for your baby to wear home from the hospital or for a special occasion. Later, you might want to pack the outfit away to give to him when he's older, maybe when he has kids someday.

⤳

My husband and I bought a special outfit for our babies to wear the first time they went to church, which was when they were around six weeks old.

—*Judy Dudum, MD, a mom of three, an ob-gyn, and a senior staff physician at Henry Ford Health System in Detroit, with interests in nutrition and adolescent gynecology*

⤳

I'm Jewish, and in Jewish tradition, we don't do a lot of preparations until the baby is born safe and healthy. Generally, we try not to bring any baby things into the house until the baby arrives.

I did go with my mom to some baby stores to choose basics such as the baby's layette. We put everything on hold with a credit card number, and then when we called, the card was charged and the stuff was shipped.

My husband set up the crib after the baby was born while I was still in the hospital. I think the guy who delivered it helped him!

I'm a little superstitious, but thank goodness I had two healthy babies.

—*Janet Lefkowitz, DO, a mother of two girls and an ob-gyn in private practice in Rhode Island*

⤳

I received an amazing amount of baby clothing as gifts and clothes passed down by my friends. But I did buy my daughter a special Christmas outfit. It was a really cute red, corduroy jumper with "Baby's First Christmas" stitched in white on the chest and a matching white shirt underneath. I took lots of photos of her wearing that!

My aunt also bought her a Christmas outfit, so my daughter wore one outfit on Christmas Eve and the other on Christmas Day.

—*Kerri A. Daniels, MD, a mom of one toddler daughter and an instructor in the department of pediatrics at the University of Arkansas for Medical Science in Little Rock*

Mommy MD Guide-Recommended Product
Lil' Dressers Drawer Labels

If it feels like your baby's socks, onesies, and shirts are multiplying like rabbits and taking over your house, you're not alone. Organizing and reorganizing all of those tiny pieces of clothing can be a joy to some moms, but a royal pain to others.

One way to help keep things straight is Lil' Dressers Drawer Labels. You place the adorable labels on the outside of drawers to indicate what's stashed inside. They come in boys' packages and girls' packages, and each pack includes 18 labels, with illustrations of items such as shirts, pants, and socks.

Who knows, they might make it easy for your partner, and someday your child, to help put away the laundry.

You can buy Lil' Dressers Drawer Labels on **www.MommyMD Guides.com** for less than $10 a pack.

Buying a Car Seat

A car seat is critical; the hospital or birth center won't let you take your baby home without one.

Every aspect of buying a car seat can be very challenging—from deciding which seat to buy to installing it and even to using it correctly. Experts agree that the best car seat is the one that fits your child properly, installs in your vehicle correctly, and is easy to use.

The website of the National Highway Traffic Safety Administration (NHTSA) is an invaluable resource. All car seats rated by NHTSA meet federal safety standards and strict crash performance standards. While all rated seats are safe, they do differ in their ease of use in four basic categories: their instructions, labels, installation features, and ease of securing the child. The NHTSA offers a new five-star rating system for car seats that evaluates these four categories. Visit www.NHTSA. gov and search for "car seat ease of use."

Purchasing your baby's car seat might feel like the easy part compared with installing it in your vehicle. The NHTSA is there to help you with this as well. On their website, you can search for a car seat inspection station. Experts there will check to make sure that your baby's car seat is installed correctly—for free. Sometimes the best things in life *are* free. Your baby's safety depends on that car seat being installed correctly and on you using it every time that he rides in the car.

～◦～

Early on, we bought one of those car seats that doubles as a carrier. We bought two bases, and my husband installed one in each of our cars.

—*Kerri A. Daniels, MD*

～◦～

My husband and I bought a Graco Travel System, which is a stroller and a car seat combination. I highly recommend them. It makes life 100 percent easier to pop that car seat into the car and into the stroller and back again. That way you don't wake your sleeping baby trying to get him into and out of the car. Those travel systems were one of the best inventions ever.

—*Dianna K. Kim, MD, a mom of three and an ob-gyn in private practice in Vernon Hills, IL, at the Midwest Center for Women's Healthcare*

～◦～

I did buy car seats—several of them, actually. At one point, I had four car seats in my vehicle at the same time. We bought a full-size Chevy express van that seats 15—one of those things you take to and from an airport. To this day, our friends call it the Bone Bus.

You need a large vehicle if you have more than two car seats because you can't put two car seats next to each other. Luckily, our nanny was thin, and she could squeeze in between two car seats!

—*Melanie Bone, MD, a mom of four "tweens" ages 15 to 12, a gynecologist, the founder of the Cancer Sensibility Foundation, and the author of the syndicated column Surviving Life and the book* Cancer, What's Next?, *in West Palm Beach, FL*

～◦～

My friends held a wonderful baby shower for me, and my coworkers surprised me with another one. I received many helpful, thoughtful gifts. But the most helpful thing for the baby, I actually bought myself.

Back in 2000, while I was reading an American Airlines magazine, I read about a car seat that has rollers that come down like Rollerblades. In essence, the car seat transforms into a stroller for traveling. I bought one before my daughter was born, and it was invaluable. My husband and I took my daughter on planes often to visit her grandparents. People would stop us all the time in airports and ask where we got that car seat.

One brand that's currently sold is called the Sit 'n' Stroll car seat. You can buy them online. We also bought and installed a traditional car seat in each of our cars for everyday use.

—*Mary Mason, MD, a mom of a nine-year-old girl and six-year-old boy, an internist, and the chief medical officer for a multi-state managed care company that coordinates care for about 70,000 pregnant Medicaid moms a year*

Preventing and Treating Preterm Labor

Preterm labor is defined as labor before you've completed 37 weeks of pregnancy. Studies show that moms older than age 35 have a 20 percent higher chance of having a baby before 37 weeks. Warning signs of preterm labor include backaches, dull cramps, and discharge.

It's reassuring to know that you can control some causes of preterm labor. First, don't smoke and stay out of secondhand smoke. Next, avoid alcohol and drugs, standing for hours at a time, and regularly lifting heavy loads. Last, use good dental hygiene to avoid gum infections.

You also have modern medicine on your side. If you're at risk for preterm labor, between weeks 24 and 34, your doctor or midwife might recommend that you have a fetal fibronectin (fFN) test. This test checks for a protein called fetal fibronectin, a protein that attaches the fetal sac to the uterine lining. The quirky thing about fFN is that it's normally present in your vaginal secretions up to around week 22, then it usually disappears from around weeks 24 to 34, and then it's usually present again after around week 38.

During an fFN test, your doctor or midwife collects a sample with a swab; it is very similar to a Pap test. After around 24 hours, you'll have the results. If fFN is present between weeks 24 and 34, it means that your body is "leaking" fetal fibronectin, and there's a possibility of preterm labor and delivery.

On the flip side, women who have a negative fFN test have a less that 1 percent chance of delivering within the next two weeks.

❧

During my second pregnancy, I was working at a grueling job. I went into early labor, with regular contractions, and so I went to the hospital. They sent me home for two days of bed rest. I wasn't very good at resting. I spent those two days cleaning and organizing my house! I continued to have contractions, and my daughter came a little early—five days before her due date.

—*Patricia S. Brown, MD, a mom of two daughters, ages nine and seven, and a three-year-old son and a psychiatrist at Columbia-New York Child and Adolescent Telepsychiatry and in private practice in Cresskill, NJ*

? When to Call Your Doctor or Midwife

Signs of preterm labor might include watery, mucous, or bloody vaginal discharge; menstrual-like cramps; low, dull backache; pelvic or lower abdominal pressure; abdominal cramps with or without diarrhea; your water breaking; or contractions every 10 minutes or more frequently.

If you experience any or all of these symptoms, stop what you are doing and call your doctor or midwife right away. Your doctor or midwife might tell you to rest on your left side for an hour and drink two or three glasses of water or juice.

I had preterm labor at about 6 months, and I was monitored in the hospital overnight. I was careful to stay hydrated. I drank something every hour or two and monitored the color of my urine and how often I went. I wanted to be sure I was peeing every three to four hours at least—and not just because the baby was pressing on my bladder, but because I was actually making urine! It's important to drink water. Dehydration is a risk factor for preterm labor.

—*Sharonne N. Hayes, MD, a mom of two and the director of the Women's Heart Clinic at Mayo Clinic in Rochester, MN*

❧

At my 21-week ultrasound, I found out I was having twins, a boy and a girl. It was the perfect dream, but soon after that I started to have the complications and began the complex journey that people often have with twins. My pregnancy quickly got difficult, and it stayed that way for a long time.

I went into preterm labor, but I didn't know it right away because I didn't know what to look for. I remember going on walks with my sisters-in-law and feeling my belly tightening. We thought it was Braxton Hicks contractions, which are often called false contractions. It didn't hurt; it just felt tight. But when I was talking with my doctor, she said that was actually labor. She put me on strict bed rest for the rest of my pregnancy.

It can be very difficult to distinguish between Braxton Hicks contractions and labor contractions. Call your doctor or midwife right away if you are having contractions.

—*Ruth D. Williams, MD, a mom of twins—a boy and a girl—and another boy, and an ophthalmologist in private practice at the Wheaton Eye Clinic in Wheaton, IL, who specializes in the diagnosis and treatment of glaucoma*

With my son, I went into labor at 31 weeks. I was treated with some medication to try to stop my labor, but it made me very sick. One day when I was in the ICU due to a reaction to the medications used to stop labor, something happened that really helped me. A nurse came in and showed me a photo of her eight-year-old son—a thriving, handsome boy. The nurse explained that he, too, had been born premature. Her gesture was so meaningful to me. And then she offered to wash my hair. I was so grateful.

It was a difficult time, and I don't think I coped any better or worse than any other woman would have. You do what you have to do for your children.

—*Julie Silver, MD, a mom of a 17-year-old son and 13- and 9-year-old daughters, a Boston-area physiatrist, and the award-winning writer of more than a dozen books, including* After Cancer Treatment: Heal Faster, Better, Stronger

During my second pregnancy, I went into labor 10 weeks early, at 30 weeks. I had been having random contractions. When my doctor checked me, he said I was around a fingertip dilated, and he sent me home.

But I still had a nagging feeling that something wasn't right. I went back to the office three times that week. Finally, they put me on the monitor to see if I was having contractions. I was on the monitor for half an hour, and I had six contractions. They said, "Okay, you're right. You need to go to labor and delivery right away." My baby was born a week later, at 31 weeks. You know your body better than anyone. If something doesn't feel right, speak up and *keep* speaking up until you're heard.

—*Kristie McNealy, MD, a mom of seven- and four-year-old daughters and a two-year-old son, who's pregnant with another son, and a blogger at www.KristieMcNealy.com, in Denver, CO*

When I was around 30 weeks pregnant with my son, my family and I had planned to fly to San Francisco to take our daughter to a museum. I asked my obstetrician ahead of time if it was okay for me to fly. She said that it was no problem. She's also a good friend, and she asked me if I wanted her to check me first to make sure I wasn't dilating. I said that I wouldn't want her to treat me any differently than any other patient, so no.

In the evening after we returned from the museum, I had a little bit of bloody discharge. I called my ob, and she told me to fly home right away. It was the first time I'd ever been wheeled through an airport; my husband pushed my wheelchair while I held our daughter on my lap.

When we got home, I went to my ob's office, and she discovered I was four centimeters dilated and having regular contractions. I hadn't even felt them! She admitted me to the hospital right away and put me on medication to stop my labor. She also gave me steroid shots to help mature my baby's lungs. She put me on strict bed rest at home for the rest of my pregnancy. My son was born at 37 weeks.

—*Diane Truong, MD, FAAP, a mom of one daughter and one son and a pediatrician in a multispecialty group practice in Southern California*

Shopping for New Shoes for Your Bigger Feet

Pregnancy truly changes everything—from the top of your head to the bottom of your feet. Many pregnant women's feet swell and flatten so much that they go up a half to a whole shoe size during pregnancy.

Don't give away all of your old shoes just yet, though. It's possible that your feet might return to their pre-pregnancy size after your baby is born.

My feet were terribly swollen during my pregnancies. Early on, I had to abandon my high heels in favor of ugly Grandma shoes. You do what you have to do for your kids.

— *Michelle Paley, MD, PA, a mom of a six-year-old daughter a two-year-old son and a psychiatrist and psychotherapist in private practice in Miami Beach, FL*

During my pregnancy, my feet swelled a lot. I was grateful that my hands didn't, and I could still wear my rings.

But my feet got to be so big that I had to buy Velcro Sketcher shoes. The Velcro allowed me to make them larger or smaller as my feet changed. The shoes were dark brown and quite ugly. They were the only shoes I could wear the last six weeks of my pregnancy.

After our daughter was born, my husband said, "I never want to see those shoes again!"

—*Kerri A. Daniels, MD*

Toward the end of my pregnancy, my feet got bigger, and I started to wear hospital-type shoes. They were roomier and wider, and they offered orthotic support. I wore them with everything. My entire outfit every day was designed around those shoes.

I believe those shoes also helped me avoid back pain because they offered a lot of support. On the few occasions when I tried to wear other shoes, my back would hurt.

—*Christy Valentine, MD, a mom of one, a specialist in pediatrics and internal medicine, and the founder of the Valentine Medical Center in Gretna, LA*

During my pregnancy, I had a tremendous amount of swelling. My feet were so swollen they looked like puffer fish. I couldn't wear any of my regular shoes. I could only wear gym shoes and flip-flops. Thankfully, I live in sunny Arizona, and so I wore flip-flops even with nice dresses.

There's no better time than pregnancy to have a pedicure. Pregnancy can make your feet feel tired and achy. Plus you might not be able to reach your feet, or even to see them right now, to take good care of them yourself.

A pregnancy pedi would be great, for many reasons. You'll feel pampered, your feet will feel less painful, and you won't have to worry about taking care of your toenails for a few weeks to boot!

Of course, now more than ever, you want to be safe. Make sure that the pedicure area looks clean, and it's a great idea to confirm that it has a good rating by the Health Department. Check out the bathrooms as well because they can be a good indication of the facilities' overall cleanliness. Make sure that the pedicure instruments look very clean and sterilized and that disposable supplies such as orangewood sticks are indeed thrown out after every client.

Don't shave your legs before having a pedicure. Shaving can cause very small nicks in the skin that can allow bacteria to enter from the whirlpool, leading to an infection.

If you have gestational diabetes, don't have a pedicure. Ask your partner to give you a good foot rub instead.

Even after my babies were born, my feet didn't quite return to their pre-pregnancy size. There are shoes I never got back into and had to give away.

—*Gina Dado, MD, a mom of two daughters and an ob-gyn with Arizona OBGYN Affiliates, Paradise Valley Branch, in Scottsdale, AZ*

During my pregnancy, my feet swelled so much I went up two shoe sizes. I bought clogs from www.Allheart.com and Lands' End. They were loose and conformed to my feet. I love clogs. As soon as I had the baby, my feet went back to their old size.

—*Sonia Ng, MD, a mom of seven-year-old and one-year-old sons and a pediatrician and expert in sedation at Children's Hospital of Philadelphia Pediatric Care at Princeton Health Care System in Princeton, NJ*

The first time I was pregnant, I remember my feet getting to be so big that none of my shoes fit. Residents wear clogs, which are very forgiving, so I was able to make it through the workday. But I remember one night I was meeting my husband for dinner after work, and I could only fit into sneakers with the laces open!

I desperately needed to get new shoes. Thankfully, it was a Friday night, and I had the time to go shopping for shoes the very next day. I bought a pair of low slingbacks with an elastic strap on the back because I believed that my feet would go back to their normal size. But they never did. I wore size 7 shoes my entire life, but now I'm an 8. It took me a while to accept that and get rid of an old pair of Doc Martens lace-ups that I had, but I finally got rid of all of my old shoes, and I've moved on.

—*Siobhan Dolan, MD, MPH, a mom of three, a consultant to the March of Dimes, and an associate professor of obstetrics and gynecology and women's health at Albert Einstein College of Medicine/Montefiore Medical Center in the Bronx, NY*

∼⌢∽

Many women's feet get a full size larger during pregnancy, and some never return to their original size. Fortunately, I was the exception to that rule!

During my first pregnancy, I pretty much wore my regular heels up until the week before delivery. Then I simply wore my comfortable, flat, operating room shoes, which are sort of like sneakers.

In my second pregnancy, I was having triplets, and I was home on bed rest after week 25. I don't wear shoes in my home, so it wasn't an issue. On the rare occasions I went out, I wore my operating room shoes. But after my babies were born, I was delighted to find that all of my old shoes still fit.

—*Sadaf T. Bhutta, MBBS, a mom of a three-year-old daughter and 18-month-old triplets and an assistant professor and the fellowship director of pediatric radiology at the University of Arkansas for Medical Sciences and Arkansas Children's Hospital, both in Little Rock*

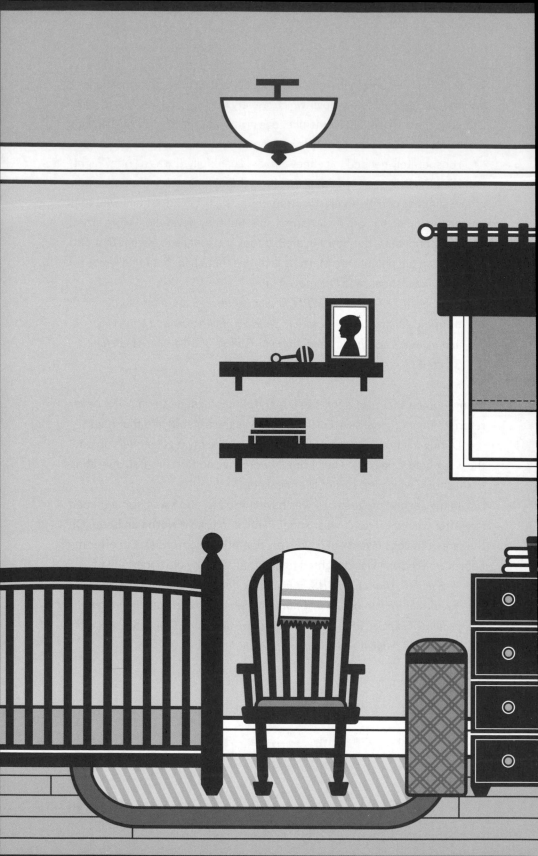

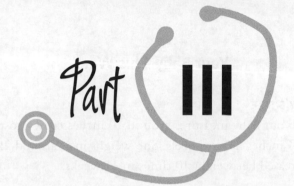

Part III

YOUR THIRD TRIMESTER

Chapter 28
Week 28

Your Baby This Week

Your baby's size

This week your baby measures around 10 inches crown to rump, and around 15¾ inches head to heels. She weighs in at around 2½ pounds, having increased her weight 10 times in 11 weeks.

Your baby's latest developments

Amazing transformations are under way in your baby's brain. Prior to now, your baby's brain appeared smooth. But around this week, your baby's brain begins to form grooves and indentations on its surface.

Your baby's hair and eyelashes continue to grow. Some babies need a haircut a few weeks after birth, while others don't need a trim for many months.

If your baby's eyes haven't already opened, around now, they will open again. Most babies have blue eyes when they're born, and their final color isn't set until they're around nine months old. Now that your baby's eyelids can open, she can blink and becomes much more aware of light differences. Around this time, your baby can start to focus her eyes. When she's born, she'll be able to focus to around eight inches away, which is about where your face will be when you cradle her in your arms.

Your baby now has clearly defined skin creases and perfectly formed fingernails.

As your baby puts on weight, she looks plumper and rounder.

You're probably wondering how your baby is lying. Around this time, some doctors and midwives start to make note of the baby's position at each office visit. The position of your baby might be oblique (lying at an angle across your uterus), longitudinal (vertical with her head down, which is called cephalic presentation, or bottom down, which is called a breech presentation), or transverse (lying horizontally across your uterus). It can still be difficult to tell just by feeling your abdomen. Plus, your baby still has enough wriggle room that she can change position. In another three or four weeks, your baby's head will be harder and it will be easier for your doctor or midwife to figure out how she is lying.

YOUR LATEST DEVELOPMENTS

Welcome to your third trimester. You're in the homestretch!

Your uterus is now around 3½ inches above your belly button. By this time, you've probably gained between 17 and 24 pounds, but more or less is probably just fine, depending on what you weighed when you began this great adventure.

There's a good chance you'll start to feel more Braxton Hicks contractions. Talk with your doctor or midwife about how to tell them apart from regular contractions.

Around now, you might actually be able to see your baby move, such as a foot or an arm pushing out.

You are probably finding it harder and harder to get comfortable, especially when you're trying to sleep. Maternity stores and websites sell products that might help, such as a wedge-shaped pillow that you slide under your belly for support.

If you are Rh-negative and your partner is Rh-positive, you'll receive an injection of RhoGAM this week, and another one after your baby is born. This prevents your immune system from attacking your baby.

JUSTIFICATION FOR A CELEBRATION

Babies born this week have a 95 percent survival rate.

Decorating Your Nursery

Perhaps you've already chosen a theme for your baby's nursery. Maybe you received some decorations as gifts. This is a great time to pull it all together and decorate your baby's nursery.

But before you go all Ty Pennington and pick up a paint scraper, consider the age of your home. Prior to 1978, many apartments and houses were painted with lead-based paint. If you live in an older home, visit www.epa.gov/lead for information on how to test for and remove lead-based paint—a task that you'll need to delegate to someone else because lead residue can cause miscarriage and low birth weight.

❧

For my first baby, my husband and I decided not to find out ahead of time if we were having a boy or a girl. We decorated the nursery in neutral colors, mainly white.

> —*Judy Dudum, MD, a mom of three, an ob-gyn, and a senior staff physician at Henry Ford Health System in Detroit, with interests in nutrition and adolescent gynecology*

❧

My husband and I decided not to find out if we were having a boy or a girl. I chose a neutral theme for the nursery and decorated around a wallpaper border of a little girl standing with her dog. It was such a hectic time in my life that I didn't finish the nursery until about two weeks before my son was due. Good thing he was born two weeks late!

> —*Karen Heald, MD, a mom of four boys and a board-certified family physician in private practice outside Atlanta, GA*

❧

I'm a total pragmatist, and I don't spend a lot of time decorating. It's not my gig.

When I was pregnant with my twins, I did paint a big picture on the wall of the nursery of my older daughter and the twins holding balloons. While I was painting it, my daughter walked into the room. She took off running, and I heard her yell, "Daddy, Mommy's painting on the wall!"

> —*Susan Wilder, MD, a mom of an older daughter and twin girls, a primary care physician, and CEO and founder of Lifescape Medical Associates in Scottsdale, AZ*

For some reason, during my pregnancy I was drawn to the color orange. I found baby bedsheets that I loved. They are light blue with orange embroidered birds. I also bought a white, wrought-iron crib. Along with a rocker glider and a cute rug, the nursery came together beautifully.

Amy J. Derick, MD, a mom of one 15-month-old son who is 17 weeks pregnant with her second son. Dr. Derick is a dermatologist in private practice at Derick Dermatology in Barrington, IL

My husband and I moved into a house a few months before our daughter was born. When we moved in, the nursery was painted beige, which was just fine with me. But one day, my husband decided that because we were having a girl, she needed a pink room, so he repainted it pink.

I bought a crib and changing table online, and I picked out a pretty pink and green bedding pattern that has flowers and bees on it. It came with matching wall art and a lamp. The room came together beautifully.

—Kerri A. Daniels, MD, a mom of one toddler daughter and an instructor in the department of pediatrics at the University of Arkansas for Medical Science in Little Rock

During my first pregnancy, I was a resident, working 110 hours a week! At that point in life, I was generally in overdrive anyway, and very organized. I find that when I have little time, I make the most of it because there's no other option. Also, like many doctors, I'm the kind of person who likes to have things in order. So I was nesting and organizing and preparing for my baby at light speed.

For each of my pregnancies, my husband and I decided not to find out our baby's gender. We liked the element of surprise, and I think a baby's gender is one of life's last great surprises.

For each baby, I'd go to the store and choose one style of bed linens if the baby was a boy, and another style if the baby was a girl. Then I'd dispatch my husband to pick them up after I had the baby.

—Kathie Bowling, MD, a mom of three grown sons and an ob-gyn in private practice in Providence, RI, who's also on the clinical faculty at the Warren Alpert School of Medicine at Brown University

Buying Baby Equipment

It's a wonderful time to become a mom. An entire industry longs to make motherhood easier for you! Stores such as Target and Walmart have expansive baby departments, and entire stores such as buybuy Baby are dedicated to baby gear.

At times it can be hard to choose because there are so many wonderful products available. You'll find websites and books that offer recommendations on baby products, and your friends and family members will likely love to share their opinions on what worked for them.

Here's one important safety precaution. Never buy baby equipment such as cribs, play yards, and car seats from yard sales or consignment shops. These used products likely don't come with safety manuals, and they could have been recalled or involved in an accident.

Several agencies and organizations test and rate products on cost, durability, and safety. Look for the Underwriters Laboratories seal, which is a sign that the product has been tested for safety. The U.S. Consumer Products Safety Commission (www.CPSC.gov) is your go-to resource for safety information and product recalls.

Happy shopping!

Mommy MD Guide-Recommended Product
White Noise Machine

For months, your baby has been lulled to sleep by the soothing—and loud!—sounds of the beating of your heart and blood rushing through your arteries. These sounds bring her comfort and make her feel safe. You can help to re-create some of this comfort in her nursery with a white noise machine.

As an added benefit, a white noise machine will help to mask some of the noise in your house. Then you won't have to tiptoe all over your home when your baby is asleep.

You can buy white noise machines in all shapes and sizes in stores and online. You can even buy them disguised as teddy bears! They can cost as little as $25.

During my first pregnancy, I was put on bed rest at 22 weeks. My husband went out by himself to buy a crib. He told me that the saleslady said it was the first time she had ever sold a crib to a man shopping all by himself!

—*Ruth D. Williams, MD, a mom of twins—a boy and a girl—and another boy, and an ophthalmologist in private practice at the Wheaton Eye Clinic in Wheaton, IL, who specializes in the diagnosis and treatment of glaucoma*

Having had three babies, I can say that the number one thing I couldn't live without is a baby swing. All three of my babies had horrible acid reflux, and the only way they slept was sitting in that swing. They wouldn't sleep for 10 minutes in their cribs, but they'd sleep for 12 hours in the swing. My second baby slept in it until she was a year old.

—*Kristie McNealy, MD, a mom of seven- and four-year-old daughters and a two-year-old son, who's pregnant with another son, and a blogger at www.KristieMcNealy.com, in Denver, CO*

One thing that was important to me to buy before my baby was born was a jogging stroller. I did a lot of research into that purchase because you aren't supposed to use a lot of jogging strollers until the baby is six months old. I found that a helpful book for product research is *Baby Bargains*.

—*Mary Mason, MD, a mom of a nine-year-old girl and six-year-old boy, an internist, and the chief medical officer for a multi-state managed care company that coordinates care for about 70,000 pregnant Medicaid moms a year*

When I was pregnant, I turned to my friends who already each had two or three kids. They were especially helpful when I had questions about baby things. As a first-time mom, it's so easy to get wrapped up in the details of which stroller to buy and what diaper bag to get. I remember feeling so overwhelmed trying to decide which of the 1,000 strollers to buy. But my friends who have kids brought me back to reality. They were past all of that nonsense, and they knew what I needed.

Regarding the stroller, a friend of mine said that you want something light and easy to fold with one hand. You want to be able to collapse it quickly and easily in the mall parking lot with baby in one hand and trying to grab your toddler who's trying to run away from you.

One thing I didn't get is the baby wipe warmer. But it's funny, my two-year-old son just told me that the wipes are too cold on his bottom!

—*Michelle Paley, MD, PA, a mom of a six-year-old daughter and a two-year-old son and a psychiatrist and psychotherapist in private practice in Miami Beach, FL*

A friend went with me to the baby supply store to pick out things for my baby, and I found so many of those purchases to be helpful. One thing that was especially great, even though it wasn't expensive, was a toy that sticks to the baby's high chair tray. It distracted my baby during meals. It only cost a few dollars, but it was very helpful.

Another thing that I found to be invaluable for my second and third babies was a white noise machine. It helped them sleep despite other noise in the house. If you don't have a white noise machine, you can just tune a radio to static and crank up the volume.

The *most* helpful item for us was our ExerSaucer. It was awesome. We

Mommy MD Guide-Recommended Product
Munchkin Baby Wipe Warmer

"When I registered for baby things, I wasn't a big fan of the baby wipe warmer," said Joanna Dolgoff, MD, a mom of a seven-year-old son and a four-year-old daughter, a board-certified pediatrician/child obesity expert with practices in Manhattan and Roslyn Heights, NY, creator of an online child weight loss program (www.DrDolgoff.com), and author of the book *Red Light, Green Light, Eat Right*. "But when the time came for my first middle-of-the-night changing, I was so happy that I had warm wipes for my baby's tushy. As a doctor, I thought a wipe warmer was silly. But as a mom, I thought it was great."

You can buy a wipe warmer, such as Munchkin Warm Glow Wipe Warmer or No More Dry Wipes Deluxe Wipe Warmer, in stores and online for around $25 to $30.

borrowed one for our first baby, and it was so helpful that we bought one for the second baby. We used it all of the time. The baby played and snacked in it in the kitchen while I was cooking Then we'd move it to the TV room while we watched a show. It was perfect for keeping the baby entertained—and safe.

—Dianna K. Kim, MD, a mom of three and an ob-gyn in private practice in Vernon Hills, IL, at the Midwest Center for Women's Healthcare

During my pregnancies, I didn't have a baby shower, but currently two of my older children are pregnant, and they are having showers. It's amazing the gadgets they have now. One of my kids got a baby wipe warmer!

When my first babies were born, I used cloth diapers. We didn't even have running water, and I drove to town once a week to wash dirty diapers. My hope is that we don't teach our children that they can buy every comfort. I hope we hold on to the real treasures of sunrises, the magic of each moment, and love—not things!

—Hana R. Solomon, MD, a mom of four, ages 35 to 19, a board-certified pediatrician, the president of BeWell Health, LLC, and the author of Clearing the Air One Nose at a Time: Caring for Your Personal Filter

When my babies were born, I was young. We didn't need much in the way of gear. It was 1973; we didn't even need car seats! We didn't need swings or breast pumps. We didn't need baby monitors because our homes were small; we were in the same room or the next room all of the time. My friends passed down clothes, cloth diapers, and plastic pants, and that was about all we needed. I crack up at what moms think they need now.

—Stacey Marie Kerr, MD, a mother of two grown daughters, a family physician with strong roots in midwifery, and the author of Homebirth in the Hospital, *in Santa Rosa, CA*

Considering a Doula

In Greek, *doula* means "female helper." A doula is a person who's been trained in childbearing and delivery. She can provide you with support during your pregnancy, during birth, and even postpartum. Some doulas also help with breastfeeding support. During labor, doulas can help with pain relief by giving moms-to-be massages and suggesting breathing techniques.

Generally, a doula will remain with you the entire time from when your labor begins until your baby is born. She can communicate your wishes to the doctors and nurses while you're in labor.

You can learn more about doulas and find one online at the website of DONA International, www.dona.org.

⁓

Even though my sons were born at home, I didn't have a doula. I had a midwife, and because her assistant and she were there during most of the labor, I didn't think I needed a doula also. There was plenty of womanhood around.

—*Lauren Feder, MD, a mom of two sons, a nationally recognized physician who specializes in homeopathic medicine, and the author of* Natural Baby and Childcare *and* The Parents' Concise Guide to Childhood Vaccinations, *in Los Angeles*

⁓

I didn't have a doula during either of my pregnancies. If I had, it would have been more for my husband than for myself. I felt that having experienced labor so many times as a physician, I didn't need the support a doula would offer.

I do think that a doula can be very helpful for a woman trying to have a natural or unmedicated labor. A doula can be really supporting of that.

—*Stephanie Ring, MD, a mom of two sons, ages six and two, and an ob-gyn at Red Rocks Ob-Gyn in Lakewood, CO*

Starting to See Your Doctor or Midwife Once a Month, or More

By now you can probably drive to your doctor's or midwife's office backward with your eyes closed. Around this time, your visits will likely become even more frequent. Many doctors and midwives schedule appointments in the third trimester once a month, or even more.

⁓

During pregnancy, I remember that there were many tests I had to take and so many doctor's visits that I had to go to. You get poked and prodded, and you lose all modesty. I just took it in stride because that's what it's all about. Perhaps it's all good training for labor—and parenthood.

—*Rebecca Kazin, MD, a mom of three girls and the medical director of the Johns Hopkins Dermatology and Cosmetic Center at Green Spring Station in Lutherville, MD*

◦◦

Toward the end of my pregnancy, I went to the doctor once a month. We were living in France at the time, and I really liked my doctor. But I did have an interesting experience: When I was around six months pregnant, I had an infection. The doctor told me that I was going to have a C-section because of it. I thought, *Hello! How can medicine be so different? Where I'm from, you let the woman go into labor, and then you decide if she needs a C-section!*

—*Lilian Morales, MD, a mom of an 11-year-old daughter and a physician in Bogotá, Colombia*

RALLIE'S TIP

In the last trimester of my second pregnancy, my ob asked me to start coming in for checkups every two weeks. I was on the internal medicine service at the hospital, and it seemed that every time he saw me there I was racing through the corridors to answer a Code Blue. He was not happy that I was working such crazy hours, and he told me more than once that I would not carry this baby to term if I didn't slow down. Of course, I thought I could handle anything, so I didn't take him seriously. But I did go in for my checkups every two weeks as instructed.

The worst part was getting weighed so frequently. I started standing backward on the scales so I wouldn't have to see how much weight I had gained in such a short period of time!

As it turns out, my ob was right: My baby was born early at 36 weeks. Fortunately, my son was strong and healthy, but if I had it to do over again, I would have listened to my doctor. When you're pregnant, the most important thing you can do is take care of yourself and your baby. Everything else can wait.

Chapter 29
Week 29

Your Baby This Week

YOUR BABY'S SIZE

By week 29, your baby weighs around 2¾ pounds. Crown to rump, your baby is almost 10½ inches long, and head to heels, he probably measures around 16¾ inches.

Your baby's accommodations are starting to feel a little cramped! Yet amazingly, in the next nine weeks or so, he will double or even triple his weight.

YOUR BABY'S LATEST DEVELOPMENTS

Your baby's head is growing now to make room for his developing brain. Around this week, your baby's brain is developing the ability to regulate his own temperature. He doesn't need this skill yet, though, because he's perfectly warm and cozy inside of you.

By around this time, your baby's smaller lung airways, which are called bronchioles, are in place. The number of little air sacs, which are called alveoli, that lie at the ends of the bronchioles is increasing. Their formation will continue up to, and even after, your baby's birth. Your child's lungs won't be completely matured until he's eight years old—a second grader!

Your baby's movements are purposeful and strong. You can feel punches, kicks, and rapid changes in his position.

Around this week, your baby's bone marrow takes over production of red blood cells, which are responsible for circulating oxygen throughout his tiny body. In another 20 years or so, your then-grown son's bone marrow will produce two million red blood cells each and every second. What will he be doing then? Imagine the places he'll go!

Amazingly, your baby might already be developing habits that he could take with him after he's born, such as sucking his thumb or two fingers.

YOUR LATEST DEVELOPMENTS

This week, the top of your uterus is about 3¾ to 4 inches above your belly button. By now, you've probably gained around 19 to 25 pounds. Your size might be making it uncomfortable to move around in tight spaces.

In the weeks ahead, as your baby grows and space becomes tight inside your uterus, you'll notice his movements will change. Instead of feeling big, sweeping kicks and flips, you'll feel more jabs and pokes from elbows, hands, and feet.

Are your moods running amok again? Earlier in your pregnancy, your body was producing more progesterone than estrogen. For a few weeks, the two hormones evened out. But now, you begin to produce more estrogen, and it's likely affecting your moods.

Right now it's a good bet you're feeling the heat. Often in the third trimester, women sweat more easily. Because of changes in your circulatory system, the blood flow to your skin and mucous membranes is increased. In response, your blood vessels dilate. This might also make the palms of your hands and the soles of your feet red and feel very hot. These changes are to help your body get rid of the extra heat. Otherwise your body would overheat, like an old car.

Ironically, as your baby's lungs are developing, around this time you might be feeling more and more short of breath. Relaxing might help as well as trying to pace yourself. (See "Breathing Easy Despite Shortness of Breath" on page 330.)

JUSTIFICATION FOR A CELEBRATION

Your baby's brain has gotten a handle on breathing. If your baby was born today, he would have an excellent chance of survival.

Getting to Know Your Baby

Right now, your baby is under your heart. Forever, your baby will be *in* your heart. What will your baby be like? Will your baby love trains, games, and picture books? Will your baby play softball, hockey, and chess?

Around the seventh month, the part of the brain that's concerned with personality and intelligence becomes far more complex. Your baby's personality is developing already.

You're getting to know your baby even now. You feel him move; you sense when he's asleep. You notice how he responds when you eat spicy foods, a dog barks, or a bright light shines on your belly. You've been through an amazing journey so far, and these months have only been the first few baby steps.

❧

When I was pregnant with my eldest daughter, I was a resident. We were often on call for long hours, and two or three times every week, we stayed in the hospital overnight. It made for a lot of time spent alone in the call room.

I clearly remember the wonderful feeling that my daughter was there with me in the call room. I wasn't alone after all. It was a really nice feeling during a very stressful time in my life.

—*Siobhan Dolan, MD, MPH, a mom of three, a consultant to the March of Dimes, and an associate professor of obstetrics and gynecology and women's health at Albert Einstein College of Medicine/Montefiore Medical Center in the Bronx, NY*

❧

I remember feeling my baby move during my pregnancy and finding it to be very reassuring. When I was around 21 weeks pregnant, I was evaluated for some worrisome contractions, but I could still feel my baby moving, and that was comforting.

I did some very casual kick countings. I didn't do them every day, but every now and then if I hadn't felt any activity for a while I would drink some juice and lie down. After I felt four or five movements, I'd go about my business.

I think if you do formal kick counts every day, you can worry yourself unnecessarily. Some kids don't move as much as others do. Ask your doctor for very specific advice on how to do kick counts and what they mean if you are going to do them.

—Katja Rowell, MD, a mom of a four-year-old daughter, a family practice physician, and a childhood feeding specialist with www. familyfeedingdynamics.com, in St. Paul, MN

My second daughter was a big baby. When she was born, she weighed 7 pounds, 15 ounces, but she was 22 inches long. I'm only 5 feet 4 inches tall, so she was one-third of my height. She was up in my rib cage most of the time. I felt nothing but her kicking against my ribs.

—Marra Francis, MD, a mom of three daughters and an ob-gyn who's based in The Woodlands, TX

It was interesting when I was pregnant with my twins. One baby was the karate kid! The other baby was very calm and mellow. In fact, she was so calm and mellow that I went in to the doctor a few times to be monitored to make sure she was okay. I tried to figure out which twin was the active one and which was the mellow one, but I never could figure it out.

—Susan Wilder, MD, a mom of an older daughter and twin girls, a primary care physician, and CEO and founder of Lifescape Medical Associates in Scottsdale, AZ

My daughter was so calm during my pregnancy that I thought she'd be a calm baby. But she didn't come out calm! She came out crying and didn't stop. She had colic, and we had a lot of challenges those first three months.

—Monica Lee-Griffith, MD, a mom of one, an ob-gyn, and senior staff, Henry Ford Health System in metropolitan Detroit

I have a daughter and two sons, and it's fascinating to see the differences between girls and boys. But what's even more fascinating to me is the difference between *human beings*. My twins were born at 29 weeks, and those tiny babies in the neonatal intensive care unit already had distinct personalities. And the personalities that I observed 14 years ago are still their personalities today. My twins would have had almost three months left in the womb, and yet when they were born, they already had their personalities. This makes me know that our babies have personalities already in the womb. It's amazing.

—Ruth D. Williams, MD, a mom of twins—a boy and a girl—and another boy, and an ophthalmologist in private practice at the Wheaton Eye Clinic in Wheaton, IL, who specializes in the diagnosis and treatment of glaucoma

∽

My third baby was very active. During my pregnancy, she was always moving around and kicking.

When she was first born, I noticed that she didn't relax and sleep the way my older children had. It's amazing how early you can discern their personalities. I always find it hard to spot personalities in other people's kids, but when you're a parent, you see your own baby's personality emerge from the moment that she's born.

I knew from the beginning that my younger daughter would be a fun, energetic kid. She keeps me on my toes!

—Julie Silver, MD, a mom of a 17-year-old son and 13- and 9-year-old daughters, a Boston-area physiatrist, and the award-winning writer of more than a dozen books, including After Cancer Treatment: Heal Faster, Better, Stronger

Coping with Leg, Hip, and Pelvic Pain

Most women experience some sort of joint discomfort when they're expecting. It can become very painful later in pregnancy. The hormone relaxin is partly to blame. It relaxes your joints so that your pelvis can expand and your baby can be born. But relaxin doesn't discriminate; it relaxes all of your joints, not just the ones in your pelvis.

Another factor contributing to joint pain is that your growing belly is changing your center of gravity, moving it forward over your legs. This affects all of your joints, putting different stress on them than usual.

Joint pain is likely to be your companion from here on out until your baby is born. The best news is that it often goes away right after your baby is born, like a light switch being turned off. For now, walking, changing positions frequently, and resting might help.

During my first pregnancy, when I was around seven months pregnant, the baby was lying in my belly crosswise. She was leaning on my right side, making it practically impossible to walk. I laid down on the floor on my back and stretched, and thank goodness the baby readjusted.

—*Erika Schwartz, MD, a mom of two and the director of www. DrErika.com, who's been in private practice for more than 30 years in New York City, specializing over the past 15 years in women's health, disease prevention, and bioidentical hormones*

∽

I had such pain in my symphysis pubis, the joint between the pubic bones, that I thought it was going to pull apart. But walking four or five days a week for around 30 minutes each day kept me sane and feeling better.

—*Sharonne N. Hayes, MD, a mom of two and the director of the Women's Heart Clinic at Mayo Clinic in Rochester, MN*

∽

During my third trimester, I had sacroileitis, causing a stabbing pain in my right gluteus muscle. Stretching and pregnancy massage were wonderful. Even though the pain was still there until after I delivered, massage gave me an hour of relief and relaxation.

—*Gina Dado, MD, a mom of two daughters and an ob-gyn with Arizona OBGYN Affiliates, Paradise Valley Branch, in Scottsdale, AZ*

∽

When I was pregnant with my triplets, my daughter was lying low in my pelvis. It was very painful. She was the smallest of the three during most of my pregnancy, but she decided to gain weight in the last four to six weeks. I felt every single ounce of her. It felt like my pelvic bones were being pulled apart by some invisible force!

There wasn't really anything to do besides change positions a lot. But the good news is, the pain went away completely as soon as my babies were born.

—*Sadaf T. Bhutta, MBBS, a mom of a three-year-old daughter and 18-month-old triplets and an assistant professor and the fellowship director of pediatric radiology at the University of Arkansas for Medical Sciences and Arkansas Children's Hospital, both in Little Rock*

With this pregnancy, I had horrible hip pain. In my three other pregnancies, I had aches and pains, but nothing like this. I'm not sure if it's something particular to this pregnancy or if it's that I'm getting older. The pain started right at the beginning of my third trimester. If I sit too long in any position or do too much activity, my hips and pubic bone get very sore.

It helps to be careful about how I sleep. I lie with a pillow between my knees, and when I roll over, I move both legs together at the same time. Otherwise I wake up and can't move! Also, I find resting with a heating pad on my hip set on low for 10 to 15 minutes loosens it up. Warm baths help it too.

—Kristie McNealy, MD, a mom of seven- and four-year-old daughters and a two-year-old son, who's pregnant with another son, and a blogger at www.KristieMcNealy.com, in Denver, CO

I was finishing my ob-gyn residency during my pregnancy, so I took call on labor and delivery 24 hours in a row. It was a busy hospital, and we delivered on average 20 babies a night!

To help with my leg pain and swelling, I wore T.E.D. support stockings. The support stockings also helped to energize me, preventing me from getting worn down as fast.

—Nancy Thomas, MD, a mom of a 22-month-old son who practices general obstetrics and gynecology in Covington, LA, with Ochsner Health System

Breathing Easy Despite Shortness of Breath

Right about now, every breath you take might be about as slow as every move you make. Shortness of breath is common during pregnancy, for a myriad of reasons. This might even have begun at the end of your first trimester. Because of the increased blood in your body, all of your organs are working harder than before. They demand more oxygen. Half of that goes to your baby, placenta, and uterus. But the other half is required to fuel your heart and kidneys, muscles, breasts, and skin.

To meet this need, your lungs take in more oxygen and expel more carbon dioxide with every single breath that you take. Amazing! Your lung capacity has increased by up to 40 percent since your baby was conceived. This allows you to overbreathe, or hyperventilate, and it's why you often feel out of breath.

Another factor making it hard for you to breathe is the fact that high levels of progesterone in your body increase your body temperature as well as your breathing rate.

Plus, as your uterus moves up and out, your ribs flare outward. This stretches your diaphragm, making it less flexible. This reduced movement forces you to breathe more deeply.

Last but not least, maybe not quite yet but between weeks 31 and 34, your uterus begins to press your stomach and liver up against your diaphragm. This leaves your lungs with less room to expand when you try to breathe. Being short of breath might also be making you dizzy and light-headed.

So if you're breathless, it's not in your imagination. Hopefully just that reassurance might help you to breathe a little easier. It also might help to practice good posture by standing and sitting up straight, move more slowly, stretch your arms above your head to take pressure off of your rib cage, and sleep propped up on pillows.

Toward the end of my pregnancy, I noticed that when I was on the phone, I was short of breath. I'd have to stop talking and take a deep breath. I could only speak in short sentences!

This is very common in pregnancy, and for good reason. There's a physiologic drive to increase your respiratory rate and breathe faster so that your body gets more oxygen—so that the baby gets more oxygen. Plus, later in your pregnancy, as your abdomen gets

When to Call Your Doctor or Midwife

Feeling short of breath and breathing more shallowly are normal during pregnancy. However, call your doctor or midwife immediately if you suddenly feel severely breathless. Also call if you have a rapid pulse, heart palpitations, chest pain, fever, or chills; if you feel dizzy or faint; or if you can't stop coughing or start coughing up blood.

distended, your baby might also be crowding your lungs, making you short of breath.

—*Diane Connelly, MD, a mom of a six-year-old daughter and an ob-gyn in HMO practice in Riverside, CA*

My pregnancy was going really smoothly until I started to gain a lot more weight in my third trimester. What was most troubling was that I had a hard time breathing. I got winded right away if I tried to take the stairs.

I think I had shortness of breath because my baby was lying very high. I felt like I couldn't get enough air. It was uncomfortable, but I found that if I sat down for a few minutes, I could breathe better.

—*Kerri A. Daniels, MD, a mom of one toddler daughter and an instructor in the department of pediatrics at the University of Arkansas for Medical Science in Little Rock*

My middle daughter was a long baby, and I carried her up high in my ribs. Toward the end I was very short of breath. It was awful. I would feel like the wind was getting knocked out of me. When I had to run in the hospital to deliver a baby, I'd have to sit down and catch my breath before I could catch the baby.

I tried to walk as much as possible, not run, and I sat down to catch my breath a lot.

—*Marra Francis, MD*

Easing Stress

Stress stinks, but it's pretty unavoidable, even in pregnancy. Or perhaps *especially* in pregnancy, which ranks in the top dozen of life's most stressful events. Changes in your hormones can cause you to act in ways that aren't normal for you, which is stressful.

Some of the stress of pregnancy will be great training for the stress of parenting. Learning how to manage stress now will pay off later after your baby is born. Exercise can help to ease stress; exercise outdoors in nature is even better. Relaxation and breathing exercises are great as well. Try to take breaks whenever you can from work—and from housework.

⤙⤚

One interesting thing about doctors is sometimes we tell our patients to do the right things, but then we do all of the wrong things.

In retrospect, during my pregnancies, I would have taken more time out of my schedule and not worked so hard. I would have done more stress-relieving activities and cut down on my workload. Hindsight is 20/20.

—*Gina Dado, MD*

⤙⤚

When my husband and I started trying to get pregnant, I was working full-time as an ophthalmologist. I love my job, and I didn't think a lot about pregnancy. The truth is, I didn't take very good care of myself. I didn't regard being pregnant as something that would change anything I was doing.

But that isn't very good advice. Instead, give your body and mind a

Mommy MD Guide-Recommended Product
Natural Calm

"After my kids were born, I heard about a product called Natural Calm," said Gina Dado, MD, a mom of two daughters and an ob-gyn with Arizona OBGYN Affiliates, Paradise Valley Branch, in Scottsdale, AZ. "It's a powder that contains magnesium. You dissolve it into a teeny bit of water, warm it, and it fizzes up. It comes in several organic flavors (sweetened with organic stevia), including raspberry-lemon, and it's like drinking raspberry lemonade. I find it to be very calming, and it helps with constipation to boot."

You can buy Natural Calm for around $20 online.

break. Give yourself some emotional space to get ready for the huge changes to come in your life. When you are carrying a baby, you're doing the most important job you will do in your entire life.

I followed this advice much more during my second pregnancy. I wised up a lot between my first and second pregnancies.

—*Ruth D. Williams, MD*

∼

During my second pregnancy, my older daughter was very ill. At times it was hard for me even to eat because I spent so many days and nights at my older daughter's bedside. I had to take her to the emergency room several times, and I was under extraordinary stress.

When my second daughter was born, she had a sucking blister on her wrist because she was under so much stress that she sucked on her own hand inside of me. That showed me the impact of stress in utero. My stress led to my daughter's stress to the point that she sucked her skin off inside of me. What you do—and even what you think—matters. It's impossible to avoid stress, but it's critical to minimize it during your pregnancy as much as you can.

—*Eva Ritvo, MD, a mom of two teenaged daughters, an associate professor and vice chairman at the Miller School of Medicine of the University of Miami, and a coauthor of* The Beauty Prescription

RALLIE'S TIP

Especially during my pregnancies, I tried to prevent stress whenever possible. One thing that always helps me to keep it at bay is to tend my little herb garden and indoor plants in my kitchen. It only takes a minute or two to take care of them—pinch off dry leaves, water them, and rotate them in the sun. But my plants give me hours of viewing pleasure (especially my African violets, which bloom year-round), and pinching a pleasant smelling leaf and smelling it is very calming and relaxing. Plus, I can use fresh herbs such as basil and spearmint in my spaghetti sauce or iced or hot tea (tea is energizing and relaxing at the same time), which adds great taste.

The herbs are also good for me and my family. They improve digestion and have antimicrobial properties. Several recent studies have shown caring for plants to be very therapeutic in terms of reducing stress, improving cognition, and providing a sense of accomplishment, which is especially important when you've got a thousand projects going on at once, and none of them seem to be nearing completion Time spent in my mini-garden is very healing.

Also, when I was pregnant, to try to reduce stress, I took five- to 10-minute breaks whenever I had the chance. I'd sit in a sunbeam or under a bright light, which has been shown to improve mood. I've created a little "time-out" corner for myself, which I have come to associate with "me" time.

To create my time-out corner, I put a really comfy chair beside a window. In a bright wicker basket beside my chair, I keep a few books that I enjoy reading in five- to 10-minute snatches, as well as my knitting. I never bring my cell phone or work to my time-out corner; it's just for relaxing. I don't spend much time there, but when I do, the break is energizing and relaxing.

Another technique I used to reduce stress even in pregnancy is to journal. It's very healing and calming. Putting stuff down on paper is an excellent way to release stress. It gets it out of you and onto the paper. Sometimes I vent, but I usually try to write about what's going right more than what's going wrong. Studies have shown that writing down the things you're grateful for at least three times a week can significantly improve your happiness. As a bonus, while I'm writing, I often stumble upon solutions to problems and occasionally, a really brilliant idea!

My journaling isn't formal at all; I doubt if anyone else could even read some of the things that I write. I just get an inexpensive notebook, write the date on the front of it, and write in it whenever I feel like it. Sometimes I fill up a notebook in a week, and other times it takes me a month or two.

The other bonus that comes with journaling is that when you write things down, you remember them better; that's a proven fact. And even if I happen to forget, I can always look back and find facts that I might have forgotten. Studies show that stress impairs memory, and this is a great tool to reduce stress and improve memory at the same time.

Chapter 30
Week 30

Your Baby This Week

YOUR BABY'S SIZE

This week, your baby weighs around three pounds. From now until your baby is born, she'll gain about ½ pound each week. Her crown-to-rump length is around 10¾ inches, and she's already around 17 inches tall.

YOUR BABY'S LATEST DEVELOPMENTS

By 30 weeks, your baby's ability to survive outside of you has improved dramatically. The vast majority of babies who are born after this week will cope extremely well, with special care.

Now that your baby's brain is able to regulate her temperature and she has put on some fat to help keep her warm, she's starting to lose her downy lanugo. Your baby still might have some lanugo when she is born, most likely patches on her back and shoulders.

The white fat that your baby is putting on is also smoothing out her skin, making her look less wrinkly than she did a few weeks ago.

Your baby's fingernails and toenails are soft because they're constantly bathed in amniotic fluid. You'll find them to be still quite soft and pliable after she's born. However, they're also razor sharp because they are so thin.

Around this time, the placenta weighs a little less than one pound. Every single minute, the placenta receives about 16 fluid ounces of blood from you.

Your latest developments

Your uterus is growing up under your ribs. The top of your uterus is now around four inches above your belly button. You're probably gaining about a pound a week.

After having a break from breast tenderness, it might return in your third trimester. Your milk ducts are filling with milk. Nursing bras might be more comfortable to wear now, but don't buy too many in case your size changes after your baby is born.

Your blood volume continues to expand in the third trimester, which might be making you more tired than ever. To make matters worse, sleep might be more and more of a challenge. Many women find it very difficult to get comfortable enough to sleep soundly.

You might find that you're waddling around quite a bit now, with your feet pointed outward. This helps to compensate for your belly and shifting center of gravity. It's pretty difficult to keep your pregnancy a secret, even from behind!

Braxton Hicks contractions often become more common around this time. Talk with your doctor or midwife if you're not sure if what you're feeling are Braxton Hicks contractions or the real thing.

The whitish vaginal discharge called leukorrhea has probably gotten heavier now. This is perfectly normal, although not at all fun.

During the third trimester, pregnancy symptoms often grow like a snowball rolling downhill. You might be feeling more anxiety, constipation, heartburn, hemorrhoids, and even nausea now. Urinary incontinence might be giving you trouble. It affects most pregnant women.

Justification for a celebration

Your baby is now capable of producing tears!

Choosing a Pediatrician

Choosing a pediatrician for your baby feels like a major milestone. It's exciting to find the doctor who will care for your baby for years to come. Pediatricians provide preventive care to healthy children, as well as medical care to children who are ill. You'll be seeing a lot of your baby's pediatrician, especially in her first year.

Pediatricians specialize in the care of infants, children, and teens, usually up to age 21. They must graduate from an approved medical school, undergo three years of pediatric residency training, pass a test administered by the American Board of Pediatrics to be board certified, and then be recertified every seven years.

It's a great idea to ask your friends, family members, and perhaps even your own doctors for referrals. Check with your health insurance company to see which pediatricians in your area accept your insurance. The American Academy of Pediatrics offers a referral service on their website, www.AAP.org, to help you find a qualified pediatrician.

You might want to visit and interview a few pediatricians and then choose the one who seems to be the best fit for your family. Many pediatricians offer these parent visits at no charge, and they're happy to answer your questions and address your concerns.

Also, you might want to find out if your baby's pediatrician will be tending to your baby in the hospital. This isn't always possible, and it will be good to know ahead of time what to expect.

❧

I practiced for several years before I had kids, but now I would never go to a pediatrician who didn't have children. This is unique because you go to a surgeon who has probably never had the surgery you're having. And many women go to male gynecologists. I think that they *can* have empathy for their patients.

But motherhood is different. The challenges motherhood brings, such as being up all night with a sick baby, make it valuable to have a pediatrician who has lived it.

—*Susan Schreiber, MD, a mom of a son and daughter in their twenties and a pediatrician in Los Angeles, CA*

My husband and I interviewed several pediatricians before our daughter was born. We asked them all the same questions so we could compare their answers. For example, my husband has allergies, so we asked their views on allergy treatment. We asked their thoughts on nursing. We asked who answers middle-of-the-night phone calls.

We didn't go with any doctors that we knew. We ended up choosing the pediatrician my ob-gyn had recommended. She definitely didn't have the fanciest office or even separate sick and well-baby waiting rooms. But my husband and I had a good feeling about her. She talked to me as both a doctor and a mom, and I really value that. When your baby is sick, being a doctor goes out the window. And when I call after hours, I get a call back from the doctor, not a nurse.

—*Michelle Paley, MD, PA, a mom of a six-year-old daughter and a two-year-old son and a psychiatrist and psychotherapist in private practice in Miami Beach, FL*

ᏝᏝ

I think it's always good to ask your friends for doctor recommendations. Because many of my friends are doctors, I was able to ask people who were both friends and doctors. However, I didn't choose a pediatrician I knew personally because I preferred not to go with a friend.

It's great to ask doctors for referrals to other doctors because in addition to knowing their bedside manner, they also know how to evaluate the doctor's clinical skills. If you don't have any friends who are doctors, consider asking your own doctors for pediatrician recommendations.

—*Ayala Laufer-Cahana, MD, a pediatrician, mother, artist, serious home cook, and the founder of Herbal Water Inc., in Wynnewood, PA*

ᏝᏝ

I went into preterm labor with my first baby. I was terrified that she would be born early, and I found a pediatrician who was also board certified in neonatology.

She's cared for my children ever since, even though we've moved twice and it's now a 45-minute drive to her office. She's awesome.

—*Ann LaBarge, MD, a mom of four children, ages 16 to six, and an ob-gyn in private practice at the Midwest Center for Women's Healthcare in Park Ridge, IL*

I decided to take my kids to one of my best friends from college who is now a pediatrician. I have the inside scoop on pediatricians because of my job; I get to know them very well, and I get to see their bedside manner. An ob-gyn might be a great person to ask for recommendations.

When choosing a pediatrician, I think it's important to find someone you feel comfortable with. It's great to get referrals from your friends, but just because your friend likes a pediatrician doesn't mean you will. Interview pediatricians and ask about their availability for urgent visits and their office hours. If it's a group of pediatricians, make sure that you like most of the doctors. When your baby is sick and you need an appointment ASAP, you might not get to choose whom you get to see. Also consider where the office is located; you don't want to have a long drive in the snow with a sick baby.

—*Jennifer Kim, MD, a mom of three girls, ages eight, five, and four; an ob-gyn in private practice in Evanston, IL, at the Midwest Center for Women's Healthcare; and a clinical assistant professor at the University of Chicago, Pritzker School of Medicine*

Getting Sleep

It's ironic that you're tossing and turning at night, having a hard time getting sleep, because your baby right now spends 95 percent of her time sleeping. At least one of you is catching some Zs!

More than 75 percent of pregnant women experience insomnia around this time in pregnancy. All sorts of factors conspire in pregnancy to prevent you from sleeping. These include aches and pains, hormonal changes, having to go to the bathroom all the time, altered respiration, your baby's movements, and your big belly.

Now more than ever, sleep is important. Studies found that women who slept fewer than six hours a night during pregnancy were four times more likely to have Cesarean sections.

It might help to strategically place pillows to support your belly and between your knees. Body pillows are especially helpful for this because they're long and flexible enough to work into the right positions. (See "Mommy MD Guide–Recommended Product: Body Pillow" on page 342.)

Sweet dreams!

Toward the end of my pregnancies, my babies were so big that I couldn't sleep. The nights tossing and turning were miserable. But strangely enough, I always had enough energy during the day. I think it was because of all those growth hormones flowing through my body.

—*Karen Heald, MD, a mom of four boys and a board-certified family physician in private practice outside Atlanta, GA*

During my pregnancy, I found it helpful to sleep curled around a full-body pillow. Even with this, it was still hard to sleep. I wish you could store sleep!

—*Michelle Paley, MD, PA*

A few weeks before the end of my pregnancy, I had a terrible time getting comfortable and sleeping at night. What was especially difficult was that I couldn't sleep on my stomach.

I bought a body pillow that you can bend into shapes. I wrapped it around me to get into a more comfortable position so I could sleep at night.

—*Kerri A. Daniels, MD, a mom of one toddler daughter and an instructor in the department of pediatrics at the University of Arkansas for Medical Science in Little Rock*

Toward the end of my first pregnancy, I was not sleeping well. I woke up eight times a night to go to the bathroom. I think that the baby was pushing on my bladder, and so it couldn't hold much.

—*Amy J. Derick, MD, a mom of one 15-month-old son who is 17 weeks pregnant with her second son. Dr. Derick is a dermatologist in private practice at Derick Dermatology in Barrington, IL*

RALLIE'S TIP

I find it easiest to fall asleep when I lie on my stomach, but as my belly grew during pregnancy, this position became virtually impossible. I knew that I should try to sleep on my left side to improve circulation to my baby, but I couldn't seem to maintain that position for any length of time at night. I'd keep rolling back onto my stomach while I slept, and each time that I did, I would wake myself up. I finally invested in a body pillow. I would lie on my left side and wedge the pillow along the length of my body. (See "Mommy

MD Guide-Recommended Product: Body Pillow" below.) It gave me the comfortable sensation of sleeping on my belly while it helped me stay positioned on my left side.

∽

One thing I wasn't expecting during pregnancy was insomnia. From my sixth month on, it was very hard for me to sleep. It was hard to get comfortable, and if my baby was moving around a lot, it kept me up.

I watched more TV during those months than I've ever watched in my life. I caught up on all the shows in syndication that I didn't get to see the first time. But I found to really get sleep, I needed to turn the TV off. Also, turning on a white noise machine helped.

—*Christy Valentine, MD, a mom of one, a specialist in pediatrics and internal medicine, and the founder of the Valentine Medical Center in Gretna, LA*

∽

Some nights, you just cannot sleep, whether from hormones, stress, or your intrusive belly. When you get big enough, sitting upright will be the most comfortable way to sleep. Lying down causes the baby to rest against the diaphragm, making it harder to breathe. My best naps were in my car with the seat reclined, waiting for my morning shift to start. We didn't have room for a rocking chair in our house, but if you do, consider one with a leg rest. (See "Mommy MD Guide-Recommended Product: Recliner" on page 202.)

—*Tyeese Gaines Reid, DO, a mom of one, an emergency medicine resident physician at Yale New Haven Hospital in Connecticut, and the author of a time management book,* The Get a Life Campaign

Mommy MD Guide-Recommended Product
Body Pillow

"A body pillow helps you to lie on your side comfortably," said Tyeese Gaines Reid, DO, a mom of one, an emergency medicine resident physician at Yale New Haven Hospital in Connecticut, and the author of a time management book, *The Get a Life Campaign*. "Put it between your knees, under your arm, and dream away."

Body pillows are available at **WWW.BEDBATHANDBEYOND.COM.**

One thing that I started using in my third pregnancy is Unisom, an over-the-counter sleep medication. It's an antihistamine, so it's not habit-forming. Ironically, it also helps ease morning sickness.

I found that when I took Unisom at night, it helped me to sleep much better, and so the next day I felt more rested and had a better day. (Talk with your doctor or midwife before taking this or any medication.)

—*Ann LaBarge, MD*

Especially as my pregnancy went along, I got very cranky and tired. I would come home from work, sit down, and pass out on the couch. I recommend taking catnaps if you can during the day because it can be hard to get good sleep at night. You can take Tylenol PM or Benadryl, but then you might feel groggy when you wake up. (Talk with your doctor or midwife before taking this or any medication.)

Natural Calm, which is a magnesium powder supplement, works good too. (See "Mommy MD Guide–Recommended Product: Natural Calm" on page 333.)

—*Gina Dado, MD, a mom of two daughters and an ob-gyn with Arizona OBGYN Affiliates, Paradise Valley Branch, in Scottsdale, AZ*

I had a really rough time in my pregnancy with insomnia. I would wake up in the middle of the night and have a hard time falling back to sleep.

I found it helped me to have a plan of action, so that I didn't just lie there trying desperately to fall asleep. The worst thing you can do is just lie there thinking about how you can't sleep. I kept a glass of water on my nightstand so if I was thirsty, I didn't have to get out of bed to get something to drink and wake up more. I also kept a book within reach so I could read and distract myself.

If I was really having a hard time, it helped to change rooms. I'd get out of bed and go lie on the couch or in the spare bedroom. The change of location helped me fall back to sleep.

—*Kelly Campbell, MD, a mom of three and an ob-gyn in private practice at Women's Healthcare Physicians in West Bloomfield, MI*

I've always had a sleep disorder because as an obstetrician I was used to being awakened at all hours. During my pregnancy was no exception: I was a lousy sleeper. But as a doctor, especially during residency, you're taught to live without sleep. So I get by on very little sleep.

—*Melanie Bone, MD, a mom of four "tweens" ages 15 to 12, a gynecologist, the founder of the Cancer Sensibility Foundation, and the author of the syndicated column Surviving Life and the book* Cancer, What's Next?, *in West Palm Beach, FL*

Dealing with Muscle Cramps

As your pregnancy goes along, you might feel more and more muscle cramps and pain. That's because your muscles shift around as your hips and rib cage expand. This pulling and stretching can make your muscles feel sore and weak.

The best Rx for this is simply rest and stretching whenever you can.

During my pregnancy, I didn't have too many muscle cramps. I think that's because I was very proactive in preventing them. I got pregnancy massages every two weeks, which helped me to relax and keep my muscles relaxed as well.

—*Debra Luftman, MD, a mom of a teenaged daughter and a teenaged son, a board-certified dermatologist in private practice, a coauthor of* The Beauty Prescription, *the developer of the skincare line of products Therapeutix, and a clinical instructor of skin surgery and general dermatology at UCLA*

RALLIE'S TIP

I had terrible muscle cramps in my legs while I was pregnant, especially when I was really tired and when I hadn't been drinking enough water. It seemed like every time I sat down to rest, my calf muscles would go into spasm.

Fortunately, the spells didn't last long, and I eventually learned how to position my legs when I sat down to keep them from cramping. You just have to do a little experimenting to see what works best for you.

Managing Maternal Amnesia

Part of pregnancy that's often the butt of jokes is maternal amnesia, which is also known by other silly names such as "baby brain," "preg head," and "nappy brain," on the other side of the pond anyway.

Pregnant women sometimes grow forgetful. Perhaps it's because you're so preoccupied with the pregnancy and upcoming birth. Stress and sleep deprivation certainly don't help. Maybe it's nature's way of training you for having kids.

But here's welcome news: You're not alone! A major study conducted a few years ago by researchers at the University of New South Wales in Sydney, Australia, found that pregnant women are so impaired on some (although not all) measures of memory that their memory deficits are similar to what you'd find if you compared a healthy 20-year-old person with a healthy 60-year-old person.

RALLIE'S TIP

I suffered a terrible case of brain drain with my last pregnancy. I was incredibly forgetful. My fellow doctors in my residency training program called it "uterine steal." They were sure my uterus was stealing all of the blood and nutrients from my brain. I started carrying a date book with me everywhere I went, and whenever I needed to remember something, I'd jot it down. I have to admit that I forgot where I left my book from time to time, but as long as I had it with me, life went a lot more smoothly.

People joke about memory changes in pregnancy. But now that I've had cancer and chemotherapy, I *really* know what it's like to have memory loss. I have short-term memory problems now, but to the best of my recollection, I didn't have "placenta head" during my pregnancies. My memory and cognitive skills were both intact.

—*Melanie Bone, MD*

Chapter 31
Week 31

Your Baby This Week

YOUR BABY'S SIZE

Around this time, your baby is almost 18 inches long, 11¾ inches crown to rump, and he weighs around 3½ pounds. Your baby is now forced into the fetal position with his legs drawn in to his chest because he's too big to stretch out.

YOUR BABY'S LATEST DEVELOPMENTS

Your baby's brain is creating billions of new cells around this time. He's becoming more and more aware of the sights and sounds around him. All five of his senses are developed. He can't yet experience his sense of smell, though, because he's surrounded by fluid, not air.

As your baby puts on more white fat, his skin is less see-through and he begins to look less red and more pink.

If you are having a boy, his testicles are continuing to descend into his scrotum. The testes are formed in the body cavity from the same tissue that forms a baby girl's ovaries. The ovaries stay in place in the body cavity, but it's too warm there for the testes' sperm-producing mechanisms. That's why they migrate into the scrotum.

If your baby is a girl, her clitoris is now clearly visible.

YOUR LATEST DEVELOPMENTS

Your uterus is now filling a large part of your abdomen. This week, it's around 4½ inches above your belly button. By now you've probably gained between 21 and 27 pounds. You'll likely continue to gain between ½ and 1 pound a week until your baby is born.

Your uterus is probably really achy because it's so stretched. Try to change position slowly to avoid those sharp round ligament pains.

Because your baby is having a growth spurt and his skeleton is hardening, continue to eat plenty of food rich in calcium. Your baby's calcium needs are greatest during the last three months of pregnancy. Dairy products such as milk and cheese are good choices. The calcium in milk and milk products is very readily absorbed and used by your body.

It's also especially important at this time to eat enough food rich in iron, such as red meat and beans.

Your breasts might itch because the skin is so stretched. Try some cocoa butter lotion to ease the discomfort.

If you feel up to having sex, you might discover that it's a very intense experience. Because all of the capillaries in your genital area are filled with extra blood, you're much more sensitive now.

At this point, you're probably seeing your doctor or midwife every other week. This gives you plenty of opportunities to ask questions and make sure your concerns are addressed.

JUSTIFICATION FOR A CELEBRATION

You're in the single digits! Less than nine weeks to go!

Choosing to Breastfeed or Bottlefeed

According to the Centers for Disease Control and Prevention, in 2006, the year the most recent stats are available, almost three-quarters of babies were breastfed at some point. By six months, only 43 percent were still breastfeeding, and by a year, that number drops to 23 percent.

The CDC breaks the breastfeeding data down by state, and moms in Utah are the most likely to breastfeed, with 92.8 percent having breastfed at some point. Least likely to breastfeed are women in Mississippi, where only 48.3 percent of moms have ever breastfed.

Statistics are interesting, but what's most important is what's best for you, your baby, and your family.

∽◦∽

Breastfeeding was something I had always wanted to do. I was committed to doing it. I know that it can be challenging for some women, but I decided that I was going to do it. And I did!

—*Christy Valentine, MD, a mom of one, a specialist in pediatrics and internal medicine, and the founder of the Valentine Medical Center in Gretna, LA*

∽◦∽

I was determined to breastfeed all four of my children, each until one year of age. I even breastfed my third baby during my residency, when I was working 110 hours a week.

For me, choosing to breastfeed was a no-brainer. There was no other option. When my first baby was born, I was living on a spiritual commune called the Farm. We weren't walking around naked, doing LSD, and sleeping with a million people. We were a monogamous spiritual commune. And everyone there assumed that breastfeeding was the normal thing to do. It's how we were made; it's what God intended.

—*Hana R. Solomon, MD, a mom of four, ages 35 to 19, a board-certified pediatrician, the president of BeWell Health, LLC, and the author of* Clearing the Air One Nose at a Time: Caring for Your Personal Filter

∽◦∽

As a pediatrician, I highly recommend breastfeeding. It has many health benefits to both the baby and the mother. However, if breastfeeding is going to be a burden on your emotional, mental, or physical health, you shouldn't feel guilty about switching to formula.

I breastfed each of my babies for a month, but I just couldn't continue after that. Nursing became a "must-do," not something I enjoyed. I think women need to be prepared that breastfeeding is time-consuming, and you need a great deal of support to do it. If you don't have that support, or if breastfeeding becomes too much of a struggle, simply switch to formula.

—*Aline T. Tanios, MD, a mom of three and a general pediatrician and hospitalist who treats medically complex children at Arkansas Children's Hospital in Little Rock*

I have a unique perspective about nursing because I wasn't able to nurse my older daughter, but I did nurse my younger daughter.

You've probably heard that experts think that nursing helps to bolster a baby's immune system. That might be true in some cases, but it didn't hold true in my family. My older daughter, who didn't nurse, has the most superb immune system. On the other hand, my second daughter, whom I nursed diligently for a year, was sick constantly.

My advice is to try to nurse if you can. Nursing is one of the most special and unique experiences in life—a way of connecting to another human being that is life-giving. The mother benefits because oxytocin, the "feel-good"

Mommy MD Guide-Recommended Product
Palmer's Cocoa Butter Nursing Butter

Ask just about any mother who has breastfed, and she'll tell you that in the beginning it can be difficult—even painful. One very helpful product is Palmer's Cocoa Butter Nursing Butter. Its easy-to-apply combination of cocoa butter and vitamin B_5 in a soothing, emollient base helps relieve sore, cracked nipples. You might try using it before your baby is born to condition your nipples for breastfeeding. Best of all: You don't have to wash it off before breastfeeding your baby.

You can buy Palmer's Cocoa Butter Nursing Butter in baby supply stores and online for around $6 for 1.1 ounces.

hormone, is released. Once nursing is established and going smoothly, the release of oxytocin causes the mom to feel relaxed and happy. It's a very time-limited experience, so try to enjoy every minute of it if possible. But if you can't nurse, don't beat yourself up about it.

—*Eva Ritvo, MD, a mom of two teenaged daughters, an associate professor and vice chairman at the Miller School of Medicine of the University of Miami, and a coauthor of* The Beauty Prescription

I nursed my daughter exclusively for nine months, but I had a different philosophy when I was pregnant with my son. I nursed him, but I also supplemented with formula early on. This made a big difference in my sleep! It's so helpful when someone else can give the baby a bottle.

To prepare, I bought the bottles and nipples ahead of time. I bought BornFree bottles that you can safely put warm liquids in.

I think it's important to make whatever choice works best for you and your family. Don't listen to too much advice. Make your decision, and don't look back. If you're a happier mom, your baby will be happier too.

—*Michelle Paley, MD, PA, a mom of a six-year-old daughter and a two-year-old son and a psychiatrist and psychotherapist in private practice in Miami Beach, FL*

I breastfed each of my babies, and I hated it. It is brutally hard, and it never stopped hurting. Every time I put my older daughter to my breast, we'd both break out in a sweat. I decided I'm simply not good at this.

I kept trying with each of my babies, thinking it would be different, but it never was. I'd try for a few days and then switch over to bottlefeeding. My logic is: You can't tell 20 years later if someone was breastfed or bottlefed! I see just as many ear infections in breastfed babies as in bottlefed babies. I think breastfeeding is great in Third-World countries where they don't have good water or formula. But I don't think our formulas are bad at all.

The decision to breastfeed is your own to make. Although La Leche League provides a wonderful service and great support, there are women for whom breastfeeding is *not* the right thing. If you are one of those women, don't feel guilty or let anyone badger you into doing it. On the other hand, if you're on the fence, try it. I often marvel at the women who are successful at breastfeeding, even those I guessed would never do it.

—Melanie Bone, MD, a mom of four "tweens" ages 15 to 12, a gynecologist, the founder of the Cancer Sensibility Foundation, and the author of the syndicated column Surviving Life *and the book* Cancer, What's Next?, *in West Palm Beach, FL*

◇◇

I decided not to nurse because it would have been too much for me with twins. I felt a tremendous amount of guilt about that, but I think you have to do what works for you.

—Jennifer Gilbert, DO, a mom of three-month-old twins and an ob-gyn at Paoli Hospital in Pennsylvania

Preventing Stretch Marks

Up to 90 percent of pregnant women develop stretch marks. Sigh. There's simply not much you can do. When you gain weight, your skin is forced to expand, and collagen breaks down and shows through the top layer of your skin as red, pink, or purple indented streaks—stretch marks. If your mom had them, you're likely to get them too. Plus, the older you are when you get pregnant, the more likely you are to get them.

You're most likely to get stretch marks on your breasts, arms, tummy, hips, and butt. They also have a medical name—striae distensae.

The one way to prevent, or at least minimize, stretch marks is to keep your weight gain steady and gradual. Drinking lots of water might help, and eating fruits and vegetables, which are high in antioxidants, might provide the nutrients that your skin needs to repair and heal. Massage can increase blood flow to the area to stimulate the healing process.

Stretch marks can be itchy. Applying some cocoa butter lotion might help to ease the itch.

Despite what you might read online and see on late-night TV, once you have a stretch mark, you can't erase it. Topical lotions and potions such as steroid creams are dangerous to use during pregnancy.

The good news is that stretch marks might fade all on their own, usually to a pale silver, after your baby is born.

? When to Call Your Doctor or Midwife

There's nothing that you can do to get rid of your stretch marks now. But after your baby is born, if they're really bothering you, you could talk with your doctor about prescription-strength creams, such as Retin-A, or laser treatments.

Your body changes and grows so quickly in pregnancy that it's common to get stretch marks. I did not want to get stretch marks, so I moisturized my skin three times a day. I used a spray-on cocoa butter lotion, which was easy to apply even late in my pregnancy. At a certain point, it's hard to bend over! The lotion worked; I didn't get any stretch marks.

—*Christy Valentine, MD*

I didn't get any stretch marks on my belly during my three pregnancies. I put a lot of lotion on my stomach. Perhaps that helped, but most likely I was just lucky.

—*Lezli Braswell, MD, a mom of one daughter and two sons and a family medicine physician currently working in an emergency room fast track in Columbus, GA*

I was determined not to get stretch marks. I put cocoa butter on my belly every night and sometimes in the morning too. I love that stuff! I didn't buy anything extravagant—just a cheap brand from a five-and-dime store. But it was great! I only got one stretch mark, and that popped out the day before I delivered, right on my belly button. It's still there.

—*Patricia S. Brown, MD, a mom of two daughters, ages nine and seven, and a three-year-old son and a psychiatrist at Columbia-New York Child and Adolescent Telepsychiatry and in private practice in Cresskill, NJ*

I have a daughter and then triplets, so stretch marks were pretty inevitable. If I look closely at my stomach, I can see some silvery streaks. But they really aren't that bad because I'm from Pakistan, and I have a darker complexion. So the stretch marks aren't that obvious.

—*Sadaf T. Bhutta, MBBS, a mom of a three-year-old daughter and 18-month-old triplets and an assistant professor and the fellowship director of pediatric radiology at the University of Arkansas for Medical Sciences and Arkansas Children's Hospital, both in Little Rock*

Soothing Your Itchy Skin

Itchiness is common in pregnancy. Around 20 percent of all pregnant women suffer from it. You might feel perplexed because you don't see any bumps or marks on your skin making you itch; it just does.

The good news is this garden-variety itchiness presents no harm to you or your baby. Your skin might be itchy and dry because it's stretching. Cocoa butter might give you some relief. Or try lotions that contain aloe. It might also help to run a humidifier in your bedroom when you sleep.

Skin changes are common in pregnancy, and one thing that often crops up in the second and third trimesters is a rash. Some women get a severe, itchy, red bumpy rash called plaques of pregnancy, toxemic rash, or pruritic urticarial papules (PUPP). The rash often begins on the belly, spreads to the lower body, and then spreads to the arms and legs.

? When to Call Your Doctor or Midwife

If the itching is driving you to distraction, you might want to talk with your doctor or midwife about it at your next appointment. He or she might suggest taking some antihistamines.

Very severe itching could be a sign for concern. Some women experience very severe itching late in their pregnancies. This is often caused by a condition called cholestasis, in which bile acids can build up in the liver and spill over into the maternal bloodstream. It occurs in about 1 out of 1,000 pregnancies, but it's more common in Swedish and Chilean ethnic groups and in women who are carrying multiples, women who have liver damage, or those whose mothers or sisters had cholestasis. Cholestasis generally happens in the last trimester, when hormones are at their peak. The itching is often on the hands or feet, but some women itch all over.

Talk with your doctor or midwife right away if you develop severe itching. It could be an indication of cholestasis, and the elevated levels of maternal bile stress the baby's liver. Your doctor or midwife can suggest treatments to help ease the itching.

PUPP is more likely in Caucasian women, women who gain a lot of weight during pregnancy, and women carrying multiples. Thankfully, it won't harm your baby, but it might make *you* nuts. The itching can be severe, especially at night.

You might try some home remedies for relief, such as soaking in a cool bath and applying witch hazel to your skin. The best remedy, though, is time. PUPP usually resolves within a week or two of delivery.

❧

During my pregnancy, I had itching on my belly. I put a lot of vitamin E and cocoa butter lotion on the area. If the itching was very intense, I put an ice pack on it, which really helped.

—*Diane Truong, MD, FAAP, a mom of one daughter and one son and a pediatrician in a multispecialty group practice in Southern California*

❧

During the last 10 weeks of my pregnancy, I developed the worst case of itching all over my body. It's usually caused by the cholestasis of pregnancy. What happens is the increased volume of blood in your body causes congestion of the liver, which causes a buildup of bile acids, which then can be released into your bloodstream, causing itching.

I itched from the top of my scalp to the tips of my toes. I scratched myself incessantly, and I asked my mom to scratch me too. Once you start scratching, there's really no end to it. It really was miserable.

I talked with my doctor about it, and he prescribed medication to ease the itch and to help me sleep. One of the first things I noticed in the recovery room after my babies were born was that I didn't itch anymore! It's amazing how quickly the body heals.

—*Sadaf T. Bhutta, MBBS*

Preventing and Treating Hemorrhoids

Almost half of all pregnant women experience hemorrhoids. It's one more consequence of the high levels of progesterone in your body. The extra hormones cause the outer part of your veins to relax, which allows them to swell. Also, the pressure of your expanding uterus reduces circulation in the blood vessels around the rectum and anus.

Hemorrhoids can develop at any time in pregnancy, but they're most common in the second and third trimesters. Although hemorrhoids often go away after the baby is born, they might get worse with each succeeding pregnancy.

Hemorrhoids are simply varicose veins in the rectum. They can cause throbbing pain, itching, and even light red bleeding. You might be able to feel a tender, swollen vein protruding from your anus.

The prevention and treatment of hemorrhoids is similar to that for constipation. Drink a lot of fluid and eat a lot of fiber. Warm baths might alleviate the pain and itching, but avoid baths over 100°F. Placing wet or dry baking soda on the area might relieve the itching. Holding an ice pack on your bottom might ease the pain and itching. Try not to lift heavy things because that can make hemorrhoids worse.

⁓

Toward the end of my pregnancy, I had terrible hemorrhoids. But I didn't actually know it until I was in labor. I had asked the nurses to move the birth mirror into my room because I wanted to see my baby being born. I was shocked to see these big, purple balls!

"What is that?" I asked my doctor.

"Don't worry; they're hemorrhoids, and they'll go away," he said.

The hemorrhoids started to hurt after my baby was born. Tucks Pads and Preparation H became my best friends. No one told me that hemorrhoids were so common in pregnancy. I wish I had known that they were coming, and that it's so normal.

—*Patricia S. Brown, MD*

During my pregnancies, I had some difficulties with constipation, which also led to some difficulties with hemorrhoids. I took an over-the-counter medication my doctor recommended called Colace. (Talk with your doctor before taking this or any medication.) It's a stool softener, and it's important to keep your stool soft so you don't strain. But women often get hemorrhoids during pregnancy anyway because of the extra pressure your baby is placing on your veins. I just did what I could to keep them from getting worse.

Fortunately, a little while after each of my babies was born, the hemorrhoids always went away.

—*Lezli Braswell, MD*

During my pregnancy, I tried to eat a lot of fiber. Fruits, vegetables, and natural grains such as wheat breads are the best source. Drink plenty of liquid to prevent difficult bowel movements, which can lead to hemorrhoids.

Mommy MD Guide-Recommended Product
Tucks Medicated Pads

Witch hazel is an odd-sounding name, but there's nothing magical about how it helps to ease hemorrhoids. Witch hazel is an astringent that will help relieve both irritation and burning. Tucks Medicated Pads contain witch hazel, and they're also dye free and safe to flush into both sewer and septic systems.

"During my first pregnancy, I had terrible constipation, which led to terrible hemorrhoids," said Sonia Ng, MD, a mom of seven-year-old and one-year-old sons and a pediatrician and expert in sedation at Children's Hospital of Philadelphia Pediatric Care at Princeton Health Care System in Princeton, NJ. "By my third trimester, they were very painful and itchy. I found that Tucks Medicated Pads really helped. I tried to use over-the-counter hemorrhoid creams as little as possible because I wasn't sure how well they had been studied in pregnant women."

You can buy a box of 100 Tucks Medicated Pads at drugstores and online for around $8.

This is also very important after you have the baby because if it hurts to go to the bathroom, you'll try to avoid going, which will make your stools harder and more difficult to pass. This in turn can aggravate hemorrhoids.

Hemorrhoids are very hard to avoid during pregnancy. Even if you're not prone to hemorrhoids, during pregnancy your anatomy is different. The baby is heavy, and the weight is pushing on your perineal floor and on the veins in your pelvis. This puts you at risk for hemorrhoids, which are swollen veins that can be internal or external.

My third baby had to be delivered early because of the unbearable pain triggered by the acute onset of hemorrhoids, mainly after the baby's head was engaged in the birth canal and it was putting extra pressure on the veins. Labor was *nothing* compared with that hemorrhoid pain.

Amazingly, after my baby was born, the pain immediately resolved. It was like turning off a switch.

—*Aline T. Tanios, MD*

Chapter 32
Week 32

Your Baby This Week

YOUR BABY'S SIZE
This week, your baby weighs almost four pounds. She's more than 11¾ inches crown to rump, and she "stands" nearly 19 inches long.

YOUR BABY'S LATEST DEVELOPMENTS
Your baby's nostrils are well developed by now. Soon your baby's lungs will be mature enough to breathe unaided if she is born early. The words *preterm* and *premature* are often used interchangeably, but a baby who is born at 32 weeks with mature lung function is more correctly called a preterm infant. The word *premature* better describes an infant who has immature lungs at birth.

Your baby continues to develop white fat under her skin. Also her skeleton is continuing to harden; right now it's still quite soft and pliable.

YOUR LATEST DEVELOPMENTS
Around this time, your uterus is almost five inches above your belly button. Your baby is pressing more on your internal organs, which is likely making breathlessness, heartburn, and urine leakage more frequent.

Your eyes might be feeling dry or irritated, and your vision might even have changed. If you wear contact lenses, you could wear your old glasses or see an eye doctor for some disposable contacts to get you through the rest of your pregnancy. Generally, your eyes will be back to normal by around six weeks after your baby's birth.

This is a common time for parents-to-be to take prenatal and breastfeeding classes. There you're likely to meet other parents to be whom you might encounter at the hospital or birth center when you're delivering. You might even make friends for future baby playdates.

JUSTIFICATION FOR A CELEBRATION
Because your baby is running out of room, she might have shifted into a head-down position, ready for birth.

Nesting with a Purpose

Even if you're not an obsessive type of person, you might suddenly feel compelled to alphabetize your spices. Nesting is a powerful urge to prepare your home for your baby by cleaning and decorating. It's not a myth! Nesting can be useful because it helps you to get tasks out of the way before your baby is born so that you can relax, recover, and nurture your baby after she arrives.

Happy organizing!

By the end of my pregnancy, I needed to keep busy and not dwell on the upcoming birth. I think that nesting is a natural reaction when you are ready for labor to start and need an outlet for your nervous energy. It might not be entirely hormonal; getting the baby's room and clothes just right is one of the few things that you can control while you're waiting.

—*Ellen Kruger, MD, a mom of two teenagers and an ob-gyn in an academic and clinical practice in New Orleans, LA, with Ochsner Health System*

I had very easy pregnancies, which was lucky because I was on my feet a lot. My energy level throughout my pregnancies was actually the opposite of what you'd expect. I had extra energy like I was euphoric. I felt like I was on steroids.

I put all of that energy to good use! I was working a very demanding job and on my feet all day long. I got lots of things accomplished, and I felt great, which was awesome!

—*Debra Luftman, MD, a mom of a teenaged daughter and a teenaged son, a board-certified dermatologist in private practice, a coauthor of* The Beauty Prescription, *the developer of the skincare line of products Therapeutix, and a clinical instructor of skin surgery and general dermatology at UCLA*

I remember with my first baby, we had an extra bedroom, and so we set up the crib in there and added a changing table and some decorations. But then one weekend toward the end of my pregnancy, I had a tremendous boost of energy. I ran around that weekend washing all of the baby's clothes and organizing everything. I clearly remember thinking to myself, *Wow! Where is all this energy coming from?*

I must have been nesting. Thinking back, I remember having a similar boost of energy in each of my pregnancies, just a bit before I went into labor.

—Patricia S. Brown, MD, a mom of two daughters, ages nine and seven, and a three-year-old son and a psychiatrist at Columbia-New York Child and Adolescent Telepsychiatry and in private practice in Cresskill, NJ

During my pregnancy, I was completely exhausted—so tired I could barely move—for around four weeks. By the second trimester, my energy levels started to rise. By the time I was 35 weeks pregnant, I was nesting like a lunatic, with more energy than I knew what to do with. At that point, the only thing weighing you down is the baby.

—Erika Schwartz, MD, a mom of two and the director of www. DrErika.com, who's been in private practice for more than 30 years in New York City, specializing over the past 15 years in women's health, disease prevention, and bioidentical hormones

Considering Circumcision

If you're having a boy, you have one major decision to make that moms-to-be of girls don't: to circumcise or not. For some families, the decision is simple because of cultural or religious beliefs. For other families, the decision isn't so clear cut.

You might be surprised to read that only 55 to 65 percent of baby boys are circumcised. This rate varies by region. The north central region of the United States has the highest rate of circumcision, and the western states have the lowest rate.

Boys are born with a foreskin, which is a hood of skin covering the head of the penis. In a circumcision, the foreskin is surgically removed to expose the end of the penis. Routine circumcision is often done within 48 hours after a baby's birth; if not, it's usually done during the first 10 days of life. Circumcision can be done after the newborn period, but it is more complicated then and usually requires general anesthesia.

Benefits of circumcision include a reduced risk of urinary tract infections and possibly of penile cancer and HIV/AIDS. Some people claim that circumcision changes the sensitivity of the tip of the penis, but this hasn't been proven. As with any surgical procedure, circumcision carries some potential risks, but complications occur in less than 3 percent of cases, and they are usually limited to minor bleeding or local infection.

The American Academy of Pediatrics recommends the use of pain control measures for circumcision, such as a topical cream or an injectable anesthetic. Giving the baby a bit of sugar water can help to reduce his stress.

For us the circumcision was important. We had a ritual circumcision.
—*Debra Luftman, MD*

My husband and I decided to have our son circumcised right at birth, with a little bit of topical anesthesia. It's a very personal choice. What I've observed in my practice is if Dad is circumcised, Baby will be circumcised.
—*Diane Truong, MD, FAAP, a mom of one daughter and one son and a pediatrician in a multispecialty group practice in Southern California*

Rallie's Tip

My husband wanted to have our boys circumcised, but I wasn't sure. I had helped circumcise several babies when I was on the ob-gyn service in my residency training, and I couldn't see how surgically removing such a teeny, tiny bit of skin could make all that much difference. Later, when I was working on the surgery service, I assisted a surgeon in the circumcision of a 36-year-old man. That was all it took to convince me that I'd have my boys circumcised when they were babies.

My family is Jewish, so my son was going to be circumcised. Because my husband's side of the family has an inherited seizure disorder, we decided to have the circumcision in the hospital rather than at a bris, which is a ceremony of circumcision performed on the male child on the eighth day after his birth.

My theory about circumcision is that what's important is that the dad and the baby match. If the dad is circumcised, I think the baby should be too.
—*Ellen Kruger, MD*

The only decision regarding circumcision was where it would be. I wanted it to be *out* of the house, so I didn't have to cook or clean. I knew I was going to be tired.

On the other hand, my husband wanted the circumcision to be *in* the house because it would be more intimate. We came to a great compromise: We held the circumcision in our home, but my husband agreed to do all of the cooking and cleaning for it.

We held it on my son's eighth day. We used a mohel who's also a pediatrician so he could give our son pain medication. He slept through the whole thing!

—*Michelle Paley, MD, PA, a mom of a six-year-old daughter and a two-year-old son and a psychiatrist and psychotherapist in private practice in Miami Beach, FL*

My older son was circumcised by one of my medical partners. It was okay, but I do a *great* circumcision, so I circumcised my second son myself. It was at home, as a bris, and we had a rabbi there as well.

I don't use any anesthetic. I've never met a man who remembers his circumcision! I use a device called a Mogan Clamp. It looks like a cigar clipper. It's over so fast that the babies rarely cry. I think if the babies cry, it's more because they don't like being held down.

I give the babies a little sugar water first, and that calms them right down. Most of the babies I've circumcised fall asleep as soon as the clamp goes on. I don't think that they feel any pain of the circumcision because the clamp is so tight that their nerve endings don't have any sensation anymore.

—*Melanie Bone, MD, a mom of four "tweens" ages 15 to 12, a gynecologist, the founder of the Cancer Sensibility Foundation, and the author of the syndicated column Surviving Life and the book* Cancer, What's Next?, *in West Palm Beach, FL*

Taking Prenatal and Breastfeeding Classes

Around now, or perhaps even earlier, you might take a prenatal and/or breastfeeding class. These are held in hospitals or birth centers, by nurses and midwives, and by organizations such as the YWCA. Some insurance companies offer inexpensive classes—even free ones.

To find a class, talk with your doctor or midwife, ask your friends and family, check the newspaper, and search online. Many hospitals publish periodicals that include calendars of events. If you don't already receive your local hospital's publication, you might want to call and ask to be added to their mailing list. In addition to the calendar of events, these publications often include interesting health articles.

Classes can be wonderful opportunities to learn, ask questions, and meet other parents-to-be. You can take classes on staying healthy in pregnancy, preparing for childbirth, baby care, breastfeeding, and more. You might want to take an infant CPR/first aid class. Childbirth education classes at hospitals often include a tour of the hospital's labor and delivery section.

One type of class is the Bradley Method. It was developed by Robert A. Bradley, MD, who believed that plenty of preparation could lead to a natural, unmedicated labor and delivery. Visit www.BradleyBirth.com for more information and to find classes near you.

Lamaze classes are another type to consider. In 1951, Dr. Fernand Lamaze introduced a method of childbirth in France by incorporating techniques that he observed in Russia. This method, consisting of childbirth education classes, relaxation, breathing techniques, and continuous emotional support from the father and a specially trained nurse, became known as the Lamaze method. Visit www.Lamaze.org for more information and to find classes near you.

Taking classes can help you to prepare for labor and breastfeeding, if you choose to nurse your baby. The better prepared you are, the more relaxed and confident you'll be.

❧

I made my husband go to a Lamaze class. Even though I felt prepared for motherhood because I worked with kids, I needed him to know what to expect too. Unfortunately, he spaced out most of the time because he didn't think he needed to listen.

—*Sonia Ng, MD, a mom of seven-year-old and one-year-old sons and a pediatrician and expert in sedation at Children's Hospital of Philadelphia Pediatric Care at Princeton Health Care System in Princeton, NJ*

My husband and I took private Lamaze classes. Because they were private classes, they were more intense—and shorter—than most classes. I think that the classes were helpful. It's important to know what you don't know.

— *Debra Luftman, MD*

&

I made my husband take classes with me at home with a private teacher because he didn't know anything about pregnancy and birth. Truth be told, the classes were boring for me, and they were pretty boring for my husband too.

—*Melanie Bone, MD*

&

During my pregnancy, I went to some birth classes that I probably could have skipped. I think I knew more than the people teaching the class! The breastfeeding one was much more helpful because it was something new to me that I had never done.

—*Patricia S. Brown, MD*

RALLIE'S TIP

With my second pregnancy, my husband and I signed up for prenatal classes, and we had every intention of attending every one of them and being really good students. But we only made it to the first two classes.

My husband is an ER doctor, and he worked a lot of crazy shifts, and I was working on call every third night, because I was still in residency. At our second (and last!) class, the health educator started talking about all the yucky things that would go on in preparation for the birth: enemas, urinary catheters, IVs, shaving of the pubic area, and so on. This was back in the day when all that was standard procedure.

I couldn't take it! I figured I'd just jump off that bridge when I came to it. Or even better, I'd arrive at the hospital so close to delivery that I wouldn't have to have all those things done to me. In the end, I arrived in plenty of time to experience most of the "necessary" preparations.

I think that it would have been wiser for us to attend every single one of the prenatal classes, but thankfully, my son and I both survived without them.

I have to admit that I didn't take a breastfeeding class. In hindsight, now I see that classes can be very helpful. Taking a class is so much better than reading a book. It allows you to network with other women who want to learn about the best techniques for successful feeding of their infants.

I breastfed each of my babies for a month, and I found through trial and error that different strategies worked with each of them. If I had taken a class, perhaps I wouldn't have needed so much trial and error!

—*Aline T. Tanios, MD, a mom of three and a general pediatrician and hospitalist who treats medically complex children at Arkansas Children's Hospital in Little Rock*

❧

During my pregnancy, I was doing my family practice residency, and part of that was an obstetrics rotation. So I basically knew what to expect for labor and delivery from watching so many babies being born. I wasn't nervous or scared about the labor and delivery process.

What I wish I had done was take a breastfeeding class. Nursing was hard! I saw a lactation consultant after my daughter was born, and I highly recommend finding one before your baby is born.

—*Lezli Braswell, MD, a mom of one daughter and two sons and a family medicine physician currently working in an emergency room fast track in Columbus, GA*

My husband and I didn't take any prenatal classes, although we had the option to do so. We talked it over, but we thought that we already knew what we needed to know.

In hindsight, I wished we had taken some classes. When I went into labor, we both panicked quite a bit!

—*Diane Truong, MD, FAAP*

Chapter 33
Week 33

Your Baby This Week

Your baby's size

Around this time, your baby measures 12 inches crown to rump and nearly 19½ inches head to heels. He weighs around 4½ pounds. He's going through a period of intense growth, gaining around ½ ounce a day. At this point, your baby is filling out more than lengthening.

Your baby's latest developments

Your baby's hearing is becoming more refined. Anecdotal evidence suggests that after babies are born, they recognize sounds that they heard in utero. It's possible that in a few weeks, your baby might be soothed by music that you've played, songs that you've sung, or stories that you've read to him in the womb.

If you and your partner have dark hair, your baby might have a very impressive head of hair by now.

In preparation for birth, your baby continues to practice breathing. This is helping his lungs to make surfactant, which keeps his lungs inflated.

Your baby's skeleton continues to harden. His skull will remain soft though so that his head can fit through the birth canal.

Your latest developments

You've probably gained between 22 and 29 pounds by now, though more or less is likely just fine too. You might be gaining weight at a faster rate right now, but keep in mind that a lot of that weight is actually being put on by your baby, not by you.

Your breasts might feel a little lumpy these days. The hormone oxytocin is stimulating your milk glands to expand and fill up with colostrum—and maybe even milk.

This week, the top of your uterus is around 5¼ inches above your belly button. Your uterus squishing your stomach might be waning your appetite. Also, you might be feeling nauseated again. Plus, your nerves might feel a little frayed. Try to eat when you can and choose the most nutritious foods possible.

Around this time, you might be feeling Braxton Hicks contractions every day. Your body is practicing for the real thing!

The hormone relaxin is helping your hips to spread wider apart and encouraging the bones in your pelvis to shift to make room for when your baby drops. If you're clumsy and drop or bump into things, you're perfectly justified to blame it on your hormones.

Start to keep a lookout for your water breaking. Some women start to leak amniotic fluid as their labor gets closer. (See "Worrying about Your Water Breaking in Public" on page 418.)

Some women start to feel pain in the vagina around now. A warm bath might ease the pain. As your bones spread apart to make way for your baby, it can affect your pubic bone and vaginal muscles.

Getting sleep is hard, but try to rest when you can. Pregnant women who are very fatigued tend to be more anxious and depressed and even feel more pain.

JUSTIFICATION FOR A CELEBRATION

Your baby's immune system has matured enough that he's now able to fight off mild infections on his own.

Planning Your Route to the Hospital or Birth Center

By now, you know which hospital or birth center you'll deliver at. Perhaps you've even taken a tour or a class there.

If not, it's a great idea to take a dry run to see exactly which is the best way to go. Consider traffic patterns and if any roads are under construction. Locate and practice an alternate route, or even two. Find out where you're supposed to park and which entrance you should use. Sometimes the door you're supposed to use differs depending on the time of day.

Ask anyone who might be driving you to the hospital to go with you so that they are familiar with the route too. When you're in labor, you won't feel much like pointing out which road to turn onto.

RALLIE'S TIP

Because my husband and I worked at the hospital where I planned to deliver, we both felt like we could drive there with our eyes closed. But when I was in labor with my second child, we made the mistake of checking in at the Emergency Department rather than going straight up to the labor and delivery floor of the hospital.

I was already in labor, and I was a little anxious and worried that I was going to have that baby any minute. The nurses in the Emergency Department were busy, and it took them a while to get me pointed in the right direction. Even though I wanted to walk, they insisted on pushing me in a wheelchair.

When you're in labor, you want to get to a safe place as quickly as possible, and you don't feel like interacting with a lot of people. In most hospitals, you can check in directly at the labor and delivery department, which will save you the time and trouble of going through the Emergency Department or Admissions.

It's a good idea to find out the policies and procedures at the hospital or birth center where your baby will be born ahead of time so you'll be able to get settled into your room as quickly as possible. When you're getting ready to deliver a baby, even a five-minute wait can seem like forever!

Preparing Your Pets for the Baby

If you have a pet, he's probably gotten pretty used to being the center of attention and the only baby in your home. He likely has no idea that a dramatic change is about to turn his world upside down.

With a few simple steps, you can ease your pet's transition, get him ready for the baby, and set the stage for a positive relationship with your child.

First, take your pet to a vet for a complete exam, and make sure he is up to date on shots. Checking on your pet's health now will save you time that you might not have once baby arrives. Ask the vet to check your pet for parasites. If your pet wasn't spayed or neutered, consider doing it now. This might help your pet be calmer and less likely to bite. Be sure to discuss any health or behavior concerns during your visit.

Second, get your pet used to baby sounds and smells. Play recordings of a baby crying, cooing, laughing, and gurgling. (Check out www.PreparingFido.com to purchase online; it also includes tips from the Humane Society of the United States.) Teach your dog to lie down or sit calmly when he hears these sounds. Turn on the baby swing, play lullaby CDs, and let your pet listen to your white noise machine. Encourage your pet to sniff the baby shampoo, baby powder, and the new toys you bring home. Offer praise and treats for calm behavior.

Consider placing a sturdy barrier such as a baby gate at the nursery room door to keep your pet out of your baby's room. If your pet doesn't already have a special place of his own, such as a bed or a crate, give him one now. And remember, never leave a pet unsupervised with a baby.

My husband and I have a rescue dog named Casey. We didn't do much to prepare him before our daughter was born, but after she was born, my husband took a blanket home with her scent on it. We had read that would help him to get used to her.

—*Kerri A. Daniels, MD, a mom of one toddler daughter and an instructor in the department of pediatrics at the University of Arkansas for Medical Science in Little Rock*

When I was in the hospital having my first baby, my husband took the baby's hat and some clothes home for our dogs to sniff. That was all the preparation they got—or seemed to need.

—*Kristie McNealy, MD, a mom of seven- and four-year-old daughters and a two-year-old son, who's pregnant with another son, and a blogger at www.KristieMcNealy.com, in Denver, CO*

RALLIE'S TIP

One of the best presents I got at my baby shower was a pair of baby gates. I didn't think I'd need them until my son started walking, but as it turned out, I used them the day we came home from the hospital. They were perfect for keeping my curious, overly enthusiastic Boston Terrier in the kitchen or out of the nursery when I needed some alone time with the baby. My dog never tried to harm the baby, but she was determined to try to lick his face whenever she got the chance!

ॐ

Our cat was our baby before our babies were born. My husband and I bought a tent for our baby's crib to keep the cat out of it. We were concerned how the cat would react to the baby because she was already five years old when our daughter was born.

We were right. When the baby came home, the cat was not very happy!

—Mary Mason, MD, a mom of a nine-year-old girl and six-year-old boy, an internist, and the chief medical officer for a multi-state managed care company that coordinates care for about 70,000 pregnant Medicaid moms a year

Preparing for a Scheduled C-Section

In the United States, almost one-third of babies are born by Cesarean sections, which are commonly called C-sections. Moms older than age 35 have a higher rate of C-section deliveries.

A C-section is a surgical procedure used to deliver your baby through an incision in your abdomen. It's often planned ahead of time due to pregnancy complications or because you've had a previous C-section.

One thing you might want to do before your scheduled C-section is talk with your anesthesiologist about any pain relief questions you have. Your doctor might send you for a hemoglobin test to check for anemia.

Because a C-section requires a longer recovery than a vaginal birth, it's a great idea to line up some help with your home, baby, and other children, if you have them.

My first son was born by C-section, and at the time, they didn't do vaginal births after C-sections, so my second baby was planned to be delivered by C-section.

It was so very planned. Everything went beautifully, especially because I knew exactly what to expect the second time around. I wasn't too concerned about having the C-sections either time because I knew it was the right thing to do for my babies. We are so fortunate today because C-sections are so common. Just a few generations ago, they weren't an option, and that must have been scary.

—*Sandra Carson, MD, a mom of two grown sons and the director of the Center for Reproduction and Infertility of Women & Infants Hospital in Providence, RI*

My husband was 10 pounds, 4 ounces when he was born, and I was almost 10 pounds. Our daughter was tracking large, and there were some other health concerns related to my unusual migraines. I talked it over with my obstetrician, and we decided the safest thing to do was a planned C-section.

My daughter weighed almost 10 pounds when she was born, and we were both healthy and happy, so I was glad the planned C-section was an option for me.

—*Katja Rowell, MD, a mom of a four-year-old daughter, a family practice physician, and a childhood feeding specialist with www. familyfeedingdynamics.com, in St. Paul, MN*

Toward the end of my first pregnancy, I had an ultrasound that indicated that my baby might weigh 11 pounds! So I scheduled a C-section. The ultrasound reading was incorrect, and my son weighed only 8 pounds, 13 ounces. My son's head size was in the 99th percentile, and I later learned that head size is a metric for estimating birth weight.

—*Amy J. Derick, MD, a mom of one 15-month-old son who is 17 weeks pregnant with her second son. Dr. Derick is a dermatologist in private practice at Derick Dermatology in Barrington, Il.*

For my first delivery, I had a C-section, so for my second, I had a scheduled one. I have to say, as a working mom, it was very nice to be able to pick the day that I was going to have my C-section. I was able to plan ahead for child care for my son during that time. Plus, I was able to work up to the day I went in for the surgery.

A lot of people don't want to have C-sections, but I liked being able to have all of my bases covered.

—*Barbara Goff, MD, a mom of two and professor of obstetrics and gynecology and the director of gynecologic oncology at the University of Washington Medical Center in Seattle*

⤝⤞

I had three C-sections. I actually wanted to have C-sections because both my mother and grandmother had difficult deliveries. I was much more comfortable having C-sections because they are very controlled, and I knew what to expect.

I was also grateful to schedule the C-sections ahead of time. That way I could arrange child care for my older daughters and let my partners in my practice know when I would be out.

With my first daughter, I was ready to have a scheduled C-section, but they had to put me on hold for an emergency C-section. In the meantime, I went into labor. I labored all the way to nine centimeters, and I remember my doctor asking me if I wanted to push.

"No, I want my C-section," I said. My doctor complied, and all went well.

—*Marra Francis, MD, a mom of three daughters and an ob-gyn who's based in The Woodlands, TX*

Reading Up on Baby Care

If you haven't already, now's a great time to pick up a book on baby care. Certainly you can find tons of information online, but there's nothing quite like a trusted book to turn to in the middle of the night.

⤝⤞

I didn't get to take any classes, but I did read lots of books when I was pregnant. Thank goodness I read all about baby care before my son was born because I sure didn't have any time to read *after* he was born. I read about breastfeeding; they don't teach that in medical school! I also read books about bringing up boys. They were very helpful.

—*Dianna K. Kim, MD, a mom of three and an ob-gyn in private practice in Vernon Hills, IL, at the Midwest Center for Women's Healthcare*

MomMy TIME

Join a Book Club

You'll find book clubs all over the country. Joining a book club is a wonderful way to meet new people, and it's a great reason to read a good book and to get out of the house.

If you can't find a book club near you, why not start one? You'll find lots of helpful information at **WWW.BOOK-CLUBS-RESOURCE.COM.**

During my pregnancy, my copy of *What to Expect When You're Expecting* went everywhere with me. I followed it every month, and I referred to it often. *The Girlfriends' Guide to Pregnancy* was great for comic relief.

Then as my due date approached, I started to read more on baby care.

—*Patricia S. Brown, MD, a mom of two daughters, ages nine and seven, and a three-year-old son and a psychiatrist at Columbia-New York Child and Adolescent Telepsychiatry and in private practice in Cresskill, NJ*

During my pregnancies, I tried not to read too much. It can kinda make you crazy. I chose one book per topic and stuck with that. I find if you read too many different books, their advice starts to conflict. I also relied on a friend who has kids for advice.

—*Michelle Paley, MD, PA, a mom of a six-year-old daughter and a two-year-old son and a psychiatrist and psychotherapist in private practice in Miami Beach, FL*

Before my first baby was born, I got a little panicky. I thought, *Oh no, the baby's coming. What am I going to do?* A few days before my due date, I started frantically reading baby books and cramming. I think it's a misconception that doctors know what to do—with the exception of pediatricians! I know all about pregnancy and birth, but once the baby was born, I didn't have any experience with that. I was just like any other new mother. So I quickly read all about feeding, bathing, changing diapers, and more.

—*Jennifer Kim, MD, a mom of three girls, ages eight, five, and four; an ob-gyn in private practice in Evanston, IL, at the Midwest Center for Women's Healthcare; and a clinical assistant professor at the University of Chicago, Pritzker School of Medicine*

Chapter 34
Week 34

Your Baby This Week

YOUR BABY'S SIZE

Your baby now weighs about five pounds. She measures around 12¾ inches crown to rump and 19¾ inches head to heels. Her living quarters are really cramped now!

YOUR BABY'S LATEST DEVELOPMENTS

The waxy vernix coating is likely to thicken at this point. It continues to protect your baby's skin, and it will also help her to move through the birth canal.

By now, your baby has shed most of her lanugo.

Your baby has better control of her movements now that her central nervous system is maturing. This is critical for her to be able to drink after she is born.

If your baby is a boy, his testicles are close to their final location in the scrotum. However, around 3 percent of baby boys' testicles don't descend until after they're born.

Between 34 and 36 weeks, your amniotic fluid reaches its peak level. Around week 37, the fluid levels will begin to decline slightly to allow more room for the baby. Where does it go? Your baby continues to swallow the fluid, and some of it's stored in her body as meconium and fat. Also, some fluid is reabsorbed by your body. As this happens, you might notice that your baby's movements feel a little different.

Your latest developments

The top of your uterus now reaches about 5½ inches above your belly button. You probably feel very big and mighty uncomfortable.

If your breasts feel heavy and full, you might find that it's more comfortable to wear a bra when you sleep. Try a soft nursing bra or sports bra, nothing with underwires.

You probably can't see your shoes, and even if you could, you wouldn't be able to reach them to tie their laces. Slip-on shoes are the way to go now. Speaking of feet, now's a great time to have a pedicure. Give your feet a treat!

If your belly button has popped out, you might feel self-conscious about it, and clothing rubbing on it might be uncomfortable. You can simply cover your "outie" with a bandage or a piece of tape. Your belly button might be very sensitive to touch these days too.

If you're having twins, this is a common time to go into labor. You've probably become quite the homebody these days, which is a great idea.

Justification for a celebration

Only six more weeks to go!

Babyproofing Your Home

Right now, babyproofing might be far from your mind. After all, when your baby comes home from the hospital, she'll stay where you put her. The days when she'll venture up the stairs, try to scale your bookcases, and open the front door to wander out seem like they're far, far in the future.

But are they? Your baby's first few months will pass in the blink of an eye. Now is the perfect time to do some babyproofing—while you have the time and brainpower.

Two critical things to do now if you haven't already are install smoke and carbon monoxide alarms. You need to have them on each floor of your home, plus outside each sleeping area. Also plan a fire escape route with your partner. It's especially important to choose a meeting place outside your home where you'll do a head count to make sure that everyone made it out safely.

You might do a few easy babyproofing things now to get them out of the way. It's simple to install outlet covers in outlets, door knob covers on doors, and cabinet locks on cabinets. Time spent now will save you time later. You'll find many websites and books with helpful babyproofing advice, such as *The Babyproofing Bible.*

My husband and I didn't babyproof our home too much in preparation for our baby's birth. We did luck out, though. We moved into our home a few months before our daughter was born, and the former owners left all of the outlet covers in place. After my daughter was mobile, we did the major babyproofing.

—*Kerri A. Daniels, MD, a mom of one toddler daughter and an instructor in the department of pediatrics at the University of Arkansas for Medical Science in Little Rock*

When I was pregnant, my husband and I did the basic babyproofing. We put covers on the electrical outlets and locks on the cabinet doors. We didn't go crazy and put bumpers on the coffee tables; we just did the usual stuff.

Kids fall down; kids get hurt. It's part of life.

—*Ann LaBarge, MD, a mom of four children, ages 16 to six, and an ob-gyn in private practice at the Midwest Center for Women's Healthcare in Park Ridge, IL*

Spend some time babyproofing while you have time and can still think. Once the baby comes, you'll be completely exhausted and have no brainpower for at least six months.

My husband and I completely babyproofed our home before our oldest was born. We even installed the baby gates. And I was so glad we did. My husband and I both knew that we wouldn't have a lot of time after the baby came, so we babyproofed as much in advance as we could. But what we didn't expect is that you just can't think right for the first six months after the baby is born.

The easiest way to start babyproofing is to go to a baby store (such as buybuy Baby) and spend some time in their babyproofing section. That'll give you lots of ideas on all the things your child can get into and how to prevent that from happening.

Before your baby is born, you'll want to cover the basics, such as installing hard-mounted baby gates at the top and bottom of stairs, covering outlets with outlet protectors, putting childproof door knob covers on doors to the rooms you'll want to keep the baby out of and doors that lead to the outside, putting locks on toilets so the baby can't play in—or fall in—the toilet, and putting latches on cabinet doors in both your kitchen and bathrooms. Also, be sure to turn down your home's hot water heater to lower than 120°F and install fire and carbon monoxide alarms at least on every level of your home if you don't already have them.

—*Kristin C. Lyle, MD, FAAP, a mom of three girls and the disaster medical director at Arkansas Children's Hospital and an assistant professor of pediatrics at University of Arkansas for Medical Sciences, both in Little Rock*

⤳

I've always had smoke detectors in my home. But I never babyproofed my house. When we grew up, our parents didn't do any of that, and we turned out just fine. Bad things can happen with and without your neuroses.

—*Melanie Bone, MD, a mom of four "tweens" ages 15 to 12, a gynecologist, the founder of the Cancer Sensibility Foundation, and the author of the syndicated column* Surviving Life *and the book* Cancer, What's Next?, *in West Palm Beach, FL*

Doing Perineal Massage

Perineal massage is an exercise where you, and/or your partner, massage the perineal area (the area between your vagina and rectum) each day, usually in the last six weeks of pregnancy.

Like so many things in pregnancy—and parenting—you'll find vastly different opinions on perineal massage. Some experts believe that perineal massage eases a woman's pain in childbirth and reduces the risk of tearing. They say that women who do massage are familiar with the stretching sensations in that area, and so they're better able to relax those muscles for birth.

One study found that doing perineal massage after 34 weeks might reduce a woman's chances of tearing during birth and reduce the need for an episiotomy, which is a procedure in which an incision is made from the vagina toward the rectum during delivery to avoid undue tearing of the area.

On the flip side, other experts believe just as strongly that perineal massage is unnecessary.

If you would like to give perineal massage a try, talk with your doctor or midwife to find out how to do it and ask for their opinion on what's best for you.

∽⟊

Around week 36, I started doing perineal massage every other day. Initially it was awkward and uncomfortable, but then I got more used to it. I believe it enabled me to be more comfortable when my babies were crowning. I didn't tear at all, even though my babies were big—8 pounds, 6 ounces and 8 pounds, 8 ounces.

—*Lauren Feder, MD, a mom of two sons, a nationally recognized physician who specializes in homeopathic medicine, and the author of* Natural Baby and Childcare *and* The Parents' Concise Guide to Childhood Vaccinations, *in Los Angeles*

∽⟊

I didn't do any perineal massage. Intuitively, it seems like you might minimize damage in delivery by encouraging the tissues to stretch. But some believe that *unstretched* tissues can actually be repaired more easily than tissues that have been broken down by massage. There's no clear evidence that perineal massage is beneficial or harmful. But if women want to be proactive and do perineal massage, then great!

—*Stephanie Ring, MD, a mom of two sons, ages six and two, and an ob-gyn at Red Rocks Ob-Gyn in Lakewood, CO*

Installing Your Baby's Car Seat

If you haven't done so already, ask your partner, or a handy friend or family member, to install your baby's car seat. He or she will need both the car seat manual and your car's manual. This isn't always an easy process, so it's helpful to get it out of the way now.

Take some time to familiarize yourself with how to use your baby's car seat. If you have an infant carrier seat with a base that remains in the car, practice getting the carrier into and out of the base. Learn how to strap the baby into the seat and how to get her out. Most of all, learn how to use the seat safely, so that you'll be able to buckle her into it correctly each and every time—starting with her trip home from the hospital.

RALLIE'S TIP

My second child came a few weeks early, and although my husband and I had bought a car seat, we hadn't even taken it out of the box when I started having labor pains. It had been over a decade since our first child was a toddler, so our skills were definitely a little rusty! My husband installed the car seat in the hospital parking lot in the middle of a snowstorm while the baby and I were inside. We both agreed it would have been a lot easier if we had been better prepared for our son's early arrival. We had enough to do without worrying about the car seat.

One of the hardest things to do is to get your car seat installed correctly and know how to put your child in it. We see so many kids in the emergency room after car accidents who were in their car seats, but the seat wasn't installed correctly or the child wasn't strapped in right. It's a challenge to install and to use car seats correctly.

Before our oldest daughter was born, I took a class on choosing and installing car seats. I was so overwhelmed with the information that I hired a certified car seat specialist to come put them in my car, and every other car the baby would be riding in. We bought enough bases for every car, so we wouldn't be trying to re-install them all the time. Then I spent time with my husband and everyone else who would be helping me with the new baby to make sure that they understood how to use the car seat correctly. We practiced strapping a baby-size doll into the seat.

Now I certainly don't think most parents would—or even could—take a 40-hour car seat class, but you could take a two-hour class. And everyone should take their car seats to a car seat inspection site. They'll check to make sure your seat is installed correctly—for free. You can visit the website www.SeatCheck.org to search the National Highway Traffic Safety Administration's (NHTSA) listing of child passenger safety seat inspection locations. Certified inspectors at these locations can provide guidance on proper child restraint use and installation. Or call them at 866-SEAT-CHECK to find a location near you.

—*Kristin C. Lyle, MD, FAAP*

Stocking Up on Diapers and Other Baby Supplies

In a newborn's first few weeks, she'll go through 11 to 14 diapers a day—that's 80 to 100 in a week. Stocking up now can save you—or your partner—panicked trips to the store later. Perhaps pick up a package or two of diapers at each trip to the store. You'll find lots of diaper coupons in the newspaper and online that can help with the cost.

Besides buying newborn-size diapers, you might want to buy some size 1 diapers as well. Your baby *will* grow into them, and depending on how big she is when she's born, that day might come sooner than you think.

❧

Because I was put on bed rest for the final two months of my pregnancy, my husband had to do a lot of the prep work. One day I sent him out to buy a breast pump, which was above and beyond the call of duty. Another day I asked him to buy diapers. He came home with one package!

"Honey, do you remember the newborn stage?" I said. "This will last us about a half a day with twins."

—*Susan Wilder, MD, a mom of an older daughter and twin girls, a primary care physician, and CEO and founder of Lifescape Medical Associates in Scottsdale, AZ*

With my first baby, I knew the baby was coming, but I was in denial. Come 38 weeks, I hadn't really done anything to prepare for her arrival! That's when I hunkered down and bought the essentials. Fortunately, at the beginning, all you need is a whole lot of clothes, washcloths, diapers, and a bassinet. Then you're good to go.

—*Ashley Roman, MD, MPH, a mom of two daughters, ages three years and six months, and a clinical assistant professor in the department of obstetrics and gynecology at the New York University School of Medicine in New York City*

We had a tradition in our family that we don't bring anything for the baby into our home until the baby is born. This really takes a lot of pressure off new parents!

My husband and I ordered the baby's furniture, but we asked the store to hold it. My mother bought all of the baby's diapers and wipes and supplies and kept them at her house. That saved me from obsessing about all of those decisions: Which type of diapers should I buy? Which brand of wipes are best? I might have spent 10 hours trying to figure out what type of thermometer to buy. But it doesn't matter when someone else picks it out for you. Whatever they've selected works, and you move on from there.

—*Michelle Paley, MD, PA, a mom of a six-year-old daughter and a two-year-old son and a psychiatrist and psychotherapist in private practice in Miami Beach, FL*

Mommy MD Guide-Recommended Product
Pampers Pop-Up Baby Wipes

It's true: Regular baby wipes cost less than pop-up wipes. But pop-up wipes allow you to pull a wipe out of the tub one-handed, and that is a very good thing.

You can buy a tub of pop-up wipes at drugstores, grocery stores, pretty much everywhere, for around $3.50 for 72 wipes. Save the tubs because refill bags are cheaper.

Chapter 35
Week 35

Your Baby This Week

YOUR BABY'S SIZE

Your baby now measures about 13¼ inches from crown to rump, and he "stands" about 20¼ inches tall.

This week, most babies weigh about 5½ pounds. This is only an average, and you're likely wondering how much *your* baby weighs. You can ask your doctor or midwife, but without an ultrasound it's very difficult to estimate a baby's weight. Truth be told, even *with* an ultrasound, the estimate can be off by as much as ½ pound.

YOUR BABY'S LATEST DEVELOPMENTS

Your baby still looks a little lean, but he's no longer as red and wrinkly as he was a few short weeks ago. By now, your baby might have put on enough weight to have precious little dimpled elbows and knees.

Around this time, your baby's ability to suck from a nipple will be fully developed.

Your baby's kidneys are by now completely developed and working. The kidneys filter out waste, toxins, and water in urine.

If your baby is a boy, his testicles have finally finished their descent into his scrotum.

YOUR LATEST DEVELOPMENTS

This week, the top of your uterus is around six inches above your belly button. You've probably gained between 24 and 29 pounds. You might lose some weight between now and your baby's birth if your appetite has taken a nosedive. Around this time, you've reached your maximum blood volume.

Because your uterus is so high, some part of your baby is probably pushing on your ribs. If you're lucky, this feels like a tickle. More likely it feels like pain.

Be certain to eat plenty of iron-rich food now In your last trimester, your baby is storing up iron in his liver. That stored iron will sustain him for his first few months after birth.

You're very likely still feeling the staple symptoms of back pain, breathlessness, constipation, and heartburn. It's best to rest whenever you can.

It's very common to feel dramatic emotions now. You might feel anxious, irritable, sensitive, and worried. This is very normal. You might have very good company in this because your partner might be feeling many of these emotions too. Around this time, you *both* might be torn between the dueling urges to prepare everything possible for your baby and to rest and relax.

Your Braxton Hicks contractions are probably more frequent now, and they might even be painful. Check with your doctor or midwife if you're ever unsure that they *are* Braxton Hicks contractions, rather than actual contractions.

By now, you might be seeing your doctor or midwife once a week. At these visits, your doctor or midwife is certainly still checking your blood pressure and weight and your urine for sugar and protein. Your doctor or midwife is probably also feeling for your baby's presentation and possibly even doing a vaginal check to see if your cervix has started to dilate (open) or efface (thin).

JUSTIFICATION FOR A CELEBRATION

Even though you might be terribly uncomfortable, your body will be back to its old self in a few months.

Coping with a Big Belly

Speaking of being uncomfortable, your belly is probably making you greatly uncomfortable. Your center of gravity is off, and your belly is pulling on muscles you didn't even know that you had. The good news is that although you won't be wearing your skinny jeans home from the hospital, your belly will be markedly decreased right after your baby is born.

～⌾～

Especially during my third pregnancy, I wore a lot of dresses to accommodate my big belly. They weren't even maternity dresses—just regular flowing, empire waist dresses. I lived in those. They were loose and flowing enough to accommodate my growing belly and breasts.

— *Lezli Braswell, MD, a mom of one daughter and two sons and a family medicine physician currently working in an emergency room fast track in Columbus, GA*

～⌾～

During my last trimester, there was not enough room for all three of us— hubby, belly, and me—in our queen-size bed. Don't be offended if you and your partner have to sleep separately during the last few weeks of your pregnancy.

— *Tyeese Gaines Reid, DO, a mom of one, an emergency medicine resident physician at Yale New Haven Hospital in Connecticut, and the author of a time management book,* The Get a Life Campaign

～⌾～

During my first pregnancy, I gained 50 pounds. I was very uncomfortable at the end of my pregnancy. Because of my belly, it was hard for me to drive. I had a little car, and I could barely sit behind the wheel. I did the best I could to squeeze myself into the tiny space and stretch my arms to reach the wheel.

— *Elissa Charbonneau, DO, a mom of an 18-year-old son and a 16-year-old daughter and the medical director of the New England Rehabilitation Hospital in Portland, ME*

～⌾～

Toward the end of my pregnancy, my belly was so big that I couldn't get it out of the way when I was checking patients. Our bellies would touch, and patients could feel my baby kicking them.

Because I carried my daughter straight out in front, you couldn't tell I was pregnant from behind. One day toward the end, I was standing in line at the grocery store. I turned to my right to pick up a candy bar, which was a big deal to me because I hardly ever eat chocolate. When the woman behind me saw my belly, she let out an audible gasp!

I looked back at her and said, "I guess I won't be getting that candy bar after all."

"Oh no," she said. "You deserve it!"

—*Marra Francis, MD, a mom of three daughters and an ob-gyn who's based in The Woodlands, TX*

Trying to operate is very challenging when you're big. Being on my feet and getting close enough to the operating field was challenging.

When you're operating, you have to lean over a lot more when your tummy's in the way. I had to give up operating on very large people because I don't have enough height. I had to limit my practice a bit in the last month of my pregnancy and not operate on anyone heavier than 250 pounds.

—*Barbara Goff, MD, a mom of two and a professor of obstetrics and gynecology and the director of gynecologic oncology at the University of Washington Medical Center in Seattle*

Making a Birth Plan

As your pregnancy goes along, you're probably getting a sense of how you would like your birth to go. A birth plan will help you to communicate your wishes to the people who will be supporting you during labor.

Some things to consider mentioning in your plan are whom you would like to be with you in labor; how you feel about being cared for by students, midwives, and intern and resident doctors; whether or not you'd like to be able to walk around in labor; how you feel about pain control options; your thoughts on episiotomies or tears; and whom you would like to cut the umbilical cord.

Whatever you plan, keep in mind that it's only a plan. Try to be as flexible and open to change as you can be.

I put together a birth plan of how I hoped my birth would go. I made it like an algorithm tree to communicate what I wanted to happen in different circumstances. For example, it said if X happens, then do Y, and then if Y happens, then do Z. Luckily, I did not have to follow the plan because there were no complications.

—*Sonia Ng, MD, a mom of seven-year-old and one-year-old sons and a pediatrician and expert in sedation at Children's Hospital of Philadelphia Pediatric Care at Princeton Health Care System in Princeton, NJ*

It's fine to create a birth plan, but at the end of the day, you can't control pregnancy and birth. You can have a vision, but be prepared to ditch it.

You just never know how these things are going to go. With my first delivery, I had an epidural and forceps. With my second, I had no medication, and I didn't even get an IV. I'm glad I didn't go into my first delivery hoping for a natural birth, and I'm glad I didn't go into my second asking for an epidural. It's best to remain flexible.

—*Ellen Kruger, MD, a mom of two teenagers and an ob-gyn in an academic and clinical practice in New Orleans, LA, with Ochsner Health System*

Dragging Yourself into Work

When you're pregnant, you're already a working mom! You might be feeling the challenge and responsibility of that with each passing day.

Because sitting or standing in one position for too long can make you uncomfortable, try to move around when you can. On the flip side, rest when you're able. Try to manage stress at work as much as possible. Right now you have plenty of pregnancy stress to contend with.

If you have any concerns about your safety—and the safety of your baby—at work, talk with your doctor or midwife and your employer.

Many women stop working two weeks before their due date, but it's just as common for women to work right up until their due dates, perhaps to save as much of their maternity leaves as possible for after their babies are born.

I worked until just a few days before my son was born. My last work day was a Friday, and he was born on a Monday.

At the time, I was on an endocrinology rotation at Good Samaritan Hospital. In that atmosphere, I had to wear nice clothing to work. But toward the end of my pregnancy, I couldn't bend over to put on my clothes! Each morning, my husband had to pull my panty hose on. I can't tell you how many pairs of panty hose he ran trying to put them on with his not-so-smooth contractor's hands. It was a running joke: How many pairs will it take today?

—*JJ Levenstein, MD, FAAP, a mom of one son in college and a pediatrician in private practice in Southern California*

❦

I worked right up to the delivery during both of my pregnancies. I saw 28 patients on the day my son was born. At 5:30 pm, I admitted a patient to the emergency room, and then I drove home, picked up my bag, went to the hospital I was supposed to deliver at, and gave birth at 11 pm.

I'm not sure how I kept up with that schedule. I think I knew that I would rather spend time with the baby after he or she was born vs. taking time off before.

—*Mary Mason, MD, a mom of a nine-year-old girl and six-year-old boy, an internist, and the chief medical officer for a multi-state managed care company that coordinates care for about 70,000 pregnant Medicaid moms a year*

❦

My first pregnancy was very complicated. I had terrible swelling that led to preeclampsia and carpal tunnel syndrome. I feel God gave me such a complicated pregnancy so I'd become a much more sympathetic doctor. Being a patient is much harder than being a physician.

My doctor tried very hard to put me on bed rest. But I was stubborn and stupid, and I refused to do it. I couldn't take time out for myself. What I didn't realize at the time was when you have a child, you know that child takes precedence before everything else. But before I had the baby, I didn't understand that.

With my second pregnancy, I took better care of myself. I stopped working at 36 weeks and did all the right things. I didn't have any swelling in that pregnancy or complications, and I felt so much better.

—*Gina Dado, MD, a mom of two daughters and an ob-gyn with Arizona OBGYN Affiliates, Paradise Valley Branch, in Scottsdale, AZ*

During my pregnancies, I worked right up until delivery. One pregnancy was during my fellowship, and I even took on-call duty the night before I delivered!

I made sure to always wear comfortable shoes. Taking breaks was important as well. It's hard to take a break during surgery, but I would try to periodically sit down, even if only for a minute or two so I could rest a tiny bit. That gave me enough stamina to get through surgery.

—*Barbara Goff, MD*

∽

During my pregnancy, I signed up for a tremendous number of moonlighting hours. I was trying to take hours for moonlighting instead of money so that if I had to leave my job early because I went into labor, I wouldn't owe any time, and I could take a longer maternity leave. I do shift work at Children's Hospital of Philadelphia, and I was induced on my last day of work. Because of all that moonlighting, I got an extra month of days off, and the month I went back, I only had about five days of work total.

That is absolutely not something I would recommend to anyone. You risk premature birth and all the associated complications. But at least I worked at the hospital, which was the safest place to be if I had a medical problem. I went 42 weeks with my first child. At 36 weeks, I figured, I could do anything and the baby's lungs would already be mature. In fact, I was out washing the car in the driveway. My husband was really embarrassed about it. He thought that the neighbors would be thinking he was an awful husband. At least I didn't do it Jessica Simpson–style.

—*Sonia Ng, MD*

Having a Group B Strep Test

Group B streptococcus (GBS) is a type of bacteria that is often transmitted person to person by sexual contact. Up to 40 percent of all pregnant women have GBS in their bodies, most often in their vaginas or rectums. Even if you have GBS, you probably have no idea because it usually doesn't cause any symptoms in you. However, if you have the bacteria, you can pass it to your baby. In a newborn, GBS can cause life-threatening infections.

Women are usually screened for GBS between 35 and 37 weeks of pregnancy. A culture is taken from your vagina and rectum. If the test shows you have the bacteria, you'll be given IV antibiotics, such as penicillin, in labor. This will cut your baby's risk of infection.

∽⟨⟩

I had a group B strep test when I was around 35 weeks pregnant with both of my babies. The test came back negative both times, so I didn't have anything to worry about.

—*Ashley Roman, MD, MPH, a mom of two daughters, ages three years and six months, and a clinical assistant professor in the department of obstetrics and gynecology at the New York University School of Medicine in New York City*

∽⟨⟩

Generally, you have a test for group B strep between weeks 35 and 37. Because my first daughter was born at 36 weeks, I didn't have my test results yet. I had to stay a few extra days in the hospital with my baby until we had the results and knew we were both negative.

With my third baby, my doctors were concerned I'd go into preterm labor again. So they gave me a group B strep test very early just in case. I ended up having the test twice because the results are only good for a certain amount of time. I didn't mind because I knew that way we wouldn't have to wait to take the baby home pending the results of the test.

—*Kristie McNealy, MD, a mom of seven- and four-year-old daughters and a two-year-old son, who's pregnant with another son, and a blogger at www.KristieMcNealy.com, in Denver, CO*

∽⟨⟩

I tested positive for group B streptococcus (aka "GBS" or "group B strep"), which is a bacteria that can colonize a normal vagina. But if it is present at or around the time of the delivery, there is a small chance that the baby can contract it while passing through the vaginal canal. It can be very dangerous for the baby, so to further reduce the risk of transmission, we test for GBS around 36 weeks gestation (vaginal and rectal). If it is present, we give IV antibiotics to the mother during labor. We also give the antibiotics if at any point during the pregnancy, the woman has had a GBS-positive urine culture.

—*Janet Lefkowitz, DO, a mother of two girls and an ob-gyn in private practice in Rhode Island*

Chapter 36
Week 36

Your Baby This Week

YOUR BABY'S SIZE

This week your baby weighs around six pounds. She's longer than 13½ inches crown to rump and 20¾ inches head to heels.

YOUR BABY'S LATEST DEVELOPMENTS

Your baby is curled up tightly, probably head down, waiting for labor to begin. By this time in pregnancy, a baby has usually gotten into the position she's going to stay in for birth. In other words, if she's head down, she's likely to stay that way.

In about 3 percent of pregnancies, the baby's bottom or legs go into the pelvis first. This is called a breech presentation.

Your baby's digestive system is now ready to accept liquid food.

Even if your baby will later have dark skin, her skin will have a pinkish cast now because of the blood vessels that are close to the surface.

YOUR LATEST DEVELOPMENTS

By now, you might have gained 25 to 30 pounds. It's not unusual for a mom-to-be's weight to hover right around here until her baby is born, or even to go down a bit.

The top of your uterus probably measures about 6 inches above your belly button, up under your ribs. Now or sometime in the next few weeks, you might be shocked to discover that the top of your uterus is actually measuring lower than it was before. This will happen when your baby's head enters the birth canal. This is called dropping, engaging, or lightening. This unusual word refers to the *lightening* of the abdominal pressure.

Lightening can happen a few weeks before labor begins, or it might not happen until labor starts. In first pregnancies, the head descent can start as early as 36 weeks, but in later pregnancies, the baby's head might not engage in the pelvis until the moment labor begins. This is because a vaginal delivery slightly alters the arrangement of the pelvic bones, and that might delay engagement.

As your baby moves lower into your birth canal, you might feel pressure and worry that your baby is going to fall out. This is almost certainly not the case, but talk with your doctor or midwife about it at your next visit.

Another clue that your baby has dropped is if you suddenly have to pee all of the time. Some women find they have to urinate more than every hour after lightening occurs. Once your baby drops into your pelvic cavity in preparation for birth, your bladder will be squished. The good news is, lightening should give you a welcome break from shortness of breath and heartburn. You might be breathing a little easier—literally. Also, when your baby drops, you might notice that your lap space has decreased.

By now, you have the maximum amount of amniotic fluid, around two pints.

This week, you might step up your doctor or midwife visits to going once a week. If you haven't done so already, now's a good time to pack a bag for your baby's birth.

You might be starting to dilate and not even feel it. It's not uncommon for women to dilate one to two centimeters in the last month of pregnancy but not be in active labor or have many noticeable contractions.

Although your baby is cramped and her movements are more subtle, with the odd jab now and then, keep alert to any changes and let your doctor or midwife know about them right away.

JUSTIFICATION FOR A CELEBRATION
Babies born at 36 weeks are almost always able to breathe unattended.

Packing Your Birth Bag

Packing your birth bag is unlike packing for any other trip. You're going to the hospital pregnant, but you'll be coming home a mom.

Grab your favorite bag and put it in a convenient place. The odds are good that you're going to be adding things to the bag and pulling them back out a lot in the next few weeks as your excitement—and nerves—grow.

Here are a few things to consider packing: insurance information and hospital preregistration forms; your camera and video recorder; a cell phone or calling card and list of family and friends' phone numbers; things to distract you in labor such as a CD player and CDs and magazines; your favorite pillow and/or Boppy nursing pillow; toiletries such as a toothbrush, toothpaste, hairbrush, ponytail holder if you have long hair, soap, shampoo, and conditioner; pajamas or a nightgown and a robe; slippers or warm socks; soft, comfy bras and nursing bras if you plan to breastfeed; several pairs of underwear; sanitary pads in case the hospital doesn't supply them or they look too uncomfortable to use; candy or lollipops to suck on in labor and snacks for afterward; and a comfortable outfit that you wore around month five for your trip home.

You'll also want to bring things for your baby, perhaps in a separate bag. Consider packing a special outfit for the ride home, baby blankets, a hat, and diapers if your hospital doesn't supply them.

Last but not least, toss in some things for your partner. This could include more snacks, change for vending machines, and something for him to do, such as magazines to read.

❧

I found it invaluable to bring my own underwear, pajamas, shampoo, and soap to the hospital. I also brought my nursing pillow.
—*Michelle Paley, MD, PA, a mom of a six-year-old daughter and a two-year-old son and a psychiatrist and psychotherapist in private practice in Miami Beach, FL*

❧

I packed my bag around a week or so before I went into labor. I packed reading materials, outfits for the baby, and my Boppy nursing pillow to help me breastfeed. I also took my computer because the hospital had wireless Internet. I was actually able to use my computer because the baby slept a lot!

—*Amy J. Derick, MD, a mom of one 15-month-old son who is 17 weeks pregnant with her second son. Dr. Derick is a dermatologist in private practice at Derick Dermatology in Barrington, IL*

You have to pack your bag long before week 36! I packed mine at 20 weeks. We see many premature babies here, and I wanted to be prepared. I needed to be ready, which was one more way to decrease the stress and preparation for the "big day." When you go into labor, it's not the time to run around your house trying to pack your bags. You'll be far too worried about your health and the health of your baby at that point.

While my sanity was still intact at 20 weeks, I started to pack my bag. Every few weeks, I reviewed what was in there and added to it as necessary. I kept two lists: what I had packed for myself and what I had packed for my baby. For myself, I packed body lotion, perfume, a mirror, a book (not that I had the chance to open it), my cell phone and charger, slippers, an outfit to go home in, and a list of people I wanted to call. For my baby, I packed diapers, a going-home outfit, receiving blankets, the car seat, and presents from the new baby brother or sister for my older children. Also, don't forget the camcorder and camera.

—*Aline T. Tanios, MD, a mom of three and a general pediatrician and hospitalist who treats medically complex children at Arkansas Children's Hospital in Little Rock*

I packed my bag when I was 38 weeks pregnant. Generally, women pack theirs earlier, but for some reason I really didn't think about it.

I packed a nightgown, underwear, toothbrush, toothpaste, and hairbrush. Some women bring a pillow, but I didn't do that. I brought a few different outfits for the baby because you don't know how big the baby will be.

I actually didn't end up wearing my own nightgown or underwear while I was in the hospital. You bleed so much after delivery, and I didn't want to mess up my things. Instead I wore the hospital gown and the mesh panties they provide.

One thing I was sure to leave at home was my jewelry. You don't want to have to worry about that when you're in labor and adjusting to motherhood.

—*Ashley Roman, MD, MPH, a mom of two daughters, ages three years and six months, and a clinical assistant professor in the department of obstetrics and gynecology at the New York University School of Medicine in New York City*

RALLIE'S TIP

My second son was born at 36 weeks, right when I had started thinking about packing my birth bag. I didn't want to pack it too early, because I thought that would only make time pass more slowly.

When my contractions hit in the night, my husband and I were so focused on getting to the hospital in the middle of a blizzard before the baby came that we completely forgot about packing a bag. After the baby was born, I sent my poor husband back home to pick up some pajamas so I wouldn't have to wear a hospital gown.

I'm not sure how my husband did it, but he returned with the most hideous pair of sweat pants that I owned. I hadn't worn them for years except to paint in them, and I wasn't about to wear them in the hospital.

When I got pregnant with my next child, I had that birth bag packed and ready to go at 26 weeks!

Enlisting Help with the Baby and Home after Delivery

Those clever folks at Johnson & Johnson are right: Having a baby changes everything. Probably nothing in life changes a person more than becoming a parent. Before you have a baby, it's hard to imagine what it's going to be like and what you might need. If you're able, try to make a list of tasks you might need help with after you get home with the baby. This way, if people ask what they can do to help, you'll have some ideas. Perhaps someone could bring over a meal, run an errand for you, or watch your baby for a few hours while you nap.

⤾

My older sister and her husband came to stay with us right when I was due. Just like clockwork, I went into labor that night. My sister and her husband took over the show and watched our daughter while our twins were born. It could not have been more perfect.

—Susan Wilder, MD, a mom of an older daughter and twin girls, a primary care physician, and CEO and founder of Lifescape Medical Associates in Scottsdale, AZ

When my daughter was born, my mother came and stayed with us for a while. Having my own mother there when I was learning how to be a mother was so comforting. She helped me so much with my new baby.

We lived in a one-bedroom apartment in New York City at the time, so it was close. But it was very nice.

—Ellen Kruger, MD, a mom of two teenagers and an ob-gyn in an academic and clinical practice in New Orleans, LA, with Ochsner Health System

When my older daughter was born, I was living on a spiritual commune called the Farm. Pregnancy was revered there, and there were plenty of people anxious to help out all pregnant women. In our community, birth was considered to be the holiest thing, and to have any interaction with the midwives or the birth process was considered a lucky thing. People volunteered, "Oh, let me watch your kids for you!" That would give them access to the whole energy of pregnancy and birth.

My three-year-old daughter went to stay with a friend the day I went into labor with my second baby, and she came back to me two days later. But even then, that didn't mean I had to *watch* her the whole time. I had plenty of support and help from friends.

—Stacey Marie Kerr, MD, a mother of two grown daughters, a family physician with strong roots in midwifery, and the author of Homebirth in the Hospital, *in Santa Rosa, CA*

When my twins were born at 29 weeks, they stayed in the neonatal intensive care unit for six weeks. I really pressured their doctors to let us bring them home, but that was a mistake. My mom came and stayed to help us for a while after they came home.

But the most help came from my husband. I just assumed that my husband and I would take care of our babies ourselves. In their early months,

I went back to work while my husband stayed home with them. It never entered my mind that a dad couldn't take care of babies just as well as a mom.

—*Ruth D. Williams, MD, a mom of twins—a boy and a girl—and another boy, and an ophthalmologist in private practice at the Wheaton Eye Clinic in Wheaton, IL, who specializes in the diagnosis and treatment of glaucoma*

My family and my husband's family both live in Pakistan, so we're pretty much on our own here. But with my older daughter, my mom, who's also a physician, flew over here a week before my baby was due and stayed with us for three months. That was awesome! As a first-time mother, I had no idea what I was doing and how to care for a baby. My mom really helped me.

The second time around, I was pregnant with triplets, and my mom reversed the procedure. She flew in from Pakistan three months prior to their birth to help me, but she only stayed for five weeks after they were born. That was just fine with me because I knew how to handle babies by that time.

—*Sadaf T. Bhutta, MBBS, a mom of a three-year-old daughter and 18-month-old triplets and an assistant professor and the fellowship director of pediatric radiology at the University of Arkansas for Medical Sciences and Arkansas Children's Hospital, both in Little Rock*

RALLIE'S TIP

When my first baby was born, my older sister was already a seasoned mom. She came to visit and to show me the ropes of caring for a newborn baby. I have never been so grateful to anyone as I was to my sister then. I was a little nervous and overwhelmed, but she was calm and confident, and eventually her attitude rubbed off on me.

Whenever possible, I think it's a great idea to have a close friend or family member come and help out the first few days—or even the first few weeks—after the baby is born. Of course you can handle it all by yourself, but why would you want to?

Planning for Your Other Children's Care during Delivery

If you have older children, no doubt you have already started to think about who will care for them when you go into labor and while you are recovering at the hospital. You'll want to plan for several different contingencies. For example, what will you do if you go into labor at night, when your child is in school, or when your partner is at work?

When my son was born, my daughter was four years old. My mom was prepared to watch her while I was in the hospital. Plus our nanny was always available to help. We had a great team lined up!
— *Michelle Paley, MD, PA*

My daughter was four when our twins were born. My husband stayed home with her, and I was able to get a lot of rest both at the hospital when my twins were born and when we came home from the hospital.

Our daughter was a very easy child, and she was easy for him to care for. She played independently a lot. We had originally tried to have a second baby much earlier, but I think God knew the right plan was to wait until our daughter was older.
— *Kelly Campbell, MD, a mom of three and an ob-gyn in private practice at Women's Healthcare Physicians in West Bloomfield, MI*

When my younger son was born, my older son was four years old. Because I was having a scheduled Cesarean section, and we knew exactly when the baby would arrive, my mom came into town around a week early. This was wonderful because she watched my son while my husband and I went out to dinner and got to spend some special time alone.

I don't recommend having your mom or another helper come early if you don't have a planned delivery, though. Otherwise, grandmas-to-be arrive early and sit and wait and put a lot of pressure on moms-to-be to have the baby already!
— *Stephanie Ring, MD, a mom of two sons, ages six and two, and an ob-gyn at Red Rocks Ob-Gyn in Lakewood, CO*

Spending Special Time with Your Partner

Now is not the time to jet away to Paris. But this *is* a wonderful time to spend some time with your partner. Snuggle on the couch, have a candlelight dinner, or go to a movie. Your life is about to change—dramatically.

❮❯

During my pregnancy, my husband and I had a lot of special dinners. We used to say, "We have to do this before the baby comes!"

—*Joanna Dolgoff, MD, a mom of a seven-year-old son and a four-year-old daughter, a board-certified pediatrician/child obesity expert with practices in Manhattan and Roslyn Heights, NY, creator of an online child weight loss program (www.DrDolgoff.com), and author of the book* Red Light, Green Light, Eat Right

❮❯

When I was pregnant, my husband and I were living in the south of France. We really enjoyed many special moments together, and we traveled all over Europe. There were so many things I wanted to do, and it was so extraordinary to be able to do them with my husband—while we were expecting our baby. It was a wonderful time.

—*Lilian Morales, MD, a mom of an 11-year-old daughter and a physician in Bogotá, Colombia*

❮❯

My husband and I were living in Germany during my second pregnancy. Because of Germany's central location, we could take day trips to four different countries. We even went to Paris for two weekends. We enjoyed lots of wonderful food. It was fantastic!

—*Ann Kulze, MD, a mother of four children, ages 20, 19, 18, and 14, a nationally recognized nutrition expert, motivational speaker, physician, and the author of the critically acclaimed book* Dr. Ann's 10-Step Diet: A Simple Plan for Permanent Weight Loss and Lifelong Vitality

❮❯

I think it is so important to stay romantic as a couple, during pregnancy and beyond. I set my mind on making sure that my husband and I would continue to be each other's most important person in the world.

When my parents asked me what I would like when my first baby was born, I asked them to give me the gift of caring for our children each year for a few days while my husband and I went away together. I knew that I wouldn't trust anyone other than my own parents to watch my baby for that long. But I knew that those few days each year—and the anticipation of them before and the memories of them after—would give my husband and me special time to recharge and to keep the romance going. Never forget that you *start* as a couple, and *then* you become parents.

—*Ayala Laufer-Cahana, MD, a pediatrician, mother, artist, serious*
home cook, and the founder of Herbal Water Inc., in Wynnewood, PA

Chapter 37
Week 37

Your Baby This Week

YOUR BABY'S SIZE

Your baby now "stands" around 21 inches tall, and he measures around 14 inches crown to rump. He weighs about 6½ pounds—only a pound or two away from what he will weigh on his birthday. This time is sometimes called "finishing growth." Your baby is now snug as a bug inside of you, and by now he can only turn from side to side.

YOUR BABY'S LATEST DEVELOPMENTS

Your baby's circulatory and immune systems are all-systems-go for birth. Interestingly, your baby's digestive system isn't fully mature, and it won't be for his first year. That's why he'll drink only breast milk or formula for his first few months.

Your baby has around 8 percent body fat now. As your baby gains weight, he's developing creases at his wrists and neck.

YOUR LATEST DEVELOPMENTS

Your weight might be holding steady now. You might not be very hungry, and plus your baby is using most of the calories that you consume as he gains weight in preparation for birth. Your basal metabolic rate increases by 25 percent late in pregnancy, which means it's much more efficient in converting stored nutrients into energy. If you're having a hard time choking down solid foods, smoothies might go down easier.

This week, your uterus is about 6½ inches above your belly button. This is about where it might stay until your baby drops or until he is born.

Your joints all might feel terribly loosy-goosy now. The pregnancy hormones are loosening all of your joints and ligaments, which hold your joints together, in preparation for birth.

Because your baby is so cramped, his movements probably feel more like pressing or pushing to you. You might see your baby's hand pressing out against your belly. It would be amazing to snap a photo of that!

Your cervix is now sensitive and engorged with blood. If you have intercourse, it might cause spotting. Report bright red discharge or persistent spotting to your doctor or midwife without delay, but some spotting following sex isn't cause for alarm. Most experts agree that intercourse is fine now, even beneficial.

Around this week, your doctor or midwife might start checking your baby's station, which describes how far your baby has descended into the birth canal. "0 station" represents a bony landmark in the pelvis, the starting point of the birth canal. The stations range from -5 to +5. If your baby is at "-5 station," he's higher inside of you, floating above the pelvis. If he's at "+5 station," his head is crowning, visible outside of the vagina.

This is a great time to start thinking about what on earth you and your partner are going to eat in the weeks after your baby is born. You might want to put together a list of take-out and delivery menus from local restaurants. More places deliver than ever these days. Tip the pizza delivery guy well because you're going to be seeing a lot of him in the weeks ahead!

JUSTIFICATION FOR A CELEBRATION
At the end of this week, your baby is full term!

Preparing for Your Pets' Care during the Delivery

If you have pets, it's important to line up someone, or even a few some-ones, to care for them while you're in labor and after your baby is born.

❧

Our plan was that while I was in the hospital giving birth, my husband would go home each day to care for our hamster. He had actually taken over hamster duties throughout my pregnancy because hamsters carry a disease that's dangerous for pregnant women. The hamster passed away a few months ago, and my husband was really sad. They got to be very close!

> —Sonia Ng, MD, a mom of seven-year-old and one-year-old sons and a pediatrician and expert in sedation at Children's Hospital of Philadelphia Pediatric Care at Princeton Health Care System in Princeton, NJ

RALLIE'S TIP

My second baby came four weeks early, so I hadn't done a thing to prepare for my dogs' care during my delivery. My husband and I left the house in the middle of the night, when my contractions were about five minutes apart. The next morning, it occurred to us that those dogs needed to go out! My husband had to run home and take care of the dogs before the baby was born. Fortunately, he made it back in time, but I'm sure he was more than a little stressed.

Because you usually can't predict exactly when your baby will be born, it's a good idea to line up someone to take care of your pets well in advance of your due date.

Easing Your Fears

As your pregnancy has progressed, your anxieties and fears might have grown along with your belly. It's perfectly natural to feel nervous and to worry about pregnancy and labor and delivery. It's all great training for parenthood.

❧

Pregnancy is overwhelming. This is probably good preparation for parenting, which is even more overwhelming. At some point during my pregnancy, I realized that I was doing my best, and then I would just fake the rest. I stopped trying to control every variable. We all muddle through. I just try to use my best judgment.

—*Ellen Kruger, MD, a mom of two teenagers and an ob-gyn in an academic and clinical practice in New Orleans, LA, with Ochsner Health System*

I am a workaholic, which kept me distracted. I was in my hospital bed, in labor, hanging onto the phone telling my "coverage" about one of my more troubled patient's difficulties. The nurse came into the room and said, "Look, madam, you're here to have a baby. You're not here to fiddle with your on-call schedule. Lose the phone."

Talking with my husband also helped ease my fears.

—*Elizabeth Berger, MD, a mom of two, a child psychiatrist, and the author of* Raising Kids with Character

I embraced my pregnancy, but I had a lot of apprehension and concerns, like any mom-to-be. My father was an ob-gyn, and so I had heard so many stories about labor and delivery that I think it increased my worries about my own health.

—*Debra Luftman, MD, a mom of a teenaged daughter and a teenaged son, a board-certified dermatologist in private practice, a coauthor of* The Beauty Prescription, *the developer of the skincare line of products* Therapeutix, *and a clinical instructor of skin surgery and general dermatology at UCLA*

It seems to me that if you have a hard pregnancy, you will have an easy birth. It doesn't always work out that way, but I had terrible pregnancies and great births. If it hadn't been for the nine months of pregnancy and a lifetime of raising kids, I would have had a dozen of them. I loved giving birth.

—*Stacey Marie Kerr, MD, a mother of two grown daughters, a family physician with strong roots in midwifery, and the author of* Homebirth in the Hospital, *in Santa Rosa, CA*

During my second pregnancy, I was very worried. I didn't know how I could possibly love another baby as much as I loved my son. I felt terrible even thinking that.

I remember calling my mom, crying and saying, "I don't know how I could ever love this baby as much."

"Don't worry," my mom said. "There's enough love in your heart for both babies!"

And of course, my mom was right.

—Elissa Charbonneau, DO, a mom of an 18-year-old son and a 16-year-old daughter and the medical director of the New England Rehabilitation Hospital in Portland, ME

∽

Don't be afraid of the baby. There's not an alien inside of you; the baby is a part of you. For example, when you get a cold, you don't think that you're going to die. If the baby is lying the wrong way, pushing on an organ, and you don't feel so good, don't worry that it's something to be afraid of.

Our society has turned pregnancy into a disease. But there's nothing more natural. Being pregnant is such an empowering time. It feels wonderful to feel life inside of you. It's a time to cherish. Forget the complaints; they're nothing compared with the beauty of being pregnant and the joy of bringing another life into the world. The more you behave like normal, the more you can enjoy your pregnancy.

—Erika Schwartz, MD, a mom of two and the director of www. DrErika.com, who's been in private practice for more than 30 years in New York City, specializing over the past 15 years in women's health, disease prevention, and bioidentical hormones

∽

Because I'm an obstetrician, people ask me if it was hard for me to be pregnant, knowing as I do all of the bad things that can happen.

I see how they could think that, but it never struck me that way. Instead, I felt very empowered by my knowledge. I felt that if something wasn't going well, we could figure out what to do to fix it, which in hindsight, may or may not have been true.

I had a very positive outlook and a strong conviction that my baby would be healthy. I never focused on the negative; only on the positive. And ultimately I was very lucky to have three amazing, healthy children.

—Siobhan Dolan, MD, MPH, a mom of three, a consultant to the March of Dimes, and an associate professor of obstetrics and

gynecology and women's health at Albert Einstein College
of Medicine/Montefiore Medical Center in the Bronx, NY

I was the youngest of six, and my mother died when I was very young. My dad didn't realize how what he said impacted me, but he told me, "Your mother was never quite right after you were born."

I was very worried how pregnancy and motherhood would change me. I think it's very important to be prepared for all those changing hormones. Especially in the first week or two after your baby is born, your hormones are crashing and shifting. The big question is: *How well are you functioning?* Sleep is not a good barometer because you will be tired. The big warning signs to watch out for are super irritability, dramatic changes in behavior, long hours of crying, and suicidal thoughts. Call your doctor right away and don't worry alone.

—*Nancy Rappaport, MD, a mother of two teenaged daughters and a teenaged son, an assistant professor of psychiatry at Harvard Medical School, an attending child and adolescent psychiatrist in the Cambridge, MA, public schools, and the author of* In Her Wake: A Child Psychiatrist Explores the Mystery of Her Mother's Suicide

Surprisingly, I found that I was more nervous with my second pregnancy than with my first. My first baby was perfectly healthy, and I worried, "How do you get so lucky a second time?"

With my second pregnancy, I was over age 35, so I had to have an amniocentesis. It helped to ease my fears a lot when that came back normal. In retrospect, I think I was relatively laid-back compared to some women. It really is a miracle when a healthy baby is born with all the parts in place. I think I just couldn't allow myself to go to the place of "what ifs." I was really busy and fortunately was easily distracted.

—*Janet Lefkowitz, DO, a mother of two girls and an ob-gyn in private practice in Rhode Island*

Preparing Your Home and Stocking Up on Food and Supplies

While you have some time, energy, and brainpower left, try to stock up on food and other things that you'll need after your baby is born. You might want to prepare some meals ahead of time and freeze them. Or buy some quick-to-prepare frozen meals at the grocery store, such as Chicken Voila or Bertolli dinners. Purchase extra supplies such as paper towels, toilet paper, and trash bags. You're going to need these things; they don't take up much space; and anything you buy now, you won't have to worry about after your baby is born.

❧

During my pregnancy, we lived in France. Every week or other week, I went to the supermarket. That's where I stocked up on things for the baby, including

MomMy TIME **Try a Meal Prep Place**

What's for dinner? To answer that question simply and easily, meal prep places have been popping up all over the country. You can go to these facilities, socialize with friends or meet new people, and assemble meals for your family in take-out-style containers—in just a few hours. This is perfect for moms-to-be: Fill up your freezer in preparation for your baby's birth.

According to the Easy Meal Prep Company, which supports meal prep businesses, as of January 2010, there were 238 different meal-prep companies and 592 outlets across the country.

One of the largest companies, Dinner by Design, has 22 stores across the country, currently in Alabama, Illinois, Indiana, New Jersey, New York, Ohio, and Wisconsin. They offer "kitchen sessions."

Upon arrival, you'll see that all of the hard work has already been done, and the recipes and ingredients are ready for you. You grab an apron, wash your hands, and spend two hours or less enjoying the meal assembly process, socializing with others while putting together your entrees in easy to store, complimentary containers. Easy to follow heating or baking directions on labels are already printed for you, ready to go.

To find a meal prep location near you, visit **www.EasyMealPrep. com** and search by your zip code.

bottles, pacifiers, and even some clothing. I wanted to have everything washed, ready, and waiting when my baby was born.

—*Lilian Morales, MD, a mom of an 11-year-old daughter and a physician in Bogotá, Colombia*

I had our babysitter start work a few weeks before my baby was born. This was so helpful because she helped me set up the nursery. She also prepared a lot of meals that we froze and then ate after we came home from the hospital.

Another thing I did ahead of time was buy thank-you cards, announcements, and stamps. I even printed out all of the address labels in advance! I didn't want to have to deal with setting that all up after I came home with the baby because setting up those spreadsheets is like speaking Chinese to me. I tried to make the process as easy as possible.

—*Michelle Paley, MD, PA, a mom of a six-year-old daughter and a two-year-old son and a psychiatrist and psychotherapist in private practice in Miami Beach, FL*

Right before I gave birth to my first baby, I bought a pressure cooker. I was convinced that I wasn't going to have any more time in my life. I figured I'd have to cook super-fast. That pressure cooker sat unused for two years because I was afraid it would blow up if I used it and forgot to turn it off.

Women worry about the time vacuum that is going to happen once the baby arrives. Yes, having a baby is an intense experience and a magical shift in your life. But you will still be able to carve out the time to do the things that keep you passionate and sustained.

—*Nancy Rappaport, MD*

Chapter 38
Week 38

Your Baby This Week

YOUR BABY'S SIZE

Your baby probably hasn't lengthened much since last week, and she still measures around 14 inches crown to rump and 21 inches head to heels. She probably weighs about 6½ pounds.

YOUR BABY'S LATEST DEVELOPMENTS

A baby born between week 38 and week 42 is called a full-term infant or a term baby. Before this time, babies are called preterm, and after this time, they're called postdate.

By now, your baby's head measures about 3½ inches around. The bones in her head haven't fused together or hardened so they'll be able to compress as she journeys through the birth canal.

Because your uterus is stretched so thin, more light gets in than before. Your baby now turns toward the light when she sees it, mainly out of curiosity.

Your baby continues to practice swallowing amniotic fluid and sucking on her thumbs and fingers. This helps to strengthen the face and throat muscles that she will use to nurse or drink from a bottle.

YOUR LATEST DEVELOPMENTS

Most women don't grow larger this week, so your size and weight might stay about the same.

Around now your pregnancy breast size peaks. Your breasts might still grow a bit more after your baby is born when your milk comes in. If you plan to breastfeed and your nipples are flattened or inverted, you might want to talk with a lactation consultant.

If it hasn't happened already, sometime in the next weeks you might pass your mucus plug, which is the buildup of cervical mucus that's been protecting your baby and uterus by keeping bacteria out.

The mucus plug might be clear, or tinged with pink, red, or brown. It might come out in small pieces or one large piece. It's thick, and it looks like clear nasal mucus or mucus tinged with blood.

When you pass your mucus plug, it's called the bloody show. It might happen when you're going to the bathroom or appear in your underwear. As your cervix thins in preparation for labor, the plug loosens and then falls out.

You could go into labor at any time after passing your mucus plug, but there's no need to grab your bag and head to the hospital just yet! Passing your mucus plug means your body is *preparing* for labor, but it doesn't necessarily mean you're going into labor right away, because it can happen up to two weeks before labor begins. It's a good idea to tell your doctor or midwife, though. You shouldn't see a lot of blood when you lose your mucus plug. If it seems like a lot of blood, call your doctor or midwife right away.

After you pass your mucus plug, some experts advise against having sex or putting anything inside your vagina that can cause infection. But on the other hand, many experts recommend sex as beneficial for relaxation and bonding with your partner. Talk with your doctor or midwife about what's best for you and your baby.

As your cervix softens, it starts to feel like a peeled kiwi. Take our word for this! If you check for yourself, you risk introducing bacteria.

JUSTIFICATION FOR A CELEBRATION

Eighty-five percent of babies are born within two weeks of their due dates, and you're now within that wonderful window!

Wanting Your Pregnancy to Be Over

Most women reach a point when they can't wait for their pregnancies to be over. You've hit the "pregnancy wall." Perhaps it's nature's way of helping you cope with fears about labor. Your wish to not be pregnant anymore and your desire to meet your baby *far* outweigh your worries about labor.

❧

By week 37 or 38, you lose your mind. Patients come to me and say, "Please get me delivered!" By the end of pregnancy, you've had it.

—*Ellen Kruger, MD, a mom of two teenagers and an ob-gyn in an academic and clinical practice in New Orleans, LA, with Ochsner Health System*

❧

In my eighth month, I was so big that I really wanted my pregnancy to be over. I remember one day, I was seeing a young man who had cancer. The exam room door was closed, and I got really hot and felt like I was going to pass out. I opened the door and sat down, and I was fine. But that was the turning point for me when I was ready to have that baby.

—*Debra Luftman, MD, a mom of a teenaged daughter and a teenaged son, a board-certified dermatologist in private practice, a coauthor of* The Beauty Prescription, *the developer of the skincare line of products Therapeutix, and a clinical instructor of skin surgery and general dermatology at UCLA*

❧

I really wanted my pregnancies to be over by 38 weeks, especially my last one. I had terrible vulvar varicose veins, and they hurt badly. It felt like I had a bowling ball hanging between my legs. I remember thinking, *It'll be so nice to get this over with.*

—*Melanie Bone, MD, a mom of four "tweens" ages 15 to 12, a gynecologist, the founder of the Cancer Sensibility Foundation, and the author of the syndicated column Surviving Life and the book* Cancer, What's Next?, *in West Palm Beach, FL*

❧

With my first pregnancy, my ob told me that I had every single possible pregnancy symptom that was normal. I had really bad morning sickness, heartburn, swelling, fatigue, and more. My doctor told me that they were all perfectly normal pregnancy symptoms; I just happened to have *all* of them.

I was so miserable, especially at the end of my pregnancy, that I thought I would never ever get pregnant again. But thankfully, I had a very easy delivery and a very healthy baby, so it was all worth it.

Amazingly enough, my second pregnancy was the complete opposite! I had hardly any symptoms at all.

—*Elissa Charbonneau, DO, a mom of an 18-year-old son and a 16-year-old daughter and the medical director of the New England Rehabilitation Hospital in Portland, ME*

RALLIE'S TIP

I tend to be a little impatient and very goal-oriented, and it drove me crazy that I didn't have more control over when I would give birth. It was totally out of my hands. I couldn't wait for my babies to arrive, and the last two weeks of every pregnancy seemed longer to me than the entire first 8½ months!

To distract myself from the agony of waiting and to give myself a sense of control over something in my life, I would work on tasks that I could complete in five or 10 minutes. There's something about completing a task, start to finish, that makes us feel so accomplished! It might be folding the laundry, or organizing a junk drawer, or tweezing my eyebrows. I would set small goals for myself to pass the time toward the end of my pregnancies.

I would decide to do something, and then I would do it. And then I could bask in the feeling of accomplishment for the rest of the day.

Supporting Your Partner and Easing His Fears

Partners often feel one step removed during pregnancy, labor and delivery, and in the early postpartum period. These feelings might intensify as pregnancy goes along.

Just as you have concerns about labor and delivery and becoming a parent, it's a good bet your partner does too. You know him better than anyone, and you're best qualified to help him through this hard time. Support him as best you can and try to allay his fears. Your partner likely has an extra worry that you don't in that he's also probably very worried about *you*, more worried than you might be about yourself.

You might also want to talk through what your expectations are for labor and delivery and also for your first weeks as parents, and your husband's expectations as well. Sometimes the greatest disappointments in life occur when our reality doesn't match our expectations, but you have the power to head this off! For example, if you wish that your partner will be in the labor and delivery room with you every minute, let him know now. If you hope that he will change all of your baby's diapers in the hospital, get him on board today. Communication is the key.

∾

I think pregnancy is very hard for husbands because they don't fully understand what you're going through. It's so foreign to them that you could be so sick, so sensitive to smells, and so emotional.

I tried to educate my husband as much as possible about how I was feeling. But that's somewhat of a losing battle.

—Ashley Roman, MD, MPH, a mom of two daughters, ages three years and six months, and a clinical assistant professor in the department of obstetrics and gynecology at the New York University School of Medicine in New York City

? When to Call Your Doctor or Midwife

Around one in four pregnant women suffers some depression during pregnancy, and one in 10 suffers major depression. Treating depression is critical for your health, and for the health of your baby. Moms-to-be with depression have more cases of placental abruption and preeclampsia. Babies born to depressed mothers might have lower birth weights or are more likely to be born prematurely. Plus, if you're depressed, you might not be taking as good care of yourself as you would usually.

If you have a family history of depression, you might be at a higher risk for it yourself. If you feel an overpowering sadness for a few days or have difficulty sleeping or the desire to sleep all of the time, no appetite, difficulty concentrating, or thoughts of harming yourself, call your doctor or midwife right away.

Involve your partner as much as possible. If the baby is moving, try to get him to feel the baby. Even if you have to pump the baby up by drinking a sugary juice, do it so that your husband can feel the baby going crazy in there.

Invite your partner to every doctor's visit so the doctor can talk to him too and address his questions. Luckily, my husband got to come to 90 to 95 percent of my visits, and I feel like it helped him to stay involved.

—Tyeese Gaines Reid, DO, a mom of one, an emergency medicine resident physician at Yale New Haven Hospital in Connecticut, and the author of a time management book, The Get a Life Campaign

Especially with our first baby, my husband and I were both very worried about how things would work out financially. The timing wasn't what we had planned. At that time, my husband was in school, and I was in my residency training.

I remember people telling us that there's never a perfect time to have a baby; you just deal with it. That advice really helped us make it through.

—Elissa Charbonneau, DO

One very important thing that I did before my first baby was born was ask my parents if they would watch my children for a few days each year while my husband and I went away together. I think it was important that my husband and I both had the knowledge that we would continue traveling together alone in a romantic way even after our babies were born. I also made sure that each day, and each week, we had special time for us to be a couple, to center on each other, not just on the kids.

We live in such a child-centric society, which is largely a good thing. But a lot of parents think that their spouses can wait. We're grown-ups; we can delay gratification. But after a few years have gone by with that attitude, you've lost valuable time building your relationship.

It was important for me during my pregnancy to make my marriage a priority. My husband and I chose to be the kind of parents who see their marriage and working on their intimacy as very important parts of family life.

—Ayala Laufer-Cahana, MD, a pediatrician, mother, artist, serious home cook, and the founder of Herbal Water Inc., in Wynnewood, PA

My first pregnancy was a twin pregnancy, and it was very complicated. I think that in some ways the pregnancy was more difficult for my husband than it was for me. I had a task to do. My job was to carry these babies, and I was willing to do whatever I needed to do. I got to withdraw from life and have this special status as the mother of these babies. People told me I was doing such a good job.

But meanwhile, my husband had to go on with normal life—seeing his patients all day and then coming home to run the house and care for me because I was on bed rest. My husband was more detached from the process of pregnancy, more removed. He was very anxious for me, and he was very anxious for our babies.

No one feels sorry for the dad-to-be in these situations. All of the concern goes toward the mom-to-be. But the dad needs at least as much emotional support as the mom.

I supported my husband as best as I could during my pregnancy. I was careful to always thank him for everything he did for me. When he needed some space and time alone, I gave it to him. And I clearly remember when our twins were being born, I thought to myself, *I have to push out these babies and support my husband all at the same time!* I remember willing myself to deliver my twins and send love to my husband simultaneously.

—*Ruth D. Williams, MD, a mom of twins—a boy and a girl—and another boy, and an ophthalmologist in private practice at the Wheaton Eye Clinic in Wheaton, IL, who specializes in the diagnosis and treatment of glaucoma*

Pampering Yourself and Resting Up for Delivery

You've come a long way, and you really deserve a break *today.* Try to take some time in these next days and weeks to treat yourself and rest up. Most labors and deliveries are marathons, not sprints. Get a massage or have your nails done. Rent a movie and put your feet up. Take a nap!

❧

I snuck in a pedicure the afternoon before my water broke. That was my last pedicure in a *very* long time, and I was so glad that I got it in just under the wire.

—*Ashley Roman, MD, MPH*

A few weeks before my due date, I withdrew a lot from the world. I was nesting, but I was also *resting*. I was saving my strength in anticipation of labor so that when I went into labor, I wasn't exhausted. I had two or three naps each day, and I took long walks in my neighborhood.

— *Lauren Feder, MD, a mom of two sons, a nationally recognized physician who specializes in homeopathic medicine, and the author of* Natural Baby and Childcare *and* The Parents' Concise Guide to Childhood Vaccinations, *in Los Angeles*

I think it's really important to take some time and try to slow down during the last weeks of pregnancy. For some reason, in our society, the goal is to work like crazy until our water breaks. Perhaps it's because we're so stingy with our maternity leaves that women don't think they can slow down in the weeks before delivery. It's not really dangerous for most women to work until their deliveries, but I think women feel better if they're able to relax a bit.

When I was pregnant with my first son, I was a chief resident. I was busy taking care of patients right until I delivered. With my second son, on the other hand, I cut back my hours after 36 weeks so I could get more rest. I felt so much better.

— *Stephanie Ring, MD, a mom of two sons, ages six and two, and an ob-gyn at Red Rocks Ob-Gyn in Lakewood, CO*

Rallie's Tip

Toward the end of my pregnancy, when I had the chance, I took a 20-minute revitalizing nap, especially when I had missed sleep the night before. Studies show that 20 minutes is the ideal length for a nap: long enough to refresh and recharge your brain, but too short to allow you to get into a very deep sleep, which would cause you to wake up in a fog. I've trained myself to take this kind of nap just about anywhere—in my car while I'm waiting for my son's basketball practice to be over or at my desk. It works wonders!

One thing that I did to pass the time and lift my spirits was pull out my box of family photos—I think everyone has one—and work on photo albums, just for a few minutes. In the vast majority of the photos, my husband, family, and friends are smiling, and it makes me smile. No matter what's going on in my life, seeing all those smiles on the faces of the people I love most lifts my spirits like nothing else can. The trick is to keep the box and all the tools you need accessible and easy to manage. This makes it more stress relieving than stress producing!

Worrying about Your Water Breaking in Public

Almost all pregnant women worry that their water will break at some awful and embarrassing time, such as standing in line at the grocery store. Despite many women's fears, when your water breaks, it's usually more of a constant wetness running down your leg, giving you plenty of time to reach a bathroom. If you're very concerned, you might want to wear a pad.

Outside of sitcoms on TV, a woman's water breaking at some inopportune moment hardly ever happens! Only 10 percent of women have their water break—medically this is called "rupture of membranes"—before their labor begins. Many women actually need to have their water broken in the hospital to move their labor along. It's done with a knitting needle–like tool. No, it doesn't hurt a bit!

If you think that your water has broken, call your midwife or doctor right away. That sac of water has been surrounding and protecting your baby from the beginning of your pregnancy. The fluid cushions your baby to keep her safe and protect her from infection. When that protection is gone, it's either time to deliver, or you'll need medical care to extend your pregnancy.

You might be able to tell on your own if you're leaking amniotic fluid or urine. Amniotic fluid is usually clear and watery, although sometimes it can have a bloody appearance or it might be yellow or green. Urine has a characteristic ammonia smell.

If you think that your water has broken, your doctor or midwife can do one of two simple tests to tell for sure. The first test is called a nitrazine test. A bit of fluid is placed on a strip of treated paper. If the color changes, it's likely amniotic fluid.

The second test is called a ferning test. Fluid is placed on a slide and examined under a microscope. Dried amniotic fluid looks like a fern or branches of a pine tree.

As my due date approached, I was very afraid to ride in anyone's car or sit on their furniture because I was worried my water would break. I wanted to carry a little piece of plastic around with me just in case, but my husband wouldn't let me. He was convinced that no one would be upset with me if my water did break on their couch. Thankfully, we didn't have to find out who was right.

—*Kerri A. Daniels, MD, a mom of one toddler daughter and an instructor in the department of pediatrics at the University of Arkansas for Medical Science in Little Rock*

RALLIE'S TIP

My husband loved to tease me about my water breaking. Every time we'd go somewhere, he'd ask me if I wanted to take a jar of pickles with me. He said if my water broke, I could just drop the jar and blame it on the pickle juice.

I don't think women should worry too much about having their water break and embarrassing themselves in public. It's not like we have any control over it!

Chapter 39
Week 39

Your Baby This Week

YOUR BABY'S SIZE

Your baby this week probably weighs around 7 pounds. He might have lengthened a bit more, to 14½ inches crown to rump and 21½ inches head to heels.

YOUR BABY'S LATEST DEVELOPMENTS

This week, your baby will continue to put on a bit of weight and even lengthen. When your baby is born, the circumference of his head, shoulders, abdomen, and hips will all roughly match.

Your baby's brain and lungs continue to develop this week. In fact, they'll continue to develop even after he's born.

Your baby has lost his pink hue. His skin has been lightened up by a thick layer of fat. In fact, he looks light-skinned and pale, even if his skin will later be dark. Shortly after birth, babies who will have darker skin develop dark skin pigmentation.

YOUR LATEST DEVELOPMENTS

If your baby hasn't dropped, your uterus might be as high as eight inches above your belly button. Your uterus now fills your pelvis and most of your abdomen, having shoved all of your organs out of its path.

Many women have *Wizard of Oz*–type dreams now: They dream that they're in labor, wake up excited, and then quickly realize it was all just a dream.

You might find that your moods go from excitement to panic and back again at the speed of sound. This will likely continue even a few weeks after your baby is born—until your hormones go back to normal.

When your baby drops, which might happen soon, especially if this is your first baby, your appetite might come back. In your last few days or weeks of pregnancy, you might want to consider what you eat. Sometimes women feel nauseated, or even vomit, in labor. Whatever you eat now could impact that!

Your hips, spine, vagina, and legs probably all ache these days. This is because your cartilage is softening to allow your pelvis to expand and let your baby through. Your pelvis will likely expand between 1 and 1½ centimeters.

If your baby is lying low in your pelvis, you might feel a very odd electric zapping sensation down your legs. This is because your baby is pressing on nerves that run from your spine down your leg. This odd feeling will pass as soon as your baby is born.

Your blood pressure might have been rising a bit. It's likely at its highest during the last week of your pregnancy.

At some point, your body will begin to release prostaglandin hormones to soften your cervix. When your cervix is thin enough for your baby to be born, it will be as thin as a sheet of paper.

JUSTIFICATION FOR A CELEBRATION
Your baby might be born any day now!

Preparing Your Other Children for the Baby

Depending on your children's ages, your process of preparing them for the baby's arrival might have begun weeks—or even months—ago. You know your kids best, but it's still hard to predict how any one child will react to becoming a big brother or sister. Some become frightened, others don't.

෨෦

My sons are four years apart. In some families, it might be difficult to prepare an older child for a new baby. But my older son wanted to have a brother; he'd asked for a brother! As a family, we all looked forward to our second son's birth. It was something we had all hoped and planned for—a family event.

—*Sandra Carson, a mom of two grown sons and the director of the Center for Reproduction and Infertility of Women & Infants Hospital in Providence, RI*

෨෦

My son was two years old when his sister was born. When the baby was first born, my son did okay. But when she was around two months old, he realized, *Hey, this kid's here to stay!*

—*Judy Dudum, MD, a mom of three, an ob-gyn, and a senior staff physician at Henry Ford Health System in Detroit, with interests in nutrition and adolescent gynecology*

෨෦

Before my second baby was born, my older daughter was Mommy's little helper. I kept her involved in getting ready for the baby so she wouldn't feel left out. She helped me with everything: washing clothes, shopping for baby supplies, and more.

—*Patricia S. Brown, MD, a mom of two daughters, ages nine and seven, and a three-year-old son and a psychiatrist at Columbia-New York Child and Adolescent Telepsychiatry and in private practice in Cresskill, NJ*

෨෦

When I was pregnant with my son, my two daughters were five and two years old. It was funny to get glimpses of what went on in the girls' heads as we talked about their new brother-to-be. They understood that I'd go to the hospital each day and deliver babies, and I was pregnant too. So they would ask me, "When are you bringing home our baby?"

The day finally came when I could tell them that, "I'm going to the hospital, and I'll be bringing home *our* baby." I remember wondering what they were thinking. Perhaps they thought I went through a drive-thru, picked up the baby, and came home! I don't think they really grasped how I was actually going to get their brother out. In any event, both of my daughters were very anxious for me to come home with their new baby brother.

—*Siobhan Dolan, MD, MPH, a mom of three, a consultant to the March of Dimes, and an associate professor of obstetrics and gynecology and women's health at Albert Einstein College of Medicine/Montefiore Medical Center in the Bronx, NY*

A few months before my baby was due, my husband and I took our older son (who was six years old at the time) on a big-brother trip. We went to California to visit one of his preschool friends who has a little brother.

That trip really helped our son get used to the idea of having a brother because his friend didn't like the idea of having a baby brother at first. But by the time of our visit, the little brother was older, and the boys were playing together very well. That set a great example for my son.

—*Sonia Ng, MD, a mom of seven-year-old and one-year-old sons and a pediatrician and expert in sedation at Children's Hospital of Philadelphia Pediatric Care at Princeton Health Care System in Princeton, NJ*

RALLIE'S TIP

My oldest son was 12 years old when I became pregnant with my second child. As the due date grew closer, he seemed to be experiencing mixed emotions about the impending arrival of his baby brother. My husband and I tried to include him in planning and preparing for the baby whenever we could.

Looking back, I believe one of the best decisions we made was to invite my oldest son into the delivery room to experience the arrival of his little brother. He sat beside me at the head of the bed and witnessed the miracle of birth. He was proud and happy to be included in the big event, and I believe it made him feel very close to his brother and helped him realize that although he had a new role in our family, he was just as special and as loved as ever.

When I was pregnant with my son, my daughter was four years old. She was very into dolls, and she was excited to have a brother because a lot of her friends had siblings. She asked for a sibling all the time. She drew pictures of me with a baby in my belly. We talked about it all the time.

My husband and I explained to our daughter numerous times that we didn't know when the baby would come. Perhaps, one morning, she would wake up and Mommy and Daddy would be at the hospital, and Grandma would be here with her. We wanted to prepare her for that possibility.

We also bought several books that talk about having a sibling. I find that reading books is a great way to communicate things to preschoolers. It's often better than talking about them directly.

During my pregnancy, my daughter and I started a tradition of going to Starbucks together for tea. We both love it, and I thought it was a good choice because it's something we can continue to do as she grows up.

A few weeks before my son was born, we took our daughter for a few days to the Florida Keys to unwind and get ready. We talked with her about having a sibling. She might not have been old enough to understand how it would change her life, but she did understand that she was getting a sibling.

One more thing I tried to do was to prepare my daughter that even though she *wanted* a sibling and she was excited to be a big sister, that there would be negative feelings too, such as anger and jealousy. It's important to warn kids of that. Otherwise when they have negative feelings, they might think that it's not okay to have those feelings. That doesn't come up too early on when the baby is first born and just lies around. But when the baby becomes a toddler, those negative feelings can crop up.

—*Michelle Paley, MD, PA, a mom of a six-year-old daughter and a two-year-old son and a psychiatrist and psychotherapist in private practice in Miami Beach, FL*

Wondering Whom Your Baby Will Look Like

It's fun to imagine whom your baby will look like. Will he favor you, your partner, or be a handsome blend of you both? You won't have to wonder much longer because very soon, you'll hold him in your arms.

I had a 3-D ultrasound at 38 weeks. It was incredible to see my baby's face so clearly. I thought that he looked a lot like my brother. And he still does.

—*Amy J. Derick, MD, a mom of one 15-month-old son who is 17 weeks pregnant with her second son. Dr. Derick is a dermatologist in private practice at Derick Dermatology in Barrington, IL.*

I don't like having huge expectations. I like for life to surprise me! So while I was pregnant, I didn't try to imagine whom my baby would look like. I figured I'd know soon enough. Also, as a pediatrician, I observe a lot of deliveries, and I know that when babies are first born, their features look compressed from labor, and you don't really see their defining features for a few weeks. I expected my baby to simply look like a newborn!

—*Ayala Laufer-Cahana, MD, a pediatrician, mother, artist, serious home cook, and the founder of Herbal Water Inc., in Wynnewood, PA*

RALLIE'S TIP

When I was pregnant with my third child, I read an article that said that babies tend to look more like their dads than their moms when they're first born, because that facilitates bonding between fathers and their newborn infants. So I always imagined that my son would be born looking just like my husband, and as it turns out, he is the spitting image of his dad!

About a week before my daughter was born, I was talking with my husband. I asked him whom he thought our baby would look like.

"I haven't really thought about it," he replied. In fact, he said he hadn't thought much about the baby or how things would be after the birth at all.

I was completely shocked! How could he have gone through 39 weeks of pregnancy and not wondered whom our daughter would look like? To me, this exchange spoke volumes about how differently my husband and I had experienced my pregnancy. I have to admit, I was disappointed that he wasn't more into it. It took me a while to be okay with that.

But after our daughter was born, I quickly learned that just because my husband wasn't as engrossed in the pregnancy as I was didn't predict how involved he would be as a father. He totally stepped up to the plate, changed all the diapers in the hospital, and has been a very hands-on dad. If your husband hasn't embraced your pregnancy the way you fantasized he would, don't worry about it. In my experience, it doesn't predict what sort of father he will be to your children.

Going back to wondering what our daughter would look like, she didn't look at all like I imagined! My husband and I both had blond hair, and our daughter was born a very big, beautiful baby—with jet black hair!

—*Katja Rowell, MD, a mom of a four-year-old daughter, a family practice physician, and a childhood feeding specialist with www. familyfeedingdynamics.com, in St. Paul, MN*

Preparing to Breastfeed or Bottlefeed

Will you breastfeed, bottlefeed, or do a combo of both? Whichever road you've chosen, here are a few things to think about.

If you've chosen to breastfeed, be prepared to drink lots of fluids after your baby is born. You need to drink at least two quarts of fluid a day to make milk and stay hydrated. You'll also need to eat about an

Mommy MD Guide-Recommended Product
Medela Pump in Style

"Because I had planned to breastfeed, I registered for a breast pump," said Joanna Dolgoff, MD, a mom of a seven-year-old son and a four-year-old daughter, a board-certified pediatrician/child obesity expert with practices in Manhattan and Roslyn Heights, NY, creator of an online child weight loss program (www.DrDolgoff.com), and author of the book *Red Light, Green Light, Eat Right*. "I got the Medela Pump in Style. It was very good."

You can buy a Medela Pump in Style for around $275 in baby supply stores and online. (Breast pumps vary dramatically in price, from $35 for a very basic manual model to $380 for a hands-free super-deluxe model.)

extra 500 calories a day to make up for the 425 to 700 calories you'll be secreting into your milk. It's especially important to eat enough foods rich in calcium, such as dairy products. Many women continue to take prenatal vitamins as they breastfeed.

If you haven't already bought them, buy a few nursing bras. They truly will make your life easier. Also, buy some nursing pads. They'll prevent the milk from leaking through your shirt. You might want to buy a breast pump and milk storage bags if you want to express milk.

If you've chosen to bottlefeed, you'll need to stock up on bottles and nipples. You might consider buying bottle brushes, a drying rack, and a warmer. You can buy all of these things at baby supply stores and online.

∽

I didn't do much to prepare to breastfeed. In those days, I didn't wear a bra, and I think that was helpful.

> —*Hana R. Solomon, MD, a mom of four, ages 35 to 19, a board-certified pediatrician, the president of BeWell Health, LLC, and the author of* Clearing the Air One Nose at a Time: Caring for Your Personal Filter

∽

I recommend nursing bras by Bravado Designs. I bought one during my last trimester. It doubles as a nursing bra, if you're gonna try to go that route. But, my boobs got *so* big (three to four cup sizes bigger), my regular bras became uncomfortable. I was buying a new size every month or so, and then I grew out of the sizes in regular stores (big bras are not cheap); the straps were burrowing into my shoulders. This bra was so comfortable—very supportive, without an underwire, and with comfy straps. You'll just have to get over wearing a nursing bra before the baby gets here.

> —*Tyeese Gaines Reid, DO, a mom of one, an emergency medicine resident physician at Yale New Haven Hospital in Connecticut, and the author of a time management book,* The Get a Life Campaign

RALLIE'S TIP

I nearly drove myself crazy worrying about breastfeeding, especially toward the end of my pregnancy. Like most women, I had to go back to work after my

Check Out a La Leche League Meeting

In 1956, breastfeeding rates in the United States had dropped to 20 percent. That year, Mary White held the first La Leche League meeting in her home in Franklin Park, IL. Since then, La Leche League has grown into an international association. Their mission is to "help mothers worldwide to breastfeed through mother-to-mother support, encouragement, information, and education, and to promote a better understanding of breast-feeding as an important element in the healthy development of the baby and mother."

If you plan to breastfeed, it's a great idea to find—and better yet reach out to—your local La Leche League chapter. There you'll likely find support-ive, caring women whom you could turn to if you encounter breastfeeding difficulties, or even if you just need support or someone to talk to about breastfeeding.

Visit **WWW.LLLI.ORG** for more information and to find a chapter near you.

baby was born, and I wanted to breastfeed.

I bought a breast pump, and I worried a lot about how I was going to pump at work. Turns out I didn't anticipate everything I could have. The first day I returned to work, I pumped (in the teeny supply closet they offered me), and I put my pumped milk in a sealed container in the office refrigera-tor. Imagine my surprise when the office administrator told me I had to move it to the biohazard refrigerator instead because milk was a body fluid. She wanted me to put my baby's milk in with the throat cultures and stool samples! The next day, I brought a cooler and plenty of ice packs to keep the milk cold.

Long before I went into labor, I made an appointment to see a lactation consultant after the baby was born. That made a big difference in my nursing success. If you have difficulty nursing, it's easy to give up. It can be painful and difficult to learn how.

Some women learn how to breastfeed as easy as 1, 2, 3. But it was very tough with my daughter. She didn't latch on correctly at first. It was a very emotional time for me. Nursing feels like one of those things you should just *know* how to do. When it's not going well, it feels like you're doing something wrong. And everyone was telling me a different way to do it.

But when I went to see my lactation consultant, she was amazing. She straightened it all out, and she made everything so much better.

—*Michelle Paley, MD, PA*

One of the things that still shocks me to this day is the lack of physician support for breastfeeding. I didn't have one lecture in medical school or during internal medicine residency on breastfeeding. As a first-time pregnant mom, I was completely unprepared when it came time to breastfeed my daughter.

While my obstetrician asked during the third trimester if I planned to breastfeed, the books I read focused more on how to give my new baby a bath. I was given all the information on breastfeeding *after* my child was born. After nine miserable days, I gave up. On the other hand, for my son, I was prepared, and all went well.

So my advice is: Do your reading and research on breastfeeding *before* you deliver. Push your doctor to discuss this topic with you. The reason your physician might not be discussing breastfeeding with you is that he or she might lack the training in this area and is leaving it up to the lactation specialist in the hospital.

One great book I have found is the *Breastfeeding Handbook for Physicians* by the American Academy of Pediatrics (AAP) and American Congress of Obstetricians and Gynecologists (ACOG). I wish every family practice physician and obstetrician would read that book.

—*Mary Mason, MD, a mom of a nine-year-old girl and six-year-old boy, an internist, and the chief medical officer for a multi-state managed care company that coordinates care for about 70,000 pregnant Medicaid moms a year*

When I was pregnant, I received lots of free information, samples, and coupons. I looked through everything, especially all of the information about formula. Even as a doctor, I hadn't realized all of the details and information about the different types of formula. The coupons were great too!

—*Dianna K. Kim, MD, a mom of three and an ob-gyn in private practice in Vernon Hills, IL, at the Midwest Center for Women's Healthcare*

I decided not to breastfeed because it would have been too much for me with twins. I didn't choose, or stock up on, formula ahead of time. My plan was to give my babies the same formula that they were given in the hospital, figuring that they were tolerating it well. But it's good to know that there are many types of formula, so if your baby is fussy, you can always try a different formula.

—*Jennifer Gilbert, DO, a mom of three-month-old twins and an ob-gyn at Paoli Hospital in Pennsylvania*

Dealing with Foot Pain

If your hair could hurt, right about now you'd be aching from the top of your hair to the bottom of your feet. Foot pain is definitely a reality in pregnancy, though it's often overlooked. Due to your weight gain, your center of gravity has shifted, which puts extra pressure on your feet, and also your knees.

Two of the most common foot problems pregnant women have are overpronation and swelling. These can cause you pain in your heels, arches, and the balls of your feet. Overpronation means that your feet roll inward when you walk. This can be caused by the extra pressure on your feet.

It might help your aching feet to wear comfy shoes, elevate your feet whenever you can, and drink water to stay hydrated and help your body retain less fluid. The good news is, your foot pain should go away soon after your baby is born.

When to Call Your Doctor or Midwife

If you notice a sudden increase in swelling in your feet, especially if it's accompanied by other symptoms of preeclampsia such as blurred vision, call your doctor or midwife right away.

RALLIE'S TIP

During the last month of my pregnancy, my feet swelled almost beyond recognition, and by the end of a long day, they were killing me. Propping my feet up helped, but I didn't always have time for that. I had a mini fridge in my office, and whenever I sat down to work at my desk, I'd pull a couple of bottles of water out of the fridge and roll them around under my feet. The cool temperature was refreshing, and the rolling motion helped improve the circulation in my feet and lower legs. It was like having a mini foot massage at work, and it felt great!

Be good to your feet, or they will make you pay. My favorite shoes during pregnancy are the brown Hush Pup-pies loafers that I still wear now. They helped me stand for hours while ob-serving surgeries then and now. Of all the orthopedic brands, Hush Puppies had the trendier styles. Before my Hush Puppies, my arches would ache endlessly. They definitely quieted my dogs.

—*Tyeese Gaines Reid, DO*

Chapter 40
Week 40 and Beyond

Your Baby This Week

YOUR BABY'S SIZE
The average baby's birth weight at full term is 7 to 7½ pounds. Her average crown-to-rump length is around 14¾ inches to 15¼ inches, and she "stands" around 21½ inches. She fills your uterus completely.

YOUR BABY'S LATEST DEVELOPMENTS
Your baby is quite squished. At this point, she's probably as ready to be born as you are to *have* her be born.

If your baby is born after her due date, she might have lost all of her vernix, and her skin might even be dry and flaky.

YOUR LATEST DEVELOPMENTS
You are probably really, really ready to have your baby. Now.

But if your baby isn't born by her due date, you have plenty of company. Around 45 percent of babies are born at 40 weeks or after. By 42 weeks, most doctors and midwives would induce labor.

JUSTIFICATION FOR A CELEBRATION
Reaching your due date is certainly cause for a celebration!

Having Tests to Check on the Baby

If your doctor or midwife is concerned about your baby or if your due date has come and gone, he or she might run a few tests.

One test commonly given is a nonstress test. It's easy and painless. You might be given a glass of juice to drink to encourage your baby to move around. Then you sit in a recliner, and you're hooked up to an external device that monitors your baby's heartbeat. Your doctor or midwife will check to make sure that your baby's heart rate increases with activity and decreases when she's not moving.

Your doctor or midwife might send you for an ultrasound. This can be important to check the baby's position and the level and distribution of amniotic fluid.

Or your doctor or midwife might combine the nonstress test and ultrasound and give you a test called a biophysical profile. It's noninvasive and safe. It lasts 35 to 45 minutes and checks for the baby's breathing, movements, and heartbeat, and it also measures the level and distribution of amniotic fluid.

Another test your doctor or midwife might run is called a fetal acoustical stimulation (FAS). A device will be placed on your abdomen that produces vibrations. Your baby should respond to these vibrations, and your doctor or midwife will carefully monitor her responses.

෴

With my first pregnancy, my due date came and went. My doctor did an ultrasound after I passed my due date to check my baby's weight and to make sure the placenta was functioning normally. He also checked to make sure she was still surrounded by the normal amount of fluid.

—*Ashley Roman, MD, MPH, a mom of two daughters, ages three years and six months, and a clinical assistant professor in the department of obstetrics and gynecology at the New York University School of Medicine in New York City*

RALLIE'S TIP

I loved having a nonstress test while I was pregnant. I just sat back and relaxed and let the monitor and the baby do the work. I found it very reassuring to know that my baby was doing just fine. It gave me tremendous peace of mind.

Keeping Yourself Distracted and Passing the Time

If your due date comes, and then goes, you might feel disappointed and frustrated. Know that this isn't at all under your control! Try to make the best of it and keep yourself as distracted as possible.

If you're able, one thing that you could do now to pass the time that might also help you in labor is doing squats. Hold onto a sturdy chair or lean your back against a wall and squat down with your knees apart. You could do this as many itmes as you'd like, as often as you'd like, several times a day even.

Energy and brainpower permitting, maybe you could work on your scrapbooks or baby book or catch up on some reading or spending time with your partner, friends, and family.

∾

My first son was two weeks late. That's not uncommon for a first pregnancy. Passing their due dates might make some women crazy, but I loved being pregnant! I felt so blessed. For me, going past my due date gave me two more weeks to enjoy myself.

—*Lauren Feder, MD, a mom of two sons, a nationally recognized physician who specializes in homeopathic medicine, and the author of* Natural Baby and Childcare *and* The Parents' Concise Guide to Childhood Vaccinations, *in Los Angeles*

∾

My first daughter was born about a week after her due date. When my due date came and went, I really just wanted her to come. I was exhausted. Plus, I was so anxious to meet my baby. For better or worse, I had my work to distract me.

—*Ashley Roman, MD, MPH*

∾

My son was born two weeks late. I remember every day seemed extra long. I tried to keep myself busy at work during the day, and I was grateful when people didn't remind me that I was still pregnant.

It was much harder at night, though. Because I wasn't distracted like at work, I felt all the reflux, back pain, and other complaints.

—*Karen Heald, MD, a mom of four boys and a board-certified family physician in private practice outside Atlanta, GA*

At the end of your pregnancy, take it easy, but stay busy. I felt my absolute worst on the weekends. Every weekend, I would threaten to induce the baby with some herbal remedy. But once Monday came, I'd be okay. The downtime let me feel every single ache, pain, and struggle to breathe.

Get your rest on the weekends, but do at least one fun baby thing, such as registry shopping, to distract you. Remember: On Monday, it will go away again.

—*Tyeese Gaines Reid, DO, a mom of one, an emergency medicine resident physician at Yale New Haven Hospital in Connecticut, and the author of a time mangagement book,* The Get a Life Campaign

Your due date is actually plus or minus two weeks. I was so miserable at the end of my pregnancy that two weeks before my due date, I decided to go on a brisk walk to try to bring on contractions. I wanted that baby out!

I went for a long walk in my neighborhood with my dog. My neighbors must have thought I was crazy, this big pregnant woman ready to burst, huffing and puffing, walking a tiny little dog. I trekked up a long hill and all the way back home, never feeling a single twinge.

Unfortunately, it did nothing to speed my delivery along, and my baby arrived two weeks later, on her due date.

—*Sharonne N. Hayes, MD, a mom of two and the director of the Women's Heart Clinic at Mayo Clinic in Rochester, MN*

My son was a little overbaked; he was born a little late. During that last week, I really wanted my pregnancy to be over. I had my suitcase packed, and I was ready to go. Every day, I woke wondering, *Is today the day?*

The last few days of pregnancy are hard. I was excited, but I was also very tired. I was so ready to go into labor. I had so much apprehension about the delivery and becoming a mother.

I tried to distract myself by taking long walks. That really helped me. I kept telling myself, *Just keep on walking, and it will happen.*

—*Elissa Charbonneau, DO, a mom of an 18-year-old son and a 16-year-old daughter and the medical director of the New England Rehabilitation Hospital in Portland, ME*

With my first pregnancy, my due date came and went. When I was around five days late, I started to believe that I was never going to have this baby. I remember distinctly looking at myself in the mirror and thinking, *That's it. This is me for the rest of my life. This child will never be born.*

Finally, 10 days after my due date, my mucus plug came out. Still nothing happened. I didn't sleep well that night, and the next day I went to see my ob.

"You're not doing much," he said. "Good-bye."

After my husband and I got home, we took a nap. I woke up with a searing, lightning-like pain that heralded the onset of labor.

—*Erika Schwartz, MD, a mom of two and the director of www. DrErika.com, who's been in private practice for more than 30 years in New York City, specializing over the past 15 years in women's health, disease prevention, and bioidentical hormones*

When my due date came and went, I passed the time exercising and eating spicy food, trying to bring on labor. My husband and I also had sex more to try to bring on labor. I did all the things people say to do to bring on labor. But nothing worked. The baby comes when she's ready to come.

—*Patricia S. Brown, MD, a mom of two daughters, ages nine and seven, and a three-year-old son and a psychiatrist at Columbia-New York Child and Adolescent Telepsychiatry and in private practice in Cresskill, NJ*

Dealing with Impatient People

As you reach—or even pass—your due date, well-meaning people might ask questions that make you uncomfortable—or even annoyed. You might want to come up with a response to gently let them know that no, your baby hasn't come yet. Or simply let calls go to voice mail!

If the impatient person is *you*, you might want to give some home remedies a try to get your labor moving along. These old wives' tales are by no means proven in scientific studies, but they're worth a try.

Eating spicy foods is traditionally thought to bring on labor. Taking a long walk might help, or at least distract you. Having sex is thought to bring on labor because semen contains prostaglandins, chemicals similar to those used to bring on labor. Nipple stimulation releases oxytocin, which stimulates the uterus.

Other old wives' tales might be dangerous. Don't drink castor oil or drink raspberry tea, unless your doctor or midwife has recommended it.

Better yet, sit back, relax, and let your baby choose her own birth date!

⟋⟍

I worked right up to the delivery with all three of my daughters. With my first, I was just thinking about scaling back my schedule at 37 weeks when I went into labor.

With my second daughter, I was more than two weeks past my due date. At 41 weeks, I was still dragging myself into the hospital to work. It was frustrating because people kept asking me, "Are you still pregnant? When are you due?"

But I tried to focus on the positive—that most people liked working with me while I was pregnant, especially the moms of my pediatrics patients. I think that when they realized that I was about to be a mom too, it put me on the same level as them.

—*Alicia Brennan, MD, a mom of three daughters and the medical director of inpatient pediatrics of Children's Hospital of Philadelphia Pediatric Care at Princeton Health Care System in Princeton, NJ*

⟋⟍

Toward the end of pregnancy, I received so many phone calls. I found it important to set boundaries with people. You don't have to pick up the phone whenever it rings! Let them leave a message and call them back. And if someone wants to stop by, you don't have to accept visitors if you don't want to.

Doing this toward the end of your pregnancy is good training for after your baby is born. People will want to call you to see how you're doing and express their congratulations. You don't need to call them back this minute. More than likely, they just want you to know they're thinking of you.

—*Michelle Paley, MD, PA, a mom of a six-year-old daughter and a two-year-old son and a psychiatrist and psychotherapist in private practice in Miami Beach, FL*

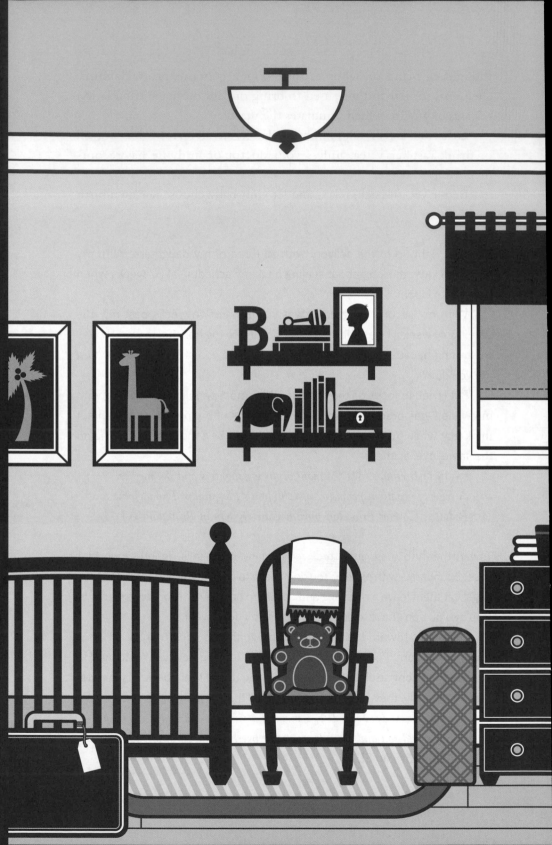

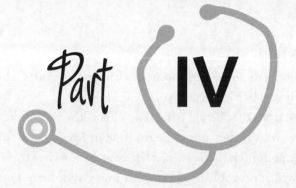

Part **IV**

YOUR BABY'S BIRTH

Chapter 41
Honey, It's Time!

Going into Labor

You'll likely remember the moment that you go into labor forever. Where will you be? How will you feel?

Contractions that herald real labor start at the top of the uterus and roll downward. Or they might begin in your lower back and spread to your lower abdomen. This is in stark contrast to Braxton Hicks contractions, which probably began in your lower abdomen. During a contraction, your uterus feels hard to the touch.

Some women describe labor as feeling like bad menstrual cramps or bad intestinal cramps. Other women experience backache. Once labor starts, you might get diarrhea and feel that you have to urinate a lot. If your water breaks, you'll feel warm fluid running down your leg.

All of these clues add up to one exciting conclusion: You're about to meet your baby!

~~

During my pregnancy with my youngest son, a dear friend of mine was pregnant at the same time. Our due dates were very close together.

We were inseparable during our pregnancies. We went everywhere together—grocery shopping, baby shopping, Christmas shopping, you name it.

I actually delivered her baby at the hospital. I had induced her because she was afraid I'd go into labor first and then be unable to deliver her baby. She delivered at 5 am on a Friday.

"You can go and have your baby now," she said.

"I think I'll do exactly that," I replied.

I had my son at 4:40 that night! I believe that women have tremendous willpower!

—Kathie Bowling, MD, a mom of three grown sons and an ob-gyn in private practice in Providence, RI, who's also on the clinical faculty at the Warren Alpert School of Medicine at Brown University

Right around my due date for my second pregnancy, I woke up in the middle of the night dreaming I was having cramps. I was actually starting labor, so I woke my husband. After three hours of fast and furious labor at home, our son was born.

—Lauren Feder, MD, a mom of two sons, a nationally recognized physician who specializes in homeopathic medicine, and the author of Natural Baby and Childcare *and* The Parents' Concise Guide to Childhood Vaccinations, *in Los Angeles*

During my second pregnancy, I started to feel cramping at 38 weeks. I thought I was going to have diarrhea because my son had recently had it. I went to the hospital as scheduled for induction. When they asked me if I was in labor, I said, "No." But when they monitored me, they found out I was in labor. The nurses couldn't believe I didn't feel it.

—Sonia Ng, MD, a mom of seven-year-old and one-year-old sons and a pediatrician and expert in sedation at Children's Hospital of Philadelphia Pediatric Care at Princeton Health Care System in Princeton, NJ

During my second pregnancy, one day at work around 1 pm, I went into labor. I didn't mention anything to anyone for the first few hours. Around 4 pm, I mentioned to someone that I was in labor and my contractions were six minutes apart.

"Get out of here!" she said.

"I have to finish my notes, and then I'll go to the maternity ward," I said.

I got there in plenty of time—and my notes were all done to boot.

—Patricia S. Brown, MD, a mom of two daughters, ages nine and seven, and a three-year-old son and a psychiatrist at Columbia-New York Child and Adolescent Telepsychiatry and in private practice in Cresskill, NJ

I'm an ob-gyn, but with my first baby, I wasn't quite sure I was in labor! I was feeling cramps, but no real pain. I was nervous because I didn't want to go in to the hospital, have them discover I wasn't really in labor, and have them send me back home. Also, I thought that my water had broken, but I wasn't sure. It felt like I was urinating all of the time without control.

I decided I'd better go to the hospital, and when I got there, they checked me. I was already dilated five centimeters, but I didn't really feel it yet. Everyone's pain tolerance and perception of pain is different. So when someone tells me she's in terrible pain at one centimeter, I believe her.

—*Judy Dudum, MD, a mom of three, an ob-gyn, and a senior staff physician at Henry Ford Health System in Detroit, with interests in nutrition and adolescent gynecology*

With my son, I went into preterm labor at 30 weeks, and I was put on bed rest for the last seven weeks or so of pregnancy. I was at home, but I had a subcutaneous terbutaline pump, which stopped my contractions and held off my labor.

My doctor told me as soon as I hit 37 weeks, I should turn off the pump. When I did, my contractions started right away. It was as if my son had been knocking at the door since 30 weeks, and we kept holding him off. The minute we opened the door, he came.

When I went into labor, my husband and I both panicked a bit. He's a cardiologist, and he started telling me to breathe.

"How do you know I need to breathe?" I asked.

"It's what they do in all of the movies," my husband said.

So we mimicked what we had seen on TV and in the movies, and it was fine. I don't remember early labor being very uncomfortable at all because it happened so quickly.

—*Diane Truong, MD, FAAP, a mom of one daughter and one son and a pediatrician in a multispecialty group practice in Southern California*

Having Your Water Break

When you go into labor, your amniotic sac, aka bag of waters, might break. Generally it's a trickle, not a gush. Your water might break on its own when you go into labor, but more likely it will need to be broken at the hospital or birth center. No worries, it doesn't hurt a bit!

☙

Right around my son's due date, I was sitting out in front of my house, doing the *LA Times* crosswords. I coughed, and I thought I had a little stress incontinence! A few seconds later, I realized that my water had broken. And then the next phase of my journey with my son began . . .

—*JJ Levenstein, MD, FAAP, a mom of one son in college and a pediatrician in private practice in Southern California*

☙

During my second pregnancy, five weeks before my due date, I suspected something. I was very tired, and I was supposed to be on call the next day, but I asked another doctor to cover for me.

My husband and I went out to dinner with friends. After we got home, we were watching TV, and my water broke. I called my doctor and explained that my water broke. He asked if I was in labor. When I said no, he said, "Take your time."

"I have no intention of getting an infection," I said. (This can happen if too much time passes after your water breaks and before your baby is born.) So I met him at the hospital. My daughter was born four hours later. Listen to your gut.

—*Erika Schwartz, MD, a mom of two and the director of www. DrErika.com, who's been in private practice for more than 30 years in New York City, specializing over the past 15 years in women's health, disease prevention, and bioidentical hormones*

☙

Despite the fact that I was worried for weeks that my water would break all over someone's car seat, my water didn't break on its own at all. They broke it at the hospital. It really wasn't a big deal. It didn't hurt. Truth be told, I had my epidural by then anyway, so I probably *couldn't* feel it.

I could feel the fluid coming out, though, and that felt strange. But it didn't hurt a bit.

—*Kerri A. Daniels, MD, a mom of one toddler daughter and an instructor in the department of pediatrics at the University of Arkansas for Medical Science in Little Rock*

I was pregnant with twins. As often is the case with multiples, my doctor was concerned that my uterus was so fatigued that I wouldn't have effective contractions, so I was induced. To get my labor started, my doctor broke my bag of waters.

I think it's common for women to worry about this. It sounds painful! But it doesn't hurt. It's a bit uncomfortable—like having a routine pelvic exam. But it's not painful.

—*Jennifer Gilbert, DO, a mom of three-month-old twins and an ob-gyn at Paoli Hospital in Pennsylvania*

During my first pregnancy, I lost all my amniotic fluid, but I didn't know it. The midwives said I might have had a slow leak and not noticed it. It wasn't scary; the baby was fine and still moving. It must have just been slowly leaking over the last week of my pregnancy. I'm proof that you don't always know when you've lost your water!

Toward the end of pregnancy, I hung out at Barnes & Noble because I knew if my water broke, my husband would not clean it up. Fortunately, my water did not break in a splash, and I am not banned from bookstores.

—*Sonia Ng, MD*

During my second pregnancy, a few days before my due date, around 11 pm, I felt a few drops. I thought that must be my water breaking. I called my midwife, and she told me to take my temperature. I wasn't running a fever, which is a sign of infection, so she told me to go to sleep. This was hard because I was so excited!

The next day, I walked around a lot to get my labor going. I felt a couple more drops, but my labor still didn't start. I intended to visit the midwife the following day, but when I went to bed that night, I woke up at 1 am dreaming of having cramps. I was going into labor! My baby was born three hours later.

—*Lauren Feder, MD*

When my water broke, I was at home relaxing. It was so subtle. I thought at first it was just heavy vaginal discharge. But after a couple of hours, I thought,

Hmm, maybe this is something more. Certainly, if fluid is running down your leg, it would be pretty obvious that your water had broken. But this was much more subtle than that.

I called my husband at work and said, "I'm not really sure, but I think my water broke."

His response was typical, "Aren't you an ob-gyn? How could you not know?"

I didn't want to call my doctor and bother him, so I drove to the hospital myself. I asked a resident there to check me.

"Yeah, your water is obviously broken," she laughed.

We called my doctor, and I was admitted to the hospital. Meanwhile, because I had left my bag at home, I sent my husband to pick it up and come back to the hospital right away.

—*Ashley Roman, MD, MPH, a mom of two daughters, ages three years and six months, and a clinical assistant professor in the department of obstetrics and gynecology at the New York University School of Medicine in New York City*

Calling Your Doctor or Midwife

If it's the middle of the night, you might have a moment of guilt thinking, *Oh no, I don't want to wake my doctor/midwife up.* That's perfectly understandable, but doctors and midwives know that middle-of-the-night calls come with the territory. If they didn't wish to receive those middle-of-the-night calls, they'd have become writers, teachers, or accountants.

Go ahead and make that call!

∝

Both of my sons were born at home, with a midwife. With my second son, we called the midwife when I went into labor, but she arrived just in the nick of time, 10 minutes before he was born.

—*Lauren Feder, MD*

I didn't know at first that I was in labor. I went across the hall to ask my friend. She put her hand on my belly.

"Yeah, this is labor," she said.

But my husband didn't believe us. He thought it was false labor. We called the doctor and told him my contractions were 10 minutes apart. His clinic was 60 miles away.

"Get your butt down here!" my doctor ordered.

—*Stacey Marie Kerr, MD, a mother of two grown daughters, a family physician with strong roots in midwifery, and the author of* Homebirth in the Hospital, *in Santa Rosa, CA*

I called my obstetrician when I went into labor, but of course the doctor was out of town that night. The doctor who was covering for her said, "I don't do twins vaginally. You have to have a C-section."

He talked with my doctor, who stood up for me and said that my first delivery was easy, the twins were head down, and that I didn't want to have surgery unless necessary. Another ob, who's a friend of mine, came in, even though she wasn't on call, and helped supervise my delivery.

—*Susan Wilder, MD, a mom of an older daughter and twin girls, a primary care physician, and CEO and founder of Lifescape Medical Associates in Scottsdale, AZ*

With my first pregnancy, when my contractions were four minutes apart, my husband said, "I think you need to call the midwives." I was reluctant to call because I didn't want to go to the hospital and be sent home. My contractions weren't hurting yet, so I didn't feel any urgency.

But now that I've had three babies, I know how vastly different each delivery can be. With my third, I had two contractions and called the midwives right away. She urged me to stay at home for an hour or two.

"No, we're in the car," I said.

When we got to the hospital, I was six centimeters dilated. It's a good thing we got in the car when we did!

—*Kristie McNealy, MD, a mom of seven- and four-year-old daughters and a two-year-old son, who's pregnant with another son, and a blogger at www.KristieMcNealy.com, in Denver, CO*

During my first pregnancy, we were living in Queens, New York, a 45-minute drive from the hospital I was to deliver at. When I went into labor, I called my ob and explained that my contractions were five to six minutes apart.

"You have plenty of time," my doctor said.

But when you're in labor, you have a strange sense of urgency—a desperate desire to be somewhere safe. The pain was so intense, I felt that I had to get to that hospital right away.

So my husband and I headed to the hospital. I remember the road was really bumpy, and every time we hit a bump, I had a contraction! I kept asking my husband to slow down. Yet I wanted him to hurry up and get to the hospital.

But the truth is, especially with a first pregnancy, labor is likely to take 12 to 24 hours, so you really don't have to rush anywhere. I didn't have my baby until 12 hours after we got to the hospital.

—*Erika Schwartz, MD*

Getting Ready to Go to the Hospital or Birth Center

Wow, can you believe it?! You're getting ready to go have your baby! This might sound like odd advice, but now's a great time to take a shower. (Although a shower might wash away evidence that your water has broken.) If you can manage it, take a few moments to reflect on the exciting journey that you're about to begin.

When you get ready to go to the hospital to have your baby, take a good look around your house. It will never be the same again. Don't get me wrong; being a mother is wonderful, but your life will never be the same.

—*Susan Schreiber, MD, a mom of a son and daughter in their twenties and a pediatrician in Los Angeles, CA*

With my first and last pregnancies, I had no need to get ready to go anywhere. I was already in the hospital working when I went into labor! That was certainly convenient. I didn't have to hurry anywhere. I just called my husband to let him know, and fortunately he made it there in time.

—*Kathie Bowling, MD*

My water broke one afternoon when I was sitting outside doing a crossword puzzle. I went inside and took a shower. I told my husband that my contractions had started and that they were the real thing. And so we headed off to the hospital, calmly—definitely not in the *I Love Lucy* panic mode.

—*JJ Levenstein, MD, FAAP*

During my first pregnancy, I went into labor on a Saturday night. My doctor had planned to induce me on Monday, but I beat him to it. I told my husband that I was in labor, and he went downstairs and watched a movie with his dad while I was in early labor. This actually was good because it let me have some time alone before the baby.

That night, the contractions weren't too painful yet, and I read and walked around the house to pass the time until it was time to go to the hospital. I also took a shower, which kept me busy and eased the pain. I dozed on and off, too, because my contractions were only 15 to 20 minutes apart.

My husband and I went to the hospital the next morning when my contractions were around five minutes apart.

—*Karen Heald, MD, a mom of four boys and a board-certified family physician in private practice outside Atlanta, GA*

Going to the Hospital or Birth Center

Most doctors and midwives tell women to head to the hospital once they have entered the active phase of labor, when contractions are around five minutes apart.

On the other hand, some doctors or midwives specify to wait until you've had an hour of contractions that are 5 to 10 minutes apart. This all varies on many factors, so it's best to talk with your doctor or midwife to find out what *you* should do when you go into labor.

What was I thinking when I left my home to go to the hospital for my babies to be born?

I don't believe I *was* thinking.

—*Elizabeth Berger, MD, a mom of two, a child psychiatrist, and the author of* Raising Kids with Character

With my second son, I probably waited a little too long to go to the hospital. I kept making my husband pull the car over so I could get out because it was painful to sit in the car during the contractions. Second babies often arrive quicker than the first, so you might consider heading to the hospital earlier the second time around.

—*Karen Heald, MD*

⌒⌒

With my first baby, as soon as I felt labor pain, I headed to the hospital. It turned out to be a good thing, because I was already four centimeters dilated. They broke my water at the hospital, and that was all it took. My baby was born a few hours later.

—*Melanie Bone, MD, a mom of four "tweens" ages 15 to 12, a gynecologist, the founder of the Cancer Sensibility Foundation, and the author of the syndicated column* Surviving Life *and the book* Cancer, What's Next?, *in West Palm Beach, FL*

⌒⌒

My second child arrived on time, in the middle of the night in a rainstorm. My husband sang the Billy Joel song *In the Middle of the Night* to me in the car on the way to the hospital. I think of that night every time I hear that song.

—*Elissa Charbonneau, DO, a mom of an 18-year-old son and a 16-year-old daughter and the medical director of the New England Rehabilitation Hospital in Portland, ME*

⌒⌒

My doctor's clinic was 60 miles south of our home. When I went into labor, we called my doctor, and then my husband, my friend, and I loaded into our big old 63 Chevy. My friend sat in the backseat, I was in front, sans seatbelts, and my husband drove. It was dark, and we took a wild drive down through the woods in the Ozarks.

During the drive, I dealt with each contraction as it came. My friend reminded me each time to open my eyes and not swirl down into the sensation of them.

My husband still wasn't convinced I was really in labor until halfway there, when he finally felt a contraction for himself.

"Oh my God, I just felt a contraction. I guess you *are* in labor," he said.

After we arrived at the birth center, I had to stop three times between the car and the clinic, right there in the parking lot, to deal with intense contractions. We barely made it to the clinic in time.

—*Stacey Marie Kerr, MD*

RALLIE'S TIP

My second baby came almost four weeks early, and my husband and I were caught completely off guard. The snow had just started falling when I went to bed, but by the time my contractions awoke me in the early morning hours, there was a foot and a half of snow on the ground.

Fortunately, my husband had a trusty SUV, and we were able to make it to the hospital without too much excitement. We never would have made it in a car without four-wheel drive.

Now I ask all of my patients who are planning to deliver in the winter months if they have a vehicle with four-wheel drive. If they don't, I encourage them to have a backup plan well in advance of their due dates.

My husband was pretty calm throughout my first pregnancy. But we didn't know what to expect when I went into labor. My husband is a physician too, and he was adamant that I needed to be in the care of my ob right away, so we went to the hospital not once, not twice, but *three times* over the course of two weeks, thinking I was in labor.

After the third time the hospital turned us away, my husband said, "Okay, we're not going to do this again. We're doctors. We should know what we're doing." So the next time we thought I was in labor, he checked my cervix to see if I was dilated. But he's a cardiologist, so I was curious how he knew what he was checking for!

"I think I feel the baby's hair," my husband said.

"That's impossible," I said. "My membrane hasn't ruptured yet."

So once again, we went to the hospital. And once again, I wasn't in labor. But by that time, the nurses felt really badly for us. They let me walk their hallways for a few hours, and then they said, "Let's break your water so we can get this done."

—*Diane Truong, MD, FAAP*

Chapter 42
Labor at the Hospital, Birth Center, or Home

Inducing Labor

Perhaps you might not have gone into labor, but instead your labor is going to be induced. Labor is induced for many reasons, such as pre-eclampsia, gestational diabetes, or a pregnancy that's gone on too long. Maybe a nonstress test has indicated that the placenta isn't functioning quite right. Or your water broke but you didn't go into labor on your own.

Many doctors use a synthetic form of the hormone oxytocin, called Pitocin, to induce labor. This drug can cause labor to move very quickly through each stage.

In any event, when your labor is induced, you'll be at the right place, at the right time, and ready to have your baby!

❦

With my daughter, I went into labor all on my own, and everything progressed normally.

Interestingly, with my sons, I was induced. I've heard many women say that labor is more painful when you're induced. In my experience, that wasn't true. I'm here to tell you that both labors felt exactly the same!

—*Kelly Campbell, MD, a mom of three and an ob-gyn in private practice at Women's Healthcare Physicians in West Bloomfield, MI*

❦

Not only is every person different, but every *delivery* is different. With my first baby, my water broke, and I went to the hospital to be induced because once your water breaks, there's an increased risk of infection if the baby isn't born soon.

But eight hours after the induction, I was going nowhere! They were going to schedule a C-section when finally my labor started, and I went from being dilated 0 centimeters to 10 centimeters in half an hour.

With my second baby, I was at full term and my blood pressure was going up, so my doctor decided to induce me. Again, nothing happened! So they told me to go home and call when I went into labor. A week later, I had my first pain, and my baby was born three hours after that. When babies are ready to come, they come.

—Susan Schreiber, MD, a mom of a son and daughter in their twenties and a pediatrician in Los Angeles, CA

∽⌒

Around two weeks before my daughter was born, I went to see my doctor. When he checked me, I was two centimeters dilated already, so he said he'd schedule an appointment for a week, but he didn't think I'd make it that long. The week went by, and nothing happened.

At my next visit, the doctor said if I didn't deliver in another week, I'd come in to be induced. Sure enough, I was still holding on, so I went in at midnight for the induction, and my daughter was born at 3:08 pm the next afternoon.

—Kerri A. Daniels, MD, a mom of one toddler daughter and an instructor in the department of pediatrics at the University of Arkansas for Medical Science in Little Rock

∽⌒

I was pregnant with twins, and I was induced around 37 weeks. That's actually quite common with multiples. I was a little disappointed because I had hoped to go into labor naturally. But the concern with multiples is your uterus is so distended that it might be too fatigued to contract effectively. Plus, my medical partner who was going to deliver my babies was going on vacation!

My water bag was broken, and I walked around the hospital floor for around three hours trying to get my labor going. Nothing happened. I ultimately needed Pitocin, and then I had beautiful contractions. They were strong and regular, every two minutes.

—Jennifer Gilbert, DO, a mom of three-month-old twins and an ob-gyn at Paoli Hospital in Pennsylvania

I'm probably one of a few women who's had three kids and never gone into labor. I was induced three times for three different reasons. With my first daughter, my belly was measuring small, so I was induced at 38 weeks. She turned out to be just fine.

My second daughter was induced at 39 weeks out of convenience. My understanding doctor knew I was swamped in residency and that I had a one-year-old at home.

My third daughter was induced at 37 weeks because she was measuring heavier. My doctor was worried she'd get to be too big. Because 37 weeks is pretty early, my doctor did an amnio to make sure her lungs were mature enough.

Truth be told, I was happy to be induced. I'm a planner, and I loved knowing when my babies were going to be born.

—*Rebecca Kazin, MD, a mom of three girls and the medical director of the Johns Hopkins Dermatology and Cosmetic Center at Green Spring Station in Lutherville, MD*

Making It through Labor

After you arrive at the hospital, the nurses will probably do a labor check to see if you are indeed in labor. They'll check your vital signs, place a monitor on your abdomen, and do a pelvic exam to see if your cervix is dilating (opening) and effacing (thinning). At this point, you might be admitted, or they might send you home. Don't feel bad if you get sent home; this happens all of the time, and you'll be back again soon.

If you tested positive for group B strep, be sure to gently remind your doctor or midwife so that they give you antibiotics to prevent transmission to your baby.

Labor is the stretching out and opening of the cervix so that the baby can pass out of the uterus. You'll go through three stages of labor. The first stage of labor is the longest and most painful one. It begins with the onset of contractions, and it goes all the way through active labor and transition from labor to pushing. The first stage of labor can take anywhere from 2 to 20 hours. Throughout this stage, your cervix is dilating and effacing. The dilation is measured in centimeters. The thinning process is called effacement, and it's measured in percentages.

When your cervix is 10 centimeters dilated and 100 percent effaced, it's time to start pushing. The first *part* of the first *stage* of labor is called early labor. This is the time when the cervix dilates from zero to three centimeters. This is the least painful time, and contractions in this early labor usually last between 30 and 60 seconds and come every five to 20 minutes apart. Many women pass this time at home.

The second stage of labor begins when you start pushing, and it lasts until your baby is born. The time varies greatly, from a few minutes to a few hours.

The third stage of labor is delivery of the placenta. This usually takes between five and 30 minutes.

Every woman is different, and every labor is different. There's no way to predict how quickly or slowly your labor will progress. You'll just have to wait and see!

~

I had a very long labor. But I just kept telling myself that it would be over soon, and that it would all be worth it. I kept my focus on the outcome—having a healthy child. It also helped a lot that my husband and good friend were in the room with me.

—*Monica Lee-Griffith, MD, a mom of one, an ob-gyn, and senior staff, Henry Ford Health System in metropolitan Detroit*

~

I had 24-hour-long labors with both of my children. During one labor, I chatted a lot with the nice young nurse. She was obviously hanging out with me just to help me pass the time. Eventually, the nice young nurse went off duty from her eight-hour shift. I remember thinking gloomily as she walked out of the room, *Uh oh! Now things are going to fall apart for sure!*

I was right.

Breathing exercises and all that stuff might help somebody out there, but I found that a really distracting conversation was the best thing.

—*Elizabeth Berger, MD, a mom of two, a child psychiatrist, and the author of* Raising Kids with Character

~

I think one of the hardest things about my labor was not being able to have anything to eat or drink. I ate as much as I could the night before I went in to be induced. But I was still quite hungry! They let me have ice chips while I was in labor, so I had a lot! Once I was allowed to eat, I asked for a Taco Bell hard taco and a Nacho Supreme. Looking back, I can't believe that, of all there was to choose from, that was the first thing I wanted after my daughter was born!

—*Kerri A. Daniels, MD*

❧

I was supposed to have a C-section, but I ended up going into labor on my own. I went from being dilated a fingertip to nine centimeters in five hours, which was very fast for a first baby. I think that it went so fast because I had been training for a marathon before I got pregnant, and so I was in great shape. I also exercised throughout the whole pregnancy, running early on and doing water aerobics and yoga later on.

The labor was painful, but I made it through with no pain medication. I think part of that was because I wasn't focused on the pain. I just kept thinking it would be over soon. I watched movies and passed the time wondering when they were going to come get me for my C-section.

When they took me to the operating room and gave me my spinal anesthesia, and the pain was gone, I started to cry because then I realized how much pain I really had been in. I think if you can focus on something other than the pain, you can trick your mind into thinking you're not in as much pain as you are.

—*Marra Francis, MD, a mom of three daughters and an ob-gyn who's based in The Woodlands, TX*

❧

I carried my son deep in my pelvis, so I didn't show all that much. Even near my due date, I only looked around 20 weeks pregnant. When I went into labor and got to the hospital, I told the nurse at the admissions desk that my water had broken. She went white and started to panic that I was in premature labor. I quickly tried to assure her, "No, my due date is tomorrow!"

I was laboring naturally, but my labor wasn't progressing. The pain got to be overwhelming, so they gave me an epidural. Unfortunately, the epidural slowed my labor even more. I was in labor for 28 hours!

I used to work at that hospital, and what helped me make it through that labor were my close friends at the hospital who came to visit and check in on me and give my husband a break. It might be helpful to take a short list of willing, close friends' phone numbers along when you go into labor.

—*JJ Levenstein, MD, FAAP, a mom of one son in college and a pediatrician in private practice in Southern California*

I think it's impossible to have a healthy, natural birth when you're lying on your back and tied up with IVs and monitors. Lying down is the wrong thing to be doing. My secret to making it through labor was walking. I walked until I didn't think I could walk anymore, and then I walked some more. Along the way, my midwife checked me. I kept walking until I thought that my poop was coming out, but in fact it was the baby. I didn't want to have the baby in the hallway, so I got into bed and pushed.

Also, I think you have to have your *mind* ready for labor. Understand that it's going to be hard, but of course you can do it.

It also helps to have someone you really trust in the room with you during labor. There's going to be a point when you'll think to yourself, *I can't do this*. That's when you look into the eyes of that person, and you put your soul in his or her hands, and you keep pushing. And *then* you have the baby.

—*Hana R. Solomon, MD, a mom of four, ages 35 to 19, a board-certified pediatrician, the president of BeWell Health, LLC, and the author of* Clearing the Air One Nose at a Time: Caring for Your Personal Filter

Even though I had epidurals with both of my deliveries, and I couldn't feel any pain, I was able to push. Epidurals affect different women differently, and many women still feel the pressure in the perineum and the sensation of needing to push even with the epidural in place.

Even if you don't feel that sensation, you can be instructed on when and how to push. The most important thing for the nurse or doctor to see is the baby's movement progressing down the birth canal.

With my first baby, I felt like I needed to be told when and how to push. I pushed for over an hour and really needed reassurance that I was making progress. For my second, though, I felt my baby come down into the birth canal. At that point, I knew I just had to cough him out!

—*Lauren Hyman, MD, a mom of two and an ob-gyn at West Hills Hospital and Medical Center in West Hills, CA*

During my first pregnancy, I was a resident on the hospital's labor and delivery floor. So I knew everyone there. My colleagues dropped in to my room to see how I was doing. I fondly remember the intern who came in to start my IV because to this date, we're still professional colleagues, and I enjoy running into her at conferences.

I wasn't worried or self-conscious about how I would look to my colleagues while I was in labor myself. A lot of women are concerned that they might have a BM or pass urine while in labor. That's understandable, but it's simply not a big deal for the average obstetrician because we see it so much; it is so normal that it happens most of the time. The baby's head is pressing on the rectum, and some stool comes out. There's a big catch pan, and they simply wipe away anything.

On the other hand, what I was worried about was pushing. I thought, *Oh my God, if I'm a bad pusher, everyone on the labor and delivery floor will know.* So when I was fully dilated, and it was time to push, I pushed very hard. I really focused and was lucky; I only had to push for around 20 minutes—not very long at all—and then my daughter was born!

—*Siobhan Dolan, MD, MPH, a mom of three, a consultant to the March of Dimes, and an associate professor of obstetrics and gynecology and women's health at Albert Einstein College of Medicine/Montefiore Medical Center in the Bronx, NY*

Communicating Your Wishes during Labor

When you're in labor, with all of the activity buzzing around you, you might feel a little lost, like you're not exactly the captain of this ship.

For example, in the United States, most women labor lying on their backs. But in most other cultures, women kneel, sit, squat, or stand. Why not work with gravity, rather than against it? This is something to think about and talk over with your doctor or midwife.

Also, don't worry: Most women aren't shaved or given an enema anymore. If you don't want to have an enema, you probably won't have to get one. Plus, many women worry about vomiting or having a bowel movement during labor, but try not to worry about it. This is very common; the medical staff sees this every day and handles it matter-of-factly.

But bear in mind that this is *your* day. Speak up until your needs are met, your questions are answered, and your wishes are heard.

ᵕ◦

Right around the time my water bag broke, I asked to have an epidural. I had done some checking into who the best anesthesia residents were, and the one I wanted was going off duty! So I figured, let's put the epidural in place and add the pain medication later.

　—*Diane Connelly, MD, a mom of a six-year-old daughter and an ob-gyn in HMO practice in Riverside, CA*

ᵕ◦

The nurses' philosophy at the hospital I delivered at was if a woman's labor is going well, don't mess with her. They gave me the freedom to labor as I wished. With my second delivery, I didn't even get an IV. I was able to walk all around, which helped me tremendously.

　—*Ellen Kruger, MD, a mom of two teenagers and an ob-gyn in an academic and clinical practice in New Orleans, LA, with Ochsner Health System*

ᵕ◦

Speak up for what you need. When I was in labor for my first pregnancy, someone came into the room that I didn't know. My labor stopped. I asked my husband to ask him to leave, and then my labor progressed.

　Another time, a nurse—my husband and I called her Rambo—wanted to put me in stirrups. We threw her out.

　—*Hana R. Solomon, MD*

ᵕ◦

When I was in labor, I had an epidural. I didn't know what to expect, but it felt a little weird! One side of my body felt numb, but the other side didn't. It took me a little while to figure out that something was wrong. Here I am a doctor, and I had no idea this could happen. After a few minutes, I asked a nurse if the epidural was correct, and she said, "No, it shouldn't be like that," and they fixed it. If something doesn't feel right to you, ask for help right away.

　—*Debra Luftman, MD, a mom of a teenaged daughter and a teenaged son, a board-certified dermatologist in private practice, a coauthor of* The Beauty Prescription, *the developer of the skincare line of products* Therapeutix, *and a clinical instructor of skin surgery and general dermatology at UCLA*

In my second pregnancy, my water broke when I was five weeks early. I had joked prior to that with my obstetrician that I was going to go into labor because he was going away on vacation, and that's exactly what happened.

My ob's father (who was also a doctor) was on call, and so he met me at the hospital. At the time, he was 60 years old, and he kept telling me to calm down and that I should relax my shoulders. That wasn't helping me at all, and so I got upset.

"How many times have you gone through this personally?" I asked. "Stop telling me what to do if you can't reassure me. Get out."

Don't let anyone tell you what to do in that delivery room unless the person supporting you has gone through it themselves and knows what you're feeling. And don't let anyone's ego get in the way. In that labor room, *you* are the focus—not anyone else, and certainly not the doctor. He's there to support you and to help you feel your best. If he doesn't, then throw him out.

—*Erika Schwartz, MD, a mom of two and the director of www. DrErika.com, who's been in private practice for more than 30 years in New York City, specializing over the past 15 years in women's health, disease prevention, and bioidentical hormones*

Birth is so intimate. You can compare a woman having a baby with a woman making love. If you could look at the face of a woman in the process of both, you'd see what I mean. Some women take a long time to get to orgasm, and other women get there really quickly. We'd never tell a woman that she needs special drugs because she's failing to progress to orgasm. Why do we have to medicalize birth to the point that we feel we can do that to women in labor?

I found that I needed to be alone for my labor to progress, and so I tried to communicate that. With my second child, when the midwives were in the room, my labor would be moving slowly. But when they stepped out of the room, I'd have huge contractions. I wouldn't be able to make love with them around either!

—*Stacey Marie Kerr, MD, a mother of two grown daughters, a family physician with strong roots in midwifery, and the author of* Homebirth in the Hospital, *in Santa Rosa, CA*

It's amazing that I had four labors and deliveries, and each one was completely different. My second labor was very different from my first, in which I was in labor for almost 24 hours. Even if you had a hard labor the first time, it might not be bad the second time, depending on the baby's position and other factors.

One thing that's very important is to communicate exactly what you need. For example, with my second son, when my husband and I arrived at the hospital, they checked me, and I was four centimeters dilated. All of a sudden, I yelled out with a huge contraction, and I asked them to please check me again.

"Oh, you're fine," they said, but they checked anyway. I had gone from 4 centimeters to 10 centimeters with two contractions. They quickly moved me into a room so that I didn't have the baby in their check-in area.

—*Karen Heald, MD, a mom of four boys and a board-certified family physician in private practice outside Atlanta, GA*

Mommy MD Guide-Recommended Product
Preggie Pops

Depending on where you're giving birth and your situation, you might have restrictions on what you can eat and drink during labor. One thing that should be fine for you to have during labor and that you might want to bring with you to the hospital is Preggie Pops. These naturally flavored and specially formulated lollipops are made for pregnant women. Preggie Pops offer relief via a combination of essential oils, aromatherapy, and a unique delivery system. They can alleviate dry mouth, provide quick calories and energy during labor, and are soothing and comforting. Preggie Pops are completely drug free.

You can buy Preggie Pops online at their website, **WWW.THREELOLLIES.COM**. A bag contains seven lollipops and costs $3.95. In addition to lollipops, they also sell Preggie Pop Drops, which are hard candies, without sticks. A container holds around 21 drops and costs $5.50. You can also buy Preggie Pops and Preggie Pop Drops at baby supply stores and maternity stores.

Both of my sons were born at home. My two labors were very different, and it was wonderful that I had my babies at home because I could do exactly what I needed to do for each labor without any medical restrictions.

For both deliveries, we moved the bed into the living room, where there is more space. For my first labor, I stayed in the bed because that was where I was comfortable laboring.

For my second delivery, I clung to a wet washcloth that I used on my belly and face, and I moved all around the house. I was in a different room of my house for each contraction. I was walking, squatting, stooping, and trying all sorts of different positions to make it through the contractions.

—*Lauren Feder, MD, a mom of two sons, a nationally recognized physician who specializes in homeopathic medicine, and the author of* Natural Baby and Childcare *and* The Parents' Concise Guide to Childhood Vaccinations, *in Los Angeles*

Controlling Pain during Labor

Labor is painful! Your uterus has to forcefully contract so that your baby can be born. But the way that you respond to that pain and how you control it is up to you. There's a whole spectrum of pain-control options, all the way from natural nonmedicated techniques up to general anesthesia.

Some women find that breathing techniques help to ease the pain, such as paced breathing. This helps you to focus on your breathing instead of the pain. To do paced breathing, think (or even say) "hah" when you inhale, and think (or even say) "hee" when you exhale.

Another type of breathing is called patterned breathing. To try this, repeat "hah" on the inhale and "hee" on the exhale four times, but then mix it up by saying "hah" on the inhale and "who" on the exhale.

One study found that women who listened to lyric-free instrumental music for three hours during early active labor felt less pain and distress.

Hypnosis and acupuncture are two other alternative methods to consider. Some hospitals and birthing centers have these practitioners available, but more likely you would need to bring in your own practitioner. Clear this ahead of time with your doctor or midwife.

Moving along the spectrum, epidurals are the most popular pain reliever because they numb the pain from your chest down, but you are still awake. After the epidural wears off, you might feel some itching and shivering.

Analgesics are sometimes given for pain relief. One common analgesic is Demerol, which can help with pain and anxiety. It can be given through an IV or via a shot. You can receive it every two to four hours, up to two to three hours before delivery. The drawbacks are that it can cause you to feel sick or depressed and lower your blood pressure. It also can cause your baby to be born drowsy and unable to suck vigorously.

If you are having a Cesarean section, you might be given a spinal block. You'll lie on your side, and a needle will be inserted into your spinal canal. You'll have to lie on your back for around eight hours after your baby is born. At the very far end of the spectrum, sometimes women are given general anesthesia for C-sections.

⁓

I think that epidurals should be used liberally. I understand that many women don't want to do that, and I'm supportive of that, but I have a hard time *understanding* it. I had epidurals with both deliveries, and I wouldn't have considered doing it otherwise. I was even able to nap some in my second delivery.

—*Kelly Campbell, MD*

⁓

With my first baby, I was induced, and after a couple of hours of painful contractions, it was a little too much for me, so I got an epidural. I wanted to see what the contractions felt like to see if I could handle natural childbirth. I loved my epidural, and I breathed a huge sigh of relief when I got it.

—*Jennifer Kim, MD, a mom of three girls, ages eight, five, and four; an ob-gyn in private practice in Evanston, IL, at the Midwest Center for Women's Healthcare; and a clinical assistant professor at the University of Chicago, Pritzker School of Medicine*

⁓

I wanted to have an epidural, but I really wanted to feel what contractions felt like first. I was induced. My mom kept saying that she thought I had been having contractions prior to going in, but I didn't feel a thing. She insisted I was having them and just didn't know!

"I've never had a contraction before," I said. "But I think I'd know it if I felt one."

Then the contractions got started.

"Nope, I didn't feel that before," I said. "I'll take that epidural now."

—*Kerri A. Daniels, MD*

When my older daughter was born, I was in the Air Force. Epidurals were hard to come by in the military, and she was born so quickly that I had a natural birth.

So after my first contraction with my twins, I asked for my epidural. I had it at midnight and slept until 6 am. They woke me when it was time to push. It was the nicest labor ever.

—*Susan Wilder, MD, a mom of an older daughter and twin girls, a primary care physician, and CEO and founder of Lifescape Medical Associates in Scottsdale, AZ*

My labors were quick. With the first, I pushed forever, but with the second, I only pushed for 10 minutes. For both of those labors, I had epidurals. I worked at the hospital where I delivered, and they put in the epidurals practically before I asked for them.

A lot of women worry that having an epidural will hurt. I didn't think it was painful at all, and it offered great pain relief.

—*Judy Dudum, MD, a mom of three, an ob-gyn, and a senior staff physician at Henry Ford Health System in Detroit, with interests in nutrition and adolescent gynecology*

When I got to the hospital in labor, I told my ob that I didn't want any pain medication. When I did my ob rotation, I thought the women asking for epidurals were largely being drama queens. My ob laughed and said, "I'll see you in about an hour."

I thought, *That was so rude!* But lo and behold, about an hour later, I asked her to please come back and give me some meds. She gave me Demerol and an epidural, and it knocked me out. My husband said I was unconscious and drooling! He passed the time playing video games on his laptop.

Several hours later (though to me it felt like just a few minutes), my ob woke me up and told me to push. It was a wonderful experience!

—*Sonia Ng, MD, a mom of seven-year-old and one-year-old sons and a pediatrician and expert in sedation at Children's Hospital of Philadelphia Pediatric Care at Princeton Health Care System in Princeton, NJ*

ᥴ᥎

My first delivery was horrendous. But truth be told, much of that was my doing. I had the misconception that I ultimately had some control over any part of the process.

Because I had tested positive for group B strep, I had to go to the hospital even before I went into labor. I refused Pitocin—a synthetic version of oxytocin, which is produced by women in labor. Pitocin is given to augment labor as well as induce it. I refused the Pitocin to induce my labor for far too long, and I ended up having a three-day-labor ordeal and eventually delivering naturally.

However, after discovering that there's no prize for delivering without an epidural, for my second delivery, I said yes to the epidural.

I think it's best to go into labor with an open mind. When your doctor or midwife asks if you'd like pain medication, it's not to threaten your experience. We ask to make sure that you are aware that it is available and can help with the pain and potentially your labor. Ultimately it is your experience, and hopefully it will be memorable and enjoyable—even though some of it will likely involve pain! Pain medication might make your birth experience more enjoyable and more memorable.

—*Janet Lefkowitz, DO, a mother of two girls and an ob-gyn in private practice in Rhode Island*

ᥴ᥎

I went into both of my deliveries thinking I would be able to do it naturally, without any anesthesia. But both times, I elected to have an epidural.

Even though I had delivered a thousand babies, being in labor myself gave me a whole new respect for the amount of pain involved! I truly didn't know what it felt like to have a baby until I went through it myself.

For my first baby, I stayed at home as long as I could stand the pain, but at 10 pm, when I could no longer take it, I had my associate call the hospital and let them know I was on my way. She told them to give me the epidural the second I got there. With false hope, I was checked first, sure I was at least eight centimeters dilated. I was only one centimeter! I got the epidural right away, and I had the baby at 6 am.

With my second baby, I thought, *Maybe I'll give this a go without the epidural.* But when I was about three centimeters, I was feeling quite a lot of pain, and I thought, *Why am I putting myself through this?* I couldn't come up with a good reason at that point, so I decided to put myself out of my misery and request an epidural.

I'm very supportive of women who decide to go through the labor process without medication. It's a very personal choice.

—*Lauren Hyman, MD*

I'm not big into pain or natural childbirth. I don't think you get a star for doing it naturally. I found as an ob that if a patient didn't have an epidural, when I touched her to stitch her up after delivery, she would scream, "Eek!" Women don't think about that bonus of epidurals: They make the after-birth process easier too.

I am a big fan of doing something for pain relief—an epidural or a spinal. I had epidurals for my first two deliveries. But I had spinals with my second two deliveries because my last two labors were so fast that I didn't have time to get epidurals. I got one-shot spinals instead. My longest labor was three hours, and my shortest was less than two hours.

—*Melanie Bone, MD, a mom of four "tweens" ages 15 to 12, a gynecologist, the founder of the Cancer Sensibility Foundation, and the author of the syndicated column* Surviving Life *and the book* Cancer, What's Next?, *in West Palm Beach, FL*

Labor pains will not earn you a Purple Heart. There are no medals for women who deliver naturally or vaginally. Do what you gotta do to get through. We live in the 21st century, where you don't have to be tortured.

Ask early if you're going to want an epidural, which is a regional anesthetic placed in the space around your spinal cord, with fewer side effects to the baby. After a certain stage of labor, you're not allowed to have an epidural anymore. So if you wait too long to ask for an epidural, you might have to have IV sedation instead, which can make the baby "groggy."

Truth be told though, I had IV sedation during my C-section because my epidural wasn't enough for the surgery, and my baby was just fine.

—*Tyeese Gaines Reid, DO, a mom of one, an emergency medicine resident physician at Yale New Haven Hospital in Connecticut, and the author of a time management book,* The Get a Life Campaign

Having a C-Section

In 1965, only 4 percent of babies in the United States were delivered by C-section. Today, nearly one-third of all babies born in the United States come into this world via a Cesarean delivery, which is also called a Cesarean section or a C-section. In a C-section, a baby is delivered through an incision in the mom's abdominal wall, uterus, and amniotic sac.

There are many reasons why C-sections are done. The most common reason is having had a prior C-section. Some women who have had C-sections elect to deliver vaginally the next time, and this is called a vaginal birth after Cesarean (VBAC). Another reason is if your baby is too big to fit through the birth canal. Fetal distress is another reason for a C-section. Also, if your baby isn't head down, but rather rear end or feet first, she's in a breech position. Vaginal delivery of breech babies can be risky, and so your doctor might recommend a C-section.

My husband and I went in to the hospital for my first son to be born on a Sunday morning, when my contractions were around five minutes apart. Even though I was having regular contractions, after 24 hours, my labor wasn't progressing. I wasn't dilating like I was supposed to. My doctor ordered a C-section, and my son was born at 9 pounds, 9 ounces.

—*Karen Heald, MD*

My first two babies were born vaginally, and I had expected the same with my third. But because I had the starting signs and symptoms of preeclampsia, my doctor immediately decided to do a C-section. It wasn't what I had planned, but it turned out okay.

—*Judy Dudum, MD*

After I had been in labor for 28 hours, I sent my exhausted husband home to take a shower. Of course, that was when both my son and I crashed, and my doctor decided to perform an emergency C-section. As they readied me for the procedure, my lovely obstetrician, whom I adored, sat next to me and held my hand. She was sick as a dog from a stomach flu, but she stayed with me during this frightening time.

The minute before the incision was made, my husband arrived. He had fainted when we had our blood drawn for our marriage license, but he stayed right by my head and never budged. I had chills and felt uncomfortable from the anesthesia and my fever. Suddenly, my son's head popped out from my belly, and he looked around! He looked like a periscope! And then my son let out a reassuring wail. What a relief!

—*JJ Levenstein, MD, FAAP*

⁓

When I was around 38 weeks pregnant with my older daughter, I was standing over a patient I was treating in my office. Suddenly, I felt a very strange shift in my belly.

Right around my due date, my water broke, and I went into labor. When my doctor examined me, he discovered my baby was breech, which means bottom first. Apparently, when I had felt that shift, the baby totally flipped! And so I went in for a C-section.

—*Julie Silver, MD, a mom of a 17-year-old son and 13- and 9-year-old daughters, a Boston-area physiatrist, and the award-winning writer of more than a dozen books, including* After Cancer Treatment: Heal Faster, Better, Stronger

⁓

I was induced at 40 weeks. My baby was facing up so to speak, so I pushed for three hours, but because of my baby's position, I ended up needing a C-section.

I tried as hard as I could to avoid that C-section, knowing the risks it posed. I think a lot of people don't realize those risks and go into labor thinking, "Maybe a C-section would be better."

The reality is, the risks of a C-section are pretty significant for babies and for moms. For example, babies often have trouble breathing after C-sections because they don't get compression of the thorax that they get when they go through the birth canal. This compression helps to clear their lungs of fluid and mucus. Babies born by C-section are more likely to have tachypnea, or fast breathing, and because of this, they are more likely to go to the intensive care unit. Also, they have longer stays in the hospital when compared to babies born vaginally.

Moms who have C-sections have more bleeding and have a greater risk of infection. They have a higher risk of deep vein thrombosis and pulmonary embolism, which can be life-threatening. They have a longer hospital stay and a much harder recovery.

There are also risks to subsequent pregnancies. Once you have that incision in the uterus, there is always a weakness and scar there. This scar can open with any subsequent labor. This can be catastrophic during future deliveries.

So as you can see, I was resistant to having a C-section. I tried as hard as I could to deliver vaginally, but some babies just don't fit through the pelvis and have to be delivered by C-section. C-section still isn't something I'd consider doing electively—only as an exception.

—*Nancy Thomas, MD, a mom of a 22-month-old son who practices general obstetrics and gynecology in Covington, LA, with Ochsner Health System*

⤳

At the hospital, my water bag was broken, and I walked around the hospital floor for around three hours to try to get my labor going. Nothing happened. I ultimately needed Pitocin, and then I had beautiful contractions. Even though they were strong and regular, every two minutes, they did nothing to dilate my cervix! How frustrating. I tried for hours, but I didn't dilate past five centimeters.

Then my doctor discovered that one of my twins was trying to come out crooked; it's called an asynclitic presentation. That's not a proper birthing position, so I ended up needing a C-section.

This wasn't what I had expected, but I was okay with that. I trusted my doctor, and I remained focused on the goal of having healthy babies.

When that decision was made, it was very overwhelming, though. Suddenly, it's like you've taken a fork in a road. Lots of new players came into my hospital room, and everyone was doing their own thing: shaving my belly, putting in a catheter, changing my IV fluid. No one was telling me what was going on. It felt very much like things were happening *to* me, and I wasn't really a part of it. But I kept telling myself that this was normal. They were all just doing their jobs and taking care of me and my babies. I tried not to lose the focus of my babies and a safe delivery.

Then I found that having a C-section itself is a very odd experience. I was lying there, hearing what was going on, but not able to see. It takes away a lot of the experience of birth. I also had a bad reaction to the medication they gave me. I felt light-headed, like I was having an out-of-body experience. I felt very disconnected from the birth. Plus, with a vaginal delivery, you're very involved—pushing and working to get the baby out. With a C-section, I felt that my babies were being *taken* from me, instead of me *giving* my babies to be born.

It's also very different when your baby is born by C-section: They hold the baby up so you can see, but you don't get to hold the baby right away like you would after a vaginal birth. I didn't get to hold my babies until around an hour later, when I was in the recovery room. Thankfully, my husband was in the operating room with me, and he went back and forth from our babies in the warmer to me, and he took pictures to show me. That helped a lot.

In the end, I knew that my doctor made the best decision, and I came to terms with it, and it all was fine.

—*Jennifer Gilbert, DO*

Chapter 43
Welcome to the World, Little One!

Seeing Your Baby for the First Time

You've waited a long time for this wonderful moment—the instant that you see your baby for the very first time!

My first baby was born at 5 am, after a long night in labor. I was groggy and tired. When I looked at my baby for the first time, it felt surreal. I remember looking at her and thinking, *Is this my baby, really?* It felt like a wonderful dream.

—*Jennifer Kim, MD, a mom of three girls, ages eight, five, and four; an ob-gyn in private practice in Evanston, IL, at the Midwest Center for Women's Healthcare; and a clinical assistant professor at the University of Chicago, Pritzker School of Medicine*

I cannot adequately describe how I felt when my babies were born. At the time, the analogy came to me forcefully that it was just as if I had died and there really was a Heaven with the Prophets and the Angels, and that you could look at them clearly and see they were like real people, with eyelashes and fingernails. My baby's eyelashes and fingernails seemed that impossible and vivid to me. Just to look at them seemed impossible.

—*Elizabeth Berger, MD, a mom of two, a child psychiatrist, and the author of* Raising Kids with Character

The three days that my babies were born were the three happiest days of my life. My wedding day—even though I enjoyed that very much—doesn't even come close.

I had short labors, and even the labors were wonderful. The fondest memories of my life are the days of my deliveries. They were the most exciting days I ever had because they were the days when I saw my babies for the first time. When they placed my babies in my arms, with my husband standing right beside me, I felt like the luckiest person in the world!

—*Ayala Laufer-Cahana, MD, a pediatrician, mother, artist, serious home cook, and the founder of Herbal Water Inc., in Wynnewood, PA*

I had an emergency C-section, and they knocked me out at the end. When I woke up a few hours later in the recovery room, the first thing I saw was my husband rocking our baby. He was stroking our son's ears and saying how hairy they were, just like his grandfather's, for whom Max was named.

I will never forget the look on my husband's face: He was so overwhelmed with love. And looking at the two of them, so was I.

—*JJ Levenstein, MD, FAAP, a mom of one son in college and a pediatrician in private practice in Southern California*

The first time I saw my baby, she was upside down as the doctor pulled her out. I can still remember how she looked. Her eyes were wide open, and she was looking all around as if in amazement at what she saw.

I remember thinking, *Wow, this is my baby.* All the time I was pregnant, I wondered what she would look like. It was amazing to find out.

—*Kerri A. Daniels, MD, a mom of one toddler daughter and an instructor in the department of pediatrics at the University of Arkansas for Medical Science in Little Rock*

I couldn't stand being pregnant, but I *loved* having my babies. I am the youngest of parents who were the youngest in their families, so I was also the youngest cousin. There weren't any babies or younger kids in my family for me to experience.

But I was amazed at how much I got from my baby simply looking at me in the first moments of his life. It was amazing how instantly I got back all of that love from my sons.

—*Sandra Carson, MD, a mom of two grown sons and the director of the Center for Reproduction and Infertility of Women & Infants Hospital in Providence, RI*

My first daughter was born in a birthing center. I remember when she was born, the doctor put her into a little incubator box. He didn't give her to me right away, but I didn't think anything of it at that time. It was 1973, and I had just given birth! I just wanted her to be safe. I figured I'd hold her soon enough.

Around a half hour later, the doctor brought my baby to me. I remember the look on his face was of great reverence, which made a huge impact on me. It was important to me that whoever brought my baby to me for the first time know how special she was, and I could tell that my doctor knew.

When I held my baby and looked into her eyes for the first time, I remember thinking, *I know you. I have known you for generations.*

—*Stacey Marie Kerr, MD, a mother of two grown daughters, a family physician with strong roots in midwifery, and the author of* Homebirth in the Hospital, *in Santa Rosa, CA*

⤳

During my second pregnancy, a good friend of mine was pregnant at the same time, a few months ahead of me. Star is very progressive, and she asked her doctor in advance if she could help deliver her own baby. Her husband videotaped it from behind her shoulder, and later we watched it together—Star with her baby in her arms and me with my baby still in my belly. We both wept.

I'm a doctor and more traditional, and so while I admired Star for helping to deliver her own baby, I didn't think it was right for me. When I was in labor at the hospital, I was shooting the breeze with my doctor, and I told him Star's birth story.

"You can do that," my doctor said. "It's no big deal."

Sure enough, my doctor guided my baby's head out. Then I reached down and grabbed her, pulled her out, and laid her on my chest. That moment set the tone for our entire relationship. She has been such a joy from the very beginning.

—*Eva Ritvo, MD, a mom of two teenaged daughters, an associate professor and vice chairman at the Miller School of Medicine of the University of Miami, and a coauthor of* The Beauty Prescription

⤳

I was so very afraid during both of my pregnancies. I worried constantly that my babies were okay. I couldn't wait for them to be born so that I would know that they were all right.

But then, once you hold your baby in your arms, that's when you realize that the easy part was when they were inside of you!

—*Kelly Campbell, MD, a mom of three and an ob-gyn in private practice at Women's Healthcare Physicians in West Bloomfield, MI*

Introducing Your Baby to Your Partner

Your partner has waited a long time for *this* wonderful moment—the moment he gets to meet the beautiful baby the two of you have created together. What an amazing time for you and your family.

When my doctor brought my baby to me, he gently set her down on the other bed next to me there in the room. The next thing I knew, my husband came in and sat on her. That was their first meeting.

—*Stacey Marie Kerr, MD*

My husband and I chose to only have the two of us in the room when our babies were born, no other family members. I think that the time when your babies are born is a huge bonding experience as a family. It should be about you, your husband, and your child. It was a very emotional moment just between us.

A little while later, we invited our other family members into the room.

—*Debra Luftman, MD, a mom of a teenaged daughter and a teenaged son, a board-certified dermatologist in private practice, a coauthor of* The Beauty Prescription, *the developer of the skincare line of products Therapeutix, and a clinical instructor of skin surgery and general dermatology at UCLA*

My first daughter was born after three hours of pushing. I was so happy to see her, but I was so tired that I handed her to my husband, who cuddled with her for a bit and then handed her off to my mom. My daughter and I bonded later.

My second daughter was born after only five minutes of pushing. That was a completely different experience. I was totally awake and not at all exhausted. I snuggled with her right away, and it was awesome!

—*Ashley Roman, MD, MPH, a mom of two daughters, ages three years and six months, and a clinical assistant professor in the department of obstetrics and gynecology at the New York University School of Medicine in New York City*

∽

My first baby was born at 5 am. My husband was so excited! He stayed with us that whole day, but I sent him home that night because there was nowhere for him to sleep.

—*Jennifer Kim, MD*

Breastfeeding for the First Time

If you choose to breastfeed and you and your baby are both doing well, you will likely be encouraged to breastfeed your baby right away. What a beautiful, tender, unforgettable time. But be prepared and patient: You're *both* new to this.

∽

I breastfed both of my daughters shortly after they were born. I was lucky; they both knew what they were doing, so it was pretty effortless on my part.

—*Ashley Roman, MD, MPH*

∽

When I breastfed my first baby for the first time, even though I was completely committed to breastfeeding, it was painful. In fact, it was painful for a day or two. But I dealt with it. I learned how to place the baby's mouth deep onto the nipple, correctly, and other tips that helped me succeed. That's what those nipples are meant for.

—*Hana R. Solomon, MD, a mom of four, ages 35 to 19, a board-certified pediatrician, the president of BeWell Health, LLC, and the author of* Clearing the Air One Nose at a Time: Caring for Your Personal Filter

∽

I wanted to nurse my son, but I found it very hard at first. He actually didn't nurse much at all for the first three days. I think he was exhausted from 28 hours of labor, and I was physically drained from lack of sleep and having a fever. I wanted to just give him a bottle, but the lactation consultants at the hospital urged me to wait, to give him more time.

I was starting to get desperate. Then during our third night in the hospital at 3 am, when all was quiet, we found each other.

After that, I felt better. I knew instinctively, though, that nursing would be easier, and more natural, once we got home. And I was right. It got better quickly after that. Once I got home, I was producing so much milk that when I walked across the hardwood floor, I'd leave two milk trails behind me.

—*JJ Levenstein, MD, FAAP*

∽

I was committed to breastfeeding. It's something I always wanted to do for my baby.

Some women have no problem doing it, and they're able to breastfeed right away with no issues. But for me, it was the opposite. I nursed my baby right away in the hospital after my C-section. It was uncomfortable because of the C-section, but I was determined to do it, and that's what carried me through.

Also, it helped me a lot to talk with the lactation consultants at the hospital. They were very supportive. After I got home, I talked with my friends who have kids, and they shared with me how difficult it was for them too in the beginning, but that it got better. That helped me push through.

So many parts of pregnancy and birth are challenging, but it's so worth it. I'd go through it all over again to be where I am today with my daughter.

—*Christy Valentine, MD, a mom of one, a specialist in pediatrics and internal medicine, and the founder of the Valentine Medical Center in Gretna, LA*

∽

Some very nice nurses cared for me while I was in the hospital, and one of the lactation consultants really helped me learn how to breastfeed. She helped me to get my daughter latched on properly for the first time, which is critical for nursing success.

During the rest of my hospital stay, I would let the nurses know when I wanted to nurse my baby, and they would come to my room and give me support and help. They even gave me a number to call after I got home if I had any questions. Nursing was harder at first than I thought it would be, but once my daughter and I got it, it was great.

—*Kerri A. Daniels, MD*

Introducing Your Baby to Your Children, Family, and Friends

Many people have been waiting for this day—the day that they get to meet your baby.

❧

When my second and third babies were born, my husband brought our older children to the hospital to meet them. To start their relationships off on the right foot, I had packed gifts for the older siblings from the new baby. This goodwill gesture went a long way! They were touched that their new brother and sister thought of them.

> —*Aline T. Tanios, MD, a mom of three and a general pediatrician and hospitalist who treats medically complex children at Arkansas Children's Hospital in Little Rock*

❧

A few hours after my third daughter was born, my husband brought our older girls to see us. They were so excited! They hopped right up on the bed and literally climbed up on top of the baby. They couldn't get close enough to her. Both girls have been completely enamored with their baby sister since day one.

> —*Rebecca Kazin, MD, a mom of three girls and the medical director of the Johns Hopkins Dermatology and Cosmetic Center at Green Spring Station in Lutherville, MD*

❧

When my son was born, my husband and our parents brought our two older daughters to the hospital to see me and meet the new baby.

My older daughter was five at the time. Like a little mommy, she picked the baby right up! My younger daughter was really still a baby herself, around 20 months old. I was really happy to see her because I felt like I had left one baby to have another baby, and it was so reassuring to hold her in my arms. Both of my daughters bonded very quickly with their new brother.

> —*Siobhan Dolan, MD, MPH, a mom of three, a consultant to the March of Dimes, and an associate professor of obstetrics and gynecology and women's health at Albert Einstein College of Medicine/Montefiore Medical Center in the Bronx, NY*

❧

When my son was born, my mom picked my daughter up from school and then took her to a store to buy her brother a stuffed animal.

Beforehand, I had bought a gift for the baby to give to my daughter. I had also brought a photo of my daughter and placed it in his bassinet at the hospital.

When my daughter came to meet her new brother, she was so excited! She asked to hold him right away, and she was on cloud nine.

—*Michelle Paley, MD, PA, a mom of a six-year-old daughter and a two-year-old son and a psychiatrist and psychotherapist in private practice in Miami Beach, FL*

I tell my patients not to have their kids come to the hospital until after the IV is out and they've freshened up. Kids don't want to see Mommy looking sick. And they certainly don't want to see the baby being born. Kids don't handle that well.

With my second and third babies, my husband brought the older kids to see me a few hours after the baby was born. In particular, when my second baby was born, I bought a gift at the hospital gift store for the baby to "give" to her older brother. That helped to ease the transition for him.

—*Judy Dudum, MD, a mom of three, an ob-gyn, and a senior staff physician at Henry Ford Health System in Detroit, with interests in nutrition and adolescent gynecology*

Even though I'm the youngest in my family, my baby was my mother's first grandchild. I knew that she would be overjoyed to meet her first grandbaby!

After my son was born, my mother drove from New York City to Philadelphia with my brother and sister to see me and meet my baby. It was a very special time. I cherish a photo that I have of my mom holding my son when he was only a few hours old.

When we had our second child, my mom came to visit so she could stay with my two-year-old. She had a hard time watching me in labor!

—*Elissa Charbonneau, DO, a mom of an 18-year-old son and a 16-year-old daughter and the medical director of the New England Rehabilitation Hospital in Portland, ME*

My two sons were born at home. We moved the bed into the living room so all 10 people who were there could appreciate the experience. When my first son was born after 13 hours of labor, including three hours of pushing, there was much rejoicing and champagne. I don't know if people were so happy because the baby was born or because the labor was finally over.

—*Lauren Feder, MD, a mom of two sons, a nationally recognized physician who specializes in homeopathic medicine, and the author of* Natural Baby and Childcare *and* The Parents' Concise Guide to Childhood Vaccinations, *in Los Angeles*

Finding Out Your Baby Isn't Well

When your baby is born, he will be given a series of tests called APGAR. They were developed in 1952 by an anesthesiologist named Virginia Apgar. The tests assign a number between 0 and 2 for each of the following: baby's heart rate, color, breathing, muscle tone, and reflexes. Those numbers are then added up. A total score between 7 and 10 indicates the baby is doing well. Scores below 7 indicate the baby needs special care, and scores below 4 require immediate medical intervention. Your baby will be tested again five minutes after he's born.

∾

When my second daughter was born, all of the nurses were gathered around her bedside, whispering with concern. They brought my baby to me, and then whisked her right away.

I found out that my baby was having a heart arrhythmia, and her heart rhythm needed to be converted. A wire would be threaded down her esophagus, and she would receive an electrical charge to put her heart into a normal rhythm. My baby was immediately transported by ambulance to Children's Hospital of Philadelphia. I was checked out of the hospital so that I could go with her.

I knew all of the doctors at the children's hospital, and they treated me with respect, but it was so different to be there with my own sick baby. It was very stressful, but on the other hand, I was happy to be able to put my baby in their very capable hands and walk away while they did the procedure.

I think that parents going through something like this go into a sort of fugue state, for self-preservation. Only a few hours after giving birth, I just checked out of the hospital. You do what you have to do and rise to any challenge for your child. Thank goodness, my baby was fine.

—*Alicia Brennan, MD, a mom of three daughters and the medical director of inpatient pediatrics of Children's Hospital of Philadelphia Pediatric Care at Princeton Health Care System in Princeton, NJ*

⚬⁄⚬

My second child was born while we were living in Germany. When he was born, he was critically ill. During my pregnancy, there were no indications that anything was wrong.

My doctor induced me because he was going to be away on my due date, and it turned out my due date was wrong. We thought my son was 39 weeks, but he was probably only 37. He developed a condition called persistent fetal circulation (PFC), which is a life-threatening condition in which a newborn baby's circulation changes back to the circulation of a fetus and much of the blood flow bypasses the lungs. My son seemed fine at first, but the doctors quickly realized he wasn't breathing well. They ran through a gamut of tests and realized it was PFC.

The doctors put my son on a ventilator and transported him to another hospital. It was traumatic. I learned that when it's your child, you want everything done, no matter what the outcome will be, no matter what the cost. You will do *anything*—no matter how heroic or costly, to preserve that life.

We were blessed that our son did fine. Today he's a sophomore at Clemson, premed, with a 4.0.

—*Ann Kulze, MD, a mother of four children, ages 20, 19, 18, a nd 14, a nationally recognized nutrition expert, motivational speaker, physician, and the author of the critically acclaimed book* Dr. Ann's 10-Step Diet: A Simple Plan for Permanent Weight Loss and Lifelong Vitality

⚬⁄⚬

My twins were born at 29 weeks. They stayed in the neonatal intensive care unit (NICU) for six weeks. It was very hard, but like other challenges in life, you have to get through it, and so you do.

Fortunately, we live and I practice very close to the hospital where our twins were. I went back to work part-time even though they were still in the

NICU, for two reasons. First, I had been on bed rest for a few months, and I knew that I would be out for a while after the babies came home. Second, I love my work; working feeds me. I would visit my babies in the hospital, then go in to work for a few hours, and then go back to visit them again.

It was a challenging time, but it wasn't as difficult as when we brought them home and had to take care of them. My husband and I brought our babies home pretty early. We are both physicians, and plus I badgered the hospital into letting us. This is not something I recommend. It was very hard.

—*Ruth D. Williams, MD, a mom of twins—a boy and a girl— and another boy, and an ophthalmologist in private practice at the WheatonEye Clinic in Wheaton, IL, who specializes in the diagnosis and treatment of glaucoma*

Making the Most Out of Your Hospital Stay

Once you have your baby in your arms, you might be itching to go home to begin your life together. But babies don't come with instruction manuals, and right now you've got the next best thing: a cadre of trained, experienced nurses and doctors who care for newborn babies each and every day. Learn as much from them as you can; they're probably very willing and eager to help.

∽

Ask as many questions as you can think of while you're in the hospital. I remember giving my first baby her first bath. She was so wriggly and slippery, and I thought to myself, *Why don't they teach us how to do this in medical school?* And truth be told, you can go to gazillions of classes, but until you hold your own baby and do things for her for the first time, you can't really know how to do them.

—*Susan Schreiber, MD, a mom of a son and daughter in their twenties and a pediatrician in Los Angeles, CA*

∽

When my daughter was born, she stayed in my room the entire time. But when my son was born, one night I sent him to the nursery so that I could sleep. I asked the nurses to please not wake me to take my blood pressure or anything else as long as the baby was fine.

That night of good sleep made a big difference in how I felt when I went home. I was a better mom for it!

—*Michelle Paley, MD, PA*

One of the most memorable meals I've had in my entire life was the dinner I ate after the delivery of my daughter. I hadn't been able to eat much during the last six weeks of my pregnancy because of horrible heartburn, and I was hungry all of the time.

They brought me roast chicken and broccoli, and I'm sure it was just average, but to me it was delicious—one of the best meals I've had in my entire life! I was sitting in my little room and savoring every bite. Life felt so different!

—*Sharonne N. Hayes, MD, a mom of two and the director of the Women's Heart Clinic at Mayo Clinic in Rochester, MN*

I had three totally different hospital stays after my three girls were born. With my first, I was able to enjoy those 48 hours sitting in my bed and being waited on!

My second baby needed critical care right after she was born and had to be transported to Children's Hospital of Philadelphia. Just a few hours after delivery, I was on my feet, trekking down to the cafeteria to get my own food. I also found with my second daughter that it's so different when you have another child at home you want to get home to. That 48-hour hospital stay is no longer relaxing.

With my third daughter, I had mixed feelings. I was anxious to get home to my other daughters, but I knew the chaos I was going home to and how busy it would be, so I tried to really enjoy that brief hospital stay.

—*Alicia Brennan, MD*

Having your first baby is so hard because you don't know anything. When my oldest daughter was born, I remember being in the hospital trying to put on her tiny little outfit. It had snaps all over the inside and the crotch. I was tired, and my mom and friend were there with me.

My mom is a doctor, and my friend is a pediatrician. The three of us struggled mightily to figure out how to put that outfit on a 6-pound, 4-ounce newborn. We didn't know what we were doing. Three Mommy MDs were standing there like it was a jigsaw puzzle. We couldn't figure it out.

It's amazing to me that I went through four years of undergraduate schooling, four years of medical school, and four years of residency before I could even sit alone in a room with an adult patient. Yet, they sent me home from the hospital with a frail baby with not a moment of instruction. They let me take that tiny baby home when I didn't know a thing.

Ask for the help of the nurses in the hospital—while you have the chance!

—*Eva Ritvo, MD*

Recovering from the Birth or C-Section

Now that your baby is born, we wish we could wave a magic wand and change you back to your pre-pregnancy self. It took your body nine months to get to this point, but the good news is, it won't take you another nine months to get your body back. Women are incredibly resilient.

After your baby is born, your uterus shrinks *immediately* from the size of a watermelon to the size of a volleyball. This causes the placenta to detach from the uterine wall and to be delivered.

Also, after your baby is born, your hormone levels quickly change. Because of their adjustments, you might feel hot and cold flashes.

You might soon notice that your breasts and nipples are sore and tender. This will happen as your milk comes in, and it might last for a few days.

It might be painful to sit or walk for a few days if your perineum was torn during birth or if you had an episiotomy. Coughing or sneezing might hurt too. This should heal in a few days. Sitting on an ice-pack for short periods of time can help.

For a few days after your baby is born, you might feel contractions. These are called after-birth pains, and they're working hard to get your uterus down to size. You'll notice them most when your baby nurses, if you're breastfeeding.

You'll likely notice a dramatic increase in vaginal discharge after your baby is born. It will begin as bleeding that's heavier than a usual period. It might contain clots of blood. Then it will taper off and fade to white and yellow discharge. It usually stops within two months.

When you try to have a bowel movement for the first time after having your baby, it might be painful. Constipation, hemorrhoids, and sore muscles are very common. You might talk with your doctor or midwife about taking a stool softener.

Up to 80 percent of new moms experience the baby blues. They feel irritable, sad, or anxious, and they can cry at the drop of a hat. This can start within days or weeks after the baby is born. More serious than the baby blues, 10 to 25 percent of new moms suffer from postpartum depression. It can cause anxiety, mood swings, guilt, and sadness. If your mood is consistently low, if you find little joy in life, or if you have trouble summoning the energy to start a new day, seek help promptly.

Having a C-section brings the added challenge of recovery from surgery. As the anesthesia wears off, you might use a pump that allows you to adjust the dose of IV pain medication.

The catheter and IVs will likely be removed within 12 to 24 hours of the C-section. Within the first 24 hours, you'll be encouraged to get up and walk. Moving around can speed your recovery and help prevent constipation and potentially dangerous blood clots.

While you're in the hospital, your incision will be monitored for signs of infection. The nurses will also monitor your appetite, how much fluid you're drinking, and your bladder and bowel function.

It's common for women to have after-birth pains after their babies are born, as the uterus contracts back to its original size. I didn't have many after-birth pains when my first son was born, but I learned all about them after my second son was born. After your second delivery, your uterus has to work harder to contract and get back to its normal size.

I didn't think the pain would be bad, but it was actually like going through labor all over again! I didn't take any pain medication. Instead, I took a homeopathic remedy called caullophylum (blue cohosh). It took the pain right away.

—Lauren Feder, MD

Both of my kids were born by C-section. My recovery was fine. I'm told that women recover more quickly following vaginal deliveries, but I don't have anything to compare my experience to. I did take some Vicodin on the first day post op, but thereafter, I found that Tylenol was as effective in relieving the pain.

—*Diane Truong, MD, FAAP, a mom of one daughter and one son and a pediatrician in a multispecialty group practice in Southern California*

For me, recovering from a C-section wasn't a big deal. In about a week, I felt fine. I think that you're 90 percent better in a week, and then it takes about four to six weeks before you feel completely back to your normal self. But the challenge is that at the time, you're taking care of a newborn, you're not sleeping, and you're exhausted, so it takes longer than it normally would to get completely back to yourself.

—*Jennifer Gilbert, DO, a mom of three-month-old twins and an ob-gyn at Paoli Hospital in Pennsylvania*

My third baby was delivered by C-section. Recovery from that was definitely harder than from my two vaginal births. The first time I got up to walk, I thought that it was painful, and I didn't want to walk initially. But, I knew that all of my patients do it, so I needed to do it as well. I simply had to do it. Standing up and walking the first few days was hard, but after you're up and moving, it gets easier.

—*Judy Dudum, MD*

I had to have a C-section. My recovery was hard because I had dilated fully during labor and had pushed for three hours. My baby was pretty close to the perineum, and the surgery was pretty intense because I had labored all that time. I had a good bit of pain after the surgery.

I believe that the most important thing is to start moving as soon as possible after surgery. I was up and out of my hospital bed around 12 hours after my surgery! Just getting up and moving around helped me to start my recovery.

I also wore an abdominal binder for support around my incision. That helped me to move around more easily. Most labor and delivery units have these. Slowly but surely, you heal and get back to normal.

—Nancy Thomas, MD, a mom of a 22-month-old son who practices general obstetrics and gynecology in Covington, LA, with Ochsner Health System

⌒∾⌒

After my baby was born, I woke in the middle of the night with night sweats. I was terrified! But night sweats after having a baby are normal. They're caused by hormone changes, similar to menopause. Your hormones are dropping very significantly and rapidly.

Another common hormone-related symptom is depression. That happened to me after my baby was born. It happens because your progesterone levels drop, and over-the-counter progesterone really helped me. Talk with your doctor before trying it.

The good news is your hormones will balance out within a few weeks, and you'll feel much better.

—Erika Schwartz, MD, a mom of two and the director of www. DrErika.com, who's been in private practice for more than 30 years in New York City, specializing over the past 15 years in women's health, disease prevention, and bioidentical hormones

RALLIE'S TIP

I delivered my third baby at the hospital where I had worked for several years. The day after my delivery, I donned a pair of hospital scrubs and took a stroll down the hall of the labor and delivery floor to get a little exercise. Having just delivered a seven-pound baby, I was feeling slimmer and lighter on my feet than I had in months! As I made my way to the nurses' station, I was greeted by one of my physician colleagues, whom I hadn't seen in a few weeks. Obviously, he didn't know I was visiting the OB floor as a patient.

"When are you going to have that baby?" he asked, pointing at my still-protuberant belly.

I was crushed!

I've had many of my patients recount similar experiences. It's important to remember that after the birth of your baby, it's highly unlikely that you'll walk out of the hospital in your favorite pair of snug-fitting, pre-pregnancy jeans. It takes a while for all the fluid you accumulated to dissipate, and for the swelling to go down. It might take a few weeks or months to lose all of the weight you gained during your pregnancy and for your abdominal muscles to regain their tone, so be patient. More important, you might have to wear maternity pants home from the hospital, so be sure to pack an extra pair!

Going Home

When you dress your baby in his going-home outfit, gently place him into his carrier for the first time, and take one last, nostalgic look around the room where you've spent your first few days together, that's when you realize that you've come to the end of one chapter. Now you're about to turn the page and begin the next and perhaps most exciting chapter of your life.

∽∽

When I left the hospital to take my babies home, what I felt most was a big rush to beat the guests.

I can't stand being a patient in a hospital, especially after those blasted 24-hour labors. I just couldn't take it! We took both babies home when they were less than a day old. All our friends phoned up on their way to visit us in the hospital, so the staff had to tell them to turn right around and drive to our house instead, because we had just left. All these people coming over, and us with a 10-hour-old infant! It sounds a little crazy, but it worked out great in the end.

—*Elizabeth Berger, MD*

∽∽

At the time I was in the hospital, there was a nursing strike. They were unbelievably short staffed. Plus the food was terrible. I was

> ## ? When to Call Your Doctor or Midwife
>
> During the postpartum period, call your doctor or midwife right away if you develop a fever of 100.4°F or higher, bleed enough to soak more than one sanitary pad per hour or pass large clots, have a new pain or swelling in your legs, have painful urination or the sudden urge to urinate, develop a foul-smelling vaginal discharge, have a C-section or episiotomy incision that becomes red or swollen, or have hot, red, sore breasts or cracking and bleeding nipples.

determined to nurse my son, but it was so hard to do. I knew instinctively that it would be easier at home, where I felt more comfortable. A day before I was officially allowed to go home, I signed myself out of the hospital to restore a more restful climate for me and my baby. I had my ob's blessing—and the help of my classmates and family once I got home.

—*JJ Levenstein, MD, FAAP*

❧

One hour after my daughter was born, my doctor came to check me.

"You're doing great!" he said. "Once you're ready to sweep the floor, you can go home."

My husband, my friend, and I waited around a half hour, and then we packed up. By then it was dawn, and we headed back through the Ozarks toward home.

—*Stacey Marie Kerr, MD*

❧

It's amazing how different my hospital experience was between my daughter's birth and my twins' birth a few years later. When my daughter was born, they encouraged me to send her to the nursery at night so I could sleep. But when my twins were born, it was all about rooming in.

There I was in this teeny hospital room with two babies with no help. I said, "Could you please take these kids?" They said no! So I asked to go home the next day.

"But you just had twins!" the nurse replied.

"Yes, but I have three people ready and waiting to help me at home. Get me out of here!"

But truth be told, the pregnancy and delivery are easy compared to the next 18 years!

—*Susan Wilder, MD, a mom of an older daughter and twin girls, a primary care physician, and CEO and founder of Lifescape Medical Associates in Scottsdale, AZ*

Index

Note: <u>Underlined</u> references indicate boxed text.

Overweight, 15, 141
Ovulation, signs of, 2
Oxytocin, 207, 349–50, 369, 437, 451, 464. *See also* Pitocin

P

Pacing yourself, 267–68
Packing birth bag, 393, 394–96
Pain. *See* Aches and pains; Pain control; *specific types of pain*
Pain control
  for circumcision, 362, 363
  for C-section, 372
  during labor, 269–73, 461-66 (*see also* Epidural)
Paley, Michelle, 8, 58, 170, 175, 187–88, 206, 216, 266, 277, 286, 309, 319–20, 339, 341, 350, 363, 375, 383, 394, 399, 408–9, 424, 428–29, 437, 476–77, 480–81
Palmer's Cocoa Butter Nursing Butter, 349
Pampered Chef Digital Pocket Thermometer, 21
Pampering, before delivery, 416–17
Pampers pop-up baby wipes, 383
Pap smear, 94, 249
Partner
  accepting help from, 179
  announcing pregnancy to, 47–48
  birth bag items for, 394
  introducing baby to, 473–74
  at prenatal visits, 96
  spending special time with, 400–401, 415
  supporting and easing fears of, 413–16
  taking vacation with, 165–68
  Pediatrician, choosing, 338–40
Pedicure, 310, 377, 416
Pelvic pain or pressure, 75, 76, 275, 306, 329
Perineal massage, 380–81
Period, missing, 41, 56
Pets, 85–88, 370–72, 404
Photos, of pregnant belly, 58–59
Physical fitness, before pregnancy, 15–16, 27

Pica, 256, 258
Pilates, prenatal, 191, 192, 193, 202–3
Pillows, 198, 200, 201, 226, 290, 315, 330, 331, 340, 341–42, 342, 394, 395
Pitocin, 37, 451, 452, 464, 468. *See also* Oxytocin
Placenta, 23, 26, 29, 40, 49, 70, 92–93, 128, 139, 150, 152, 153, 173, 195, 203, 210, 240, 275, 281, 330, 336, 451
  delivery of, 454, 482
Placenta abruption, 22, 110, 414
Placenta previa, 22–23, 110
Planning pregnancy, 27
Position of baby. *See* Baby's position
Postpartum depression, 483
Preeclampsia, 125, 145, 216, 231, 235–37, 252, 389, 414, 430, 451, 466
Preggie Pops, 460
Pregnancy journal or scrapbook, 5–7, 434
Pregnancy mask, 119, 135–36, 137
Pregnancy test. *See* Home pregnancy test
Premature. See also Birth, premature
  meaning of, 358
Prenatal classes, 209, 297, 359, 363–65, 366, 367
Prenatal doctor visits. *See* Doctor or midwife, prenatal visits to
Prenatal vitamins, 7–9, 10, 24, 72, 94, 157, 258, 259, 427
Preparing for pregnancy, 27–29
Preterm. See also Labor, preterm
  meaning of, 305, 358, 410
Progesterone, 41, 49, 60, 77, 88, 119, 125, 135, 139, 153, 156, 173, 180, 241, 288, 293, 301, 325, 331, 354, 485
Pruritic urticarial papules (PUPP), 353–54
Pushing, during labor, 454, 456, 457, 463, 473

Q

Quickening. *See* Baby's movements, feeling
Quicken Willmaker Software, 287

Weight gain, 41, 71, 139, 141–45, 183,
    199, 241, 263, 292, 315, 323, 325,
    332, 337, 347, 351, 368–69, 384,
    392
Weight loss, 110, 145, 384–85, 392,
    485
White noise machine, 318, 320, 342, 371
Wilder, Susan, 27, 46, 50, 90, 108–9,
    121, 169, 184–85, 204, 212, 242,
    252, 316, 327, 382, 396–97, 446,
    463, 487
Will, writing, 287–88

Williams, Ruth D., 7, 102–3, 114, 121,
    125, 175, 238, 268, 306–7, 319,
    327–28, 333–34, 397–98, 416,
    479–80
Work, 154–56, 268, 388–90
Worry, 37, 38, 101–3, 114. *See also*
    Anxiety; Fears

Y

Yeast infections, 168, 247, 248–49
Yoga, prenatal, 38, 191–92, 193, 202,
    227

About the Authors

Rallie McAllister, MD, MPH

Dr. McAllister is a nationally recognized health expert. Her syndicated newspaper column, *Your Health*, appears in more than 30 newspapers in the United States and Canada and is read by more than a million people each week. She has been the featured medical expert on hundreds of radio and television shows, and her healthy-eating tips and interviews have been featured in dozens of popular magazines.

A dynamic public speaker, Dr. McAllister delivers informative and entertaining presentations at conventions, seminars, and workshops around the country. Dr. McAllister is the author of several health-related books, including *Healthy Lunchbox: The Working Mom's Guide to Keeping You and Your Kids Trim*. She lives in Lexington, KY, with her husband, Robin, and sons, Oakley and Gatlin. Her oldest son, Chad, proudly serves in the United States Marine Corps.

Jennifer Bright Reich

Jennifer is a writer and editor with more than 15 years of publishing experience. She has contributed to more than 150 books and published more than 100 magazine and newspaper articles.

Jennifer proudly served as a Lieutenant in the U.S. Army for four years, including one year working directly for the three Commanding Generals of I Corps at Fort Lewis, Washington.

After that, Jennifer worked for seven years on staff at Rodale Inc. before launching her own editorial services business, Bright Communications LLC, in 2004.

Jennifer lives in Allentown, PA, with her husband, Mike, and their sons, Tyler and Austin.